SCHEMA THERAPY

SCHEMA THERAPY

A Practitioner's Guide

JEFFREY E. YOUNG
JANET S. KLOSKO
MARJORIE E. WEISHAAR

THE GUILFORD PRESS
New York   London

To Debbie, Sarah, and Jacob
—J. E. Y.

To my mentor, Dr. David H. Barlow.
All these words can't express my gratitude.
—J. S. K.

To my parents
—M. E. W.

© 2003 The Guilford Press
A Division of Guilford Publications, Inc.
370 Seventh Avenue, Suite 1200, New York, NY 10001
www.guilford.com

Paperback edition 2006

Printed in the United States of America

This book is printed on acid-free paper.

Last digit is print number: 19   18   17   16   15   14   13   12   11   10

Library of Congress Cataloging-in-Publication Data

Young, Jeffrey E., 1950–
  Schema therapy : a practitioner's guide / Jeffrey E. Young,
Janet S. Klosko, Marjorie E. Weishaar.
        p. cm.
  Includes bibliographical references and index.
  ISBN 978-1-57230-838-1 (hardcover : alk. paper)
  ISBN 978-1-59385-372-3 (paperback : alk. paper)
    1. Schema-focused cognitive therapy. 2. Personality disorders—
Treatment.   I. Klosko, Janet S. II. Weishaar, Marjorie E. III. Title.
RC455.4.S36 Y68 2003
616.85′8—dc21

                                                    2002153858

ABOUT THE AUTHORS

Jeffrey E. Young, PhD, is on the faculty in the Department of Psychiatry at Columbia University. He is also the Founder and Director of the Cognitive Therapy Centers of New York and Connecticut, as well as the Schema Therapy Institute (*institute@schematherapy.com*). Dr. Young has lectured internationally on cognitive and schema therapies for the past 20 years. He has trained thousands of mental health professionals and is widely acclaimed for his outstanding teaching skills.

He is the founder of schema therapy, an integrative approach for longer-term disorders and for treatment resistant patients, and has published widely in the fields of both cognitive and schema therapies, including two major books—*Cognitive Therapy for Personality Disorders: A Schema-Focused Approach,* written for mental health professionals, and *Reinventing Your Life* (with Janet S. Klosko), a popular self-help book written for the general public. Dr. Young has also served as a consultant on several cognitive and schema therapy research grants, including the National Institute of Mental Health Collaborative Study of Depression, and on the editorial boards of the following journals: *Cognitive Therapy and Research* and *Cognitive and Behavioral Practice.*

Janet S. Klosko, PhD, is Codirector of the Cognitive Therapy Center of Long Island in Great Neck, New York (516-466-8485), and is a senior psychologist at the Schema Therapy Institute in Manhattan and Woodstock Women's Health in Woodstock, New York (845-679-6699). She received her PhD in clinical psychology from the State University of New York (SUNY) at Albany and interned at Brown University Medical School.

While at SUNY, she worked with David H. Barlow, researching and treating anxiety disorders. Dr. Klosko has won the Albany Award for Excellence in Research and the Dissertation Award from the American Psychological Association Section on Clinical Psychology as a Science. She has numerous academic publications and is coauthor (with William Sanderson) of *Cognitive-Behavioral Treatment of Depression,* and (with Jeffrey E. Young) of the popular book *Reinventing Your Life.* She also has a master's degree in English literature.

Marjorie E. Weishaar, PhD, is Clinical Professor of Psychiatry and Human Behavior at Brown University Medical School (*Marjorie_Weishaar@brown.edu*), where she teaches cognitive therapy to psychiatry residents and to psychology interns and postdoctoral fellows. She has also received two teaching awards from Brown Medical School. Dr. Weishaar graduated from the University of Pennsylvania and earned three graduate degrees from The Pennsylvania State University. She was trained in cognitive therapy by Aaron T. Beck, and in schema therapy by Jeffrey E. Young. She is the author of *Aaron T. Beck*, a book on cognitive therapy and its founder, which was recently translated into Chinese. Dr. Weishaar lectures widely and has written numerous articles and book chapters on cognitive therapy, particularly in the area of suicide risk. She is currently in private practice in Providence, Rhode Island.

For general information about schema therapy:
Schema Therapy Institute
36 West 44th Street, Suite 1007
New York, NY 10036
Phone: 212-221-1818, ext. 5
E-mail: *institute@schematherapy.com*
Website: *www.schematherapy.com*

PREFACE

It is difficult to believe that it has been 9 years since we wrote our last major book on schema therapy. During this decade of burgeoning interest in this therapy approach, we continually have been asked, "When are you going to write an up-to-date, comprehensive treatment manual?" With some embarrassment, we had to admit that we had not found the time to take on such a major project.

After 3 years of intensive work, however, we have finally written what we hope will become "the bible" for the practice of schema therapy. We have attempted to include in this volume all the additions and refinements from the past decade, including our revised conceptual model, detailed treatment protocols, case vignettes, and patient transcripts. In particular, we have written extended chapters that describe a major expansion of schema therapy for borderline and narcissistic personality disorders.

During the past 10 years, many changes in the mental health field have had an impact on schema therapy. As practitioners from many orientations have become dissatisfied with the limitations of orthodox therapies, there has been a corresponding interest in psychotherapy integration. As one of the first comprehensive, integrative approaches, schema therapy has attracted many new clinicians and researchers who have been searching for both "permission" and guidance to go beyond the confines of existing models.

One clear sign of this heightened interest in schema therapy has been the widespread use of the Young Schema Questionnaire (YSQ) by clinicians and researchers around the world. The YSQ has already been translated into Spanish, Greek, Dutch, French, Japanese, Norwegian, German, and Finnish, to indicate just a few of the countries that have adopted elements of this model. The extensive research on the YSQ offers substantial support for the schema model.

Another indication of the appeal of schema therapy has been the success of our two earlier books on schema therapy, even 10 years after their publication: *Cognitive Therapy for Personality Disorders: A Schema-Focused Approach* is now in its third edition, and *Reinventing Your Life,* which has sold more than 125,000 copies, is still available at most major bookstores and has been translated into several languages.

The past decade has also seen the extension of schema therapy beyond personality disorders. The approach has been applied to a wide variety of clinical problems, populations, and disorders, including, among others, chronic depression, childhood trauma, criminal offenders, eating disorders, couple work, and relapse prevention for substance abuse. Often schema therapy is being used to treat predisposing characterological issues in patients with Axis I disorders, once the acute symptoms have abated.

Another important development has been the combining of schema therapy with spirituality. Three books (*Emotional Alchemy* by Tara Bennett-Goleman; *Praying Through Our Lifetraps: A Psycho-Spiritual Path to Freedom* by John Cecero; and *The Myth of More* by Joseph Novello) that blend the schema approach with mindfulness meditation or with traditional religious practices have already been published.

One disappointing development, that we hope will change in the decade to come, is the impact of managed care and cost containment on the treatment of personality disorders in the United States. It has become increasingly difficult for practitioners to get insurance reimbursement and for researchers to obtain federal grants for personality disorders because Axis II treatment generally takes longer and thus does not fit a short-term, managed care model. As a result, the United States has fallen behind many other countries in supporting work on personality disorders.

The result of this reduced support has been a paucity of well-designed outcome studies with personality disorders. (The notable exception is Marsha Linehan's dialectical behavior therapy approach to borderline personality disorder.) This has made it extremely difficult for us to obtain funding for studies that might demonstrate empirical support for schema therapy.

Thus we are turning now to other countries to fund this important research area. We are particularly excited about a major outcome study, directed by Arnoud Arntz, nearing completion in the Netherlands. This large-scale, multisite study compares schema therapy with Otto Kernberg's approach in treating borderline personality disorder. We are eagerly awaiting the results.

For readers who are unfamiliar with schema therapy, we will review what we consider the major advantages of schema therapy over other commonly practiced therapies. Compared to most other therapy approaches, schema therapy is more integrative, combining aspects of cognitive, behavioral, psychodynamic (especially object relations), attachment, and Gestalt models. Schema therapy regards cognitive and behavioral components as vital to treatment, yet gives equal weight to emotional change, experiential techniques, and the therapy relationship.

Another key benefit of the schema model is its parsimony and seeming simplicity, on the one hand, combined with depth and complexity, on the other. It is easy for both therapists and patients to understand. The schema model incorporates complex ideas, many of which seem convoluted and confusing to patients receiving other forms of therapy, and presents them in simple and straightforward ways. Thus schema therapy has the commonsense appeal of cognitive-behavioral therapy (CBT), combined with the depth of psychodynamic and related approaches.

Schema therapy retains two vital characteristics of CBT: It is both structured and systematic. The therapist follows a sequence of assessment and treatment procedures. The assessment phase includes the administration of a number of inventories that measure schemas and coping styles. Treatment is active and directive, going beyond insight to cognitive, emotive, interpersonal, and behavioral change. Schema therapy is also valuable in the treatment of couples, helping both partners to understand and heal their schemas.

Another advantage of the schema model is its specificity. The model delineates specific schemas, coping styles, and modes. In addition, schema therapy is notable for the specificity of the treatment strategies, including guidelines about providing the appropriate form of limited reparenting for each patient. Schema therapy provides a similarly accessible method for understanding and working with the therapy relationship. Therapists monitor their own schemas, coping styles, and modes as they work with patients.

Finally, and perhaps most important, we believe that the schema approach is unusually compassionate and humane, in comparison with "treatment as usual." Schema therapy normalizes rather than pathologizes psychological disorders. Everyone has schemas, coping styles, and modes—they are just more extreme and rigid in the patients we treat. The approach is also sympathetic and respectful, especially toward the most severe patients, such as those with borderline personality disorder, who are often treated with minimal compassion and much blame in other therapies. The concepts of "empathic confrontation" and "limited reparenting" ground therapists in a caring attitude toward patients. The use of modes eases the process of confrontation, allowing the therapist to aggressively confront rigid, maladaptive behaviors, while still retaining an alliance with the patient.

In closing, we highlight some of the new developments in schema therapy during the past decade: First, there is a revised and much more comprehensive list of schemas, containing 18 schemas in five domains. Second, we have developed new, detailed protocols for the treatment of borderline and narcissistic patients. These protocols have expanded the scope of schema therapy, primarily with the addition of the schema mode concept. Third, there is a much greater emphasis on coping styles, especially avoidance and overcompensation, and on altering coping styles through pattern-breaking. Our goal is to replace maladaptive coping styles with healthier ones that enable patients to meet their core emotional needs.

As schema therapy has developed and matured, we have placed much more emphasis on limited reparenting with all patients, but especially those with more severe disorders. Within the appropriate bounds of the therapeutic relationship, the therapist attempts to fulfill the patient's unmet childhood needs. Finally, there is more focus on the therapist's own schemas and coping styles, especially in regard to the therapy relationship.

We hope that this volume will provide therapists with a new way of approaching patients with chronic, longer-term themes and patterns, and that schema therapy will provide significant benefits for those extremely difficult and needy patients whom our approach is designed to treat.

ACKNOWLEDGMENTS

From All the Authors

We want to thank the people at The Guilford Press who supported us throughout this long and difficult project: Kitty Moore, Executive Editor, who gave us invaluable editorial advice and helped shape the book; Anna Nelson, Production Editor, who oversaw the production of the book so diligently and was such a pleasure to work with; Elaine Kehoe, who edited the book so beautifully; and all the other staff who worked with us.

We would like to give special thanks to Dr. George Lockwood, who provided us with so many valuable insights and historical anecdotes about psychoanalytic approaches and who donated much of the material in Chapter 1 on other integrative therapies. You are a joy to work with, and we look forward to future collaborative efforts.

We would like to thank the staff at the Schema Therapy Institute in Manhattan, especially Nancy Ribeiro and Sylvia Tamm. Thank you for doing so much of the work that supported our efforts. You are warm and reliable ports in a storm.

Finally, we thank our patients, who have taught us about the transformation of tragedy into hope and healing.

Jeffrey E. Young

There are many individuals I want to thank who have played important roles in the development of schema therapy, in the writing of this book, and in supporting me through this grueling process.

To my close friends, for their love and caring over many years, and for their help in developing this approach. You have been like family: Wendy Behary, Pierre Cousineau, Cathy Flanagan, Vivian Francesco, George Lockwood, Marty Sloane, Bob Sternberg, Will Swift, Dick and Diane Wattenmaker, and William Zangwill.

To my colleagues, who have advanced schema therapy in many different ways, both in the United States and abroad: Arnoud Arntz, Sam Ball, Jordi Cid, Michael First, Vartouhi Ohanian, Bill Sanderson, Glenn Waller, and David Weinberger.

To Nancy Ribeiro, my Executive Administrator, for her devotion in helping me with every project, while putting up with my quirks on a daily basis.

To my father, whose unconditional love provided me with the model for parenting and reparenting.

And, to my mentor, Tim Beck, who has been both a personal friend and a guide throughout my career.

Janet S. Klosko

In addition to the above, I would like to thank my colleagues for their support, especially Dr. Jayne Rygh, Dr. Ken Appelbaum, Dr. David Bricker, Dr. William Sanderson, and Jenna Smith, CM. I would also like to thank my family and friends—especially Michael and Molly—for providing the secure base upon which I have built my career.

Marjorie E. Weishaar

I thank my teachers, especially Aaron T. Beck, MD, for their wisdom and guidance. I thank my colleagues and students for their considerable help, and I thank my family—all four generations—for their humor, optimism, probity, and sustaining love.

CONTENTS

Chapter 1

SCHEMA THERAPY: CONCEPTUAL MODEL

Schema therapy is an innovative, integrative therapy developed by Young and colleagues (Young, 1990, 1999) that significantly expands on traditional cognitive-behavioral treatments and concepts. The therapy blends elements from cognitive-behavioral, attachment, Gestalt, object relations, constructivist, and psychoanalytic schools into a rich, unifying conceptual and treatment model.

Schema therapy provides a new system of psychotherapy that is especially well suited to patients with entrenched, chronic psychological disorders who have heretofore been considered difficult to treat. In our clinical experience, patients with full-blown personality disorders, as well as those with significant characterological issues that underlie their Axis I disorders, typically respond extremely well to schema-focused treatment (sometimes in combination with other treatment approaches).

THE EVOLUTION FROM COGNITIVE TO SCHEMA THERAPY

A look at the field of cognitive-behavioral therapy[1] helps to explain the reason Young felt that the development of schema therapy was so impor-

---

[1]In this section, we use the term "cognitive-behavioral therapy" to refer to various protocols that have been developed by writers such as Beck (Beck, Rush, Shaw, & Emery, 1979) and Barlow (Craske, Barlow, & Meadows, 2000) to treat Axis I disorders.

(*continued on page 2*)

tant. Cognitive-behavioral researchers and practitioners have made excellent progress in developing effective psychological treatments for Axis I disorders, including many mood, anxiety, sexual, eating, somatoform, and substance abuse disorders. These treatments have traditionally been short term (roughly 20 sessions) and have focused on reducing symptoms, building skills, and solving problems in the patient's current life.

However, although many patients are helped by these treatments, many others are not. Treatment outcome studies usually report high success rates (Barlow, 2001). For example, in depression, the success rate is over 60% immediately after treatment, but the relapse rate is about 30% after 1 year (Young, Weinberger, & Beck, 2001)—leaving a significant number of patients unsuccessfully treated. Often patients with underlying personality disorders and characterological issues fail to respond fully to traditional cognitive-behavioral treatments (Beck, Freeman, & Associates, 1990). One of the challenges facing cognitive-behavioral therapy today is developing effective treatments for these chronic, difficult-to-treat patients.

Characterological problems can reduce the effectiveness of traditional cognitive-behavioral therapy in a number of ways. Some patients present for treatment of Axis I symptoms, such as anxiety or depression, and either fail to progress in treatment or relapse once treatment is withdrawn. For example, a female patient presents for cognitive-behavioral treatment of agoraphobia. Through a program consisting of breathing training, challenging catastrophic thoughts, and graduated exposure to phobic situations, she significantly reduces her fear of panic symptoms and overcomes her avoidance of numerous situations. Once treatment ends, however, the patient lapses back into her agoraphobia. A lifetime of dependence, along with feelings of vulnerability and incompetence—what we call her Dependence and Vulnerability schemas—prevent her from venturing out into the world on her own. She lacks the self-confidence to make decisions and has failed to acquire such practical skills as driving, navigating her surroundings, managing money, and selecting proper destinations. She prefers instead to let significant others make the necessary arrangements. Without the guidance of the therapist, the patient cannot orchestrate the public excursions necessary to maintain her treatment gains.

Other patients come initially for cognitive-behavioral treatment of Axis I symptoms. After these symptoms have been resolved, their characterological problems become a focus of treatment. For example, a male patient undergoes cognitive-behavioral therapy for his obsessive–compulsive disor-

---

Some cognitive-behavioral therapists have adapted these protocols to work with difficult patients in ways that are consistent with schema therapy (c.f. Beck, Freeman, & Associates, 1990). We discuss some of these modifications later in this chapter (see pp. 48–53). For the most part, however, current treatment protocols within cognitive-behavioral therapy do not reflect these adaptations.

der. Through a short-term behavioral program of exposure combined with response prevention, he largely eliminates the obsessive thoughts and compulsive rituals that had consumed most of his waking life. Once his Axis I symptoms have abated, however, and he has time to resume other activities, he must face the almost complete absence of a social life that is a result of his solitary lifestyle. The patient has what we call a "Defectiveness schema," with which he copes by avoiding social situations. He is so acutely sensitive to perceived slights and rejections that, since childhood, he has avoided most personal interaction with others. He must grapple with his lifelong pattern of avoidance if he is ever to develop a rewarding social life.

Still other patients who come for cognitive-behavioral treatment lack specific symptoms to serve as targets of therapy. Their problems are vague or diffuse and lack clear precipitants. They feel that something vital is wrong or missing from their lives. These are patients whose presenting problems *are* their characterological problems: They come seeking treatment for chronic difficulties in their relationships with significant others or in their work. Because they either do not have significant Axis I symptoms or have so many of them, traditional cognitive-behavioral therapy is difficult to apply to them.

Assumptions of Traditional Cognitive-Behavioral Therapy Violated by Characterological Patients

Traditional cognitive-behavioral therapy makes several assumptions about patients that often prove untrue of those patients with characterological problems. These patients have a number of psychological attributes that distinguish them from straightforward Axis I cases and make them less suitable candidates for cognitive-behavioral treatment.

One such assumption is that patients will comply with the treatment protocol. Standard cognitive-behavioral therapy assumes that patients are motivated to reduce symptoms, build skills, and solve their current problems and that, therefore, with some prodding and positive reinforcement, they will comply with the necessary treatment procedures. However, for many characterological patients, their motivations and approaches to therapy are complicated, and they are often unwilling or unable to comply with cognitive-behavioral therapy procedures. They may not complete homework assignments. They may demonstrate great reluctance to learn self-control strategies. They may appear more motivated to obtain consolation from the therapist than to learn strategies for helping themselves.

Another such assumption in cognitive-behavioral therapy is that, with brief training, patients can access their cognitions and emotions and report them to the therapist. Early in therapy, patients are expected to observe and record their thoughts and feelings. However, patients with characterological problems are often unable to do so. They often seem out of touch with their cognitions or emotions. Many of these patients engage in cognitive and affective avoidance. They block disturbing thoughts and images. They avoid looking deeply into themselves. They avoid their own disturbing memories and negative feelings. They also avoid many of the behaviors and situations that are essential to their progress. This pattern of avoidance probably develops as an instrumental response, learned because it is reinforced by the reduction of negative affect. Negative emotions such as anxiety or depression are triggered by stimuli associated with childhood memories, prompting avoidance of the stimuli in order to avoid the emotions. Avoidance becomes a habitual and exceedingly difficult to change strategy for coping with negative affect.

Cognitive-behavioral therapy also assumes that patients can change their problematic cognitions and behaviors through such practices as empirical analysis, logical discourse, experimentation, gradual steps, and repetition. However, for characterological patients, this is often not the case. In our experience, their distorted thoughts and self-defeating behaviors are extremely resistant to modification solely through cognitive-behavioral techniques. Even after months of therapy, there is often no sustained improvement.

Because characterological patients usually lack psychological flexibility, they are much less responsive to cognitive-behavioral techniques and frequently do not make meaningful changes in a short period of time. Rather, they are psychologically rigid. Rigidity is a hallmark of personality disorders (American Psychiatric Association, 1994, p. 633). These patients tend to express hopelessness about changing. Their characterological problems are ego-syntonic: Their self-destructive patterns seem to be so much a part of who they are that they cannot imagine altering them. Their problems are central to their sense of identity, and to give them up can seem like a form of death—a death of a part of the self. When challenged, these patients rigidly, reflexively, and sometimes aggressively cling to what they already believe to be true about themselves and the world.

Cognitive-behavioral therapy also assumes that patients can engage in a collaborative relationship with the therapist within a few sessions. Difficulties in the therapeutic relationship are typically not a major focus of cognitive-behavioral treatments. Rather, such difficulties are viewed as obstacles to be overcome in order to attain the patient's compliance with treatment procedures. The therapist–patient relationship is not generally regarded as an "active ingredient" of the treatment. However, patients with characterological disorders often have difficulty forming a therapeutic alliance, thus mirroring their difficulties in relating to others outside of therapy. Many difficult-to-treat patients have had dysfunctional interpersonal relationships that began early in life. Lifelong disturbances in relationships with significant others are another hallmark of personality disorders (Millon, 1981). These patients often find it difficult to form secure therapeutic relationships. Some of these patients, such as those with borderline or dependent personality disorders, frequently become so absorbed in trying to get the therapist to meet their emotional needs that they are unable to focus on their own lives outside of therapy. Others, such as those with narcissistic, paranoid, schizoid, or obsessive–compulsive personality disorders, are frequently so disengaged or hostile that they are unable to collaborate with the therapist. Because interpersonal issues are often the core problem, the therapeutic relationship is one of the best areas for assessing and treating these patients—a focus that is most often neglected in traditional cognitive-behavioral therapy.

Finally, in cognitive-behavioral treatment, the patient is presumed to have problems that are readily discernible as targets of treatment. In the case of patients with characterological problems, this presumption is often not met. These patients commonly have presenting problems that are vague, chronic, and pervasive. They are unhappy in major life areas and have been dissatisfied for as long as they can remember. Perhaps they have been unable to establish a long-term romantic relationship, have failed to reach their potential in their work, or experience their lives as empty. They are fundamentally dissatisfied in love, work, or play. These very broad, hard-to-define life themes usually do not make easy-to-address targets for standard cognitive-behavioral treatment.

Later we look at how specific schemas can make it difficult for patients to benefit from standard cognitive-behavioral therapy.

THE DEVELOPMENT OF SCHEMA THERAPY

For the many reasons just described, Young (1990, 1999) developed schema therapy to treat patients with chronic characterological problems who were not being adequately helped by traditional cognitive-behavioral therapy: the "treatment failures." He developed schema therapy as a systematic approach that expands on cognitive-behavioral therapy by integrating techniques drawn from several different schools of therapy. Schema therapy can be brief, intermediate, or longer term, depending on the patient. It expands on traditional cognitive-behavioral therapy by placing much greater emphasis on exploring the childhood and adolescent origins of psychological problems, on emotive techniques, on the therapist–patient relationship, and on maladaptive coping styles.

Once acute symptoms have abated, schema therapy is appropriate for the treatment of many Axis I and Axis II disorders that have a significant basis in lifelong characterological themes. Therapy is often undertaken in conjunction with other modalities, such as cognitive-behavioral therapy and psychotropic medication. Schema therapy is designed to treat the chronic characterological aspects of disorders, not acute psychiatric symptoms (such as full-blown major depression or recurring panic attacks). Schema therapy has proven useful in treating chronic depression and anxiety, eating disorders, difficult couples problems, and long-standing difficulties in maintaining satisfying intimate relationships. It has also been helpful with criminal offenders and in preventing relapse among substance abusers.

Schema therapy addresses the core psychological themes that are typical of patients with characterological disorders. As we discuss in detail in the next section, we call these core themes Early Maladaptive Schemas. Schema therapy helps patients and therapists to make sense of chronic, pervasive problems and to organize them in a comprehensible manner. The model traces these schemas from early childhood to the present, with particular emphasis on the patient's interpersonal relationships. Using the model, patients gain the ability to view their characterological problems as ego-dystonic and thus become more empowered to give them up. The therapist allies with patients in fighting their schemas, utilizing cognitive, affective, behavioral, and interpersonal strategies. When patients repeat dysfunctional patterns based on their schemas, the therapist empathically confronts them with the reasons for change. Through "limited reparenting," the therapist supplies many patients with a partial antidote to needs that were not adequately met in childhood.

EARLY MALADAPTIVE SCHEMAS

History of the Schema Construct

We now turn to a detailed look at the basic constructs that make up schema theory. We begin with the history and development of the term "schema."

The word "schema" is utilized in many fields of study. In general terms, a schema is a structure, framework, or outline. In early Greek philosophy, Stoic logicians, especially Chrysippus (ca. 279–206 B.C.), presented principles of logic in the form of "inference schemata" (Nussbaum, 1994). In Kantian philosophy, a schema is a conception of what is common to all members of a class. The term is also used in set theory, algebraic geometry, education, literary analysis, and computer programming, to name just some of the diverse fields in which the concept of a "schema" is used.

The term "schema" has an especially rich history within psychology, most widely in the area of cognitive development. Within cognitive development, a schema is a pattern imposed on reality or experience to help individuals explain it, to mediate perception, and to guide their responses. A schema is an abstract representation of the distinctive characteristics of an event, a kind of blueprint of its most salient elements. In psychology the term is probably most commonly associated with Piaget, who wrote in detail about schemata in different stages of childhood cognitive development. Within cognitive psychology, a schema can also be thought of as an abstract cognitive plan that serves as a guide for interpreting information and solving problems. Thus we may have a linguistic schema for understanding a sentence or a cultural schema for interpreting a myth.

Moving from cognitive psychology to cognitive therapy, Beck (1967) referred in his early writing to schemas. However, in the context of psychology and psychotherapy, a schema can be thought of generally as any broad organizing principle for making sense of one's life experience. An important concept with relevance for psychotherapy is the notion that schemas, many of which are formed early in life, continue to be elaborated and then superimposed on later life experiences, even when they are no longer applicable. This is sometimes referred to as the need for "cognitive consistency," for maintaining a stable view of oneself and the world, even if it is, in reality, inaccurate or distorted. By this broad definition, a schema can be positive or negative, adaptive or maladaptive; schemas can be formed in childhood or later in life.

Young's Definition of a Schema

Young (1990, 1999) hypothesized that some of these schemas—especially schemas that develop primarily as a result of toxic childhood experiences—might be at the core of personality disorders, milder characterological problems, and many chronic Axis I disorders. To explore this idea, he defined a subset of schemas that he labeled Early Maladaptive Schemas.

Our revised, comprehensive definition of an Early Maladaptive Schema is:

- a broad, pervasive theme or pattern
- comprised of memories, emotions, cognitions, and bodily sensations
- regarding oneself and one's relationships with others
- developed during childhood or adolescence
- elaborated throughout one's lifetime and
- dysfunctional to a significant degree

Briefly, Early Maladaptive Schemas are self-defeating emotional and cognitive patterns that begin early in our development and repeat throughout life. Note that, according to this definition, an individual's behavior is not part of the schema itself; Young theorizes that maladaptive behaviors develop as *responses* to a schema. Thus behaviors are *driven* by schemas but are not part of schemas. We explore this concept more when we discuss coping styles later in this chapter.

CHARACTERISTICS OF EARLY MALADAPTIVE SCHEMAS

Let us now examine some of the main characteristics of schemas. (From this point on, we use the terms "schema" and "Early Maladaptive Schema" virtually interchangeably.) Consider patients who have one of the four most powerful and damaging schemas from our list of 18 (see Figure 1.1 on pp. 14–17): Abandonment/Instability, Mistrust/Abuse, Emotional Deprivation, and Defectiveness/Shame. As young children, these patients were abandoned, abused, neglected, or rejected. In adulthood their schemas are triggered by life events that they perceive (unconsciously) as similar to the traumatic experiences of their childhood. When one of these schemas is triggered, they experience a strong negative emotion, such as grief, shame, fear, or rage.

Not all schemas are based in childhood trauma or mistreatment. Indeed, an individual can develop a Dependence/Incompetence schema without experiencing a single instance of childhood trauma. Rather, the individual might have been completely sheltered and overprotected throughout childhood. However, although not all schemas have trauma as their origin, all of them are destructive, and most are caused by noxious experiences that are repeated on a regular basis throughout childhood and adolescence. The effect of all these related toxic experiences is cumulative, and together they lead to the emergence of a full-blown schema.

Early Maladaptive Schemas fight for survival. As we mentioned earlier, this is the result of the human drive for consistency. The schema is what the individual knows. Although it causes suffering, it is comfortable and familiar. It feels "right." People feel drawn to events that trigger their schemas. This is one reason schemas are so hard to change. Patients regard schemas as a priori truths, and thus these schemas influence the processing of later experiences. They play a major role in how patients think, feel, act, and relate to others and paradoxically lead them to inadvertently recreate in their adult lives the conditions in childhood that were most harmful to them.

Schemas begin in early childhood or adolescence as reality-based representations of the child's environment. It has been our experience that individuals' schemas fairly accurately reflect the tone of their early environment. For example, if a patient tells us that his family was cold and unaffectionate when he was young, he is usually correct, even though he may not understand *why* his parents had difficulty showing affection or expressing feelings. His attributions for their behavior may be wrong, but his basic sense of the emotional climate and how he was treated is almost always valid.

The dysfunctional nature of schemas usually becomes most apparent later in life, when patients continue to perpetuate their schemas in their interactions with other people even though their perceptions are no longer accurate. Early Maladaptive Schemas and the maladaptive ways in which patients learn to cope with them often underlie chronic Axis I symptoms, such as anxiety, depression, substance abuse, and psychosomatic disorders.

Schemas are dimensional, meaning they have different levels of severity and pervasiveness. The more severe the schema, the greater the number of situations that activate it. So, for example, if an individual experiences criticism that comes early and frequently, that is extreme, and that is given by both parents, then that individual's contact with almost anyone is likely to trigger a Defectiveness schema. If an individual experiences criticism that comes later in life and is occasional, milder, and given by only one parent, then that individual is less likely to activate the schema later in life; for example, the schema may be triggered only by demanding authority figures of the critical parent's gender. Furthermore, in general, the more severe the schema, the more intense the negative affect when the schema is triggered and the longer it lasts.

As we mentioned earlier, there are positive and negative schemas, as well as early and later schemas. Our focus is almost exclusively on Early Maladaptive Schemas, so we do not spell out these positive, later schemas in our theory. However, some writers have argued that, for each of our Early Maladaptive Schemas, there is a corresponding adaptive schema (see Elliott's polarity theory; Elliott & Lassen, 1997). Alternatively, considering Erikson's (1950) psychosocial stages, one could argue that the successful resolution of each stage results in an adaptive schema, whereas the failure to resolve a stage leads to a maladaptive schema. Nevertheless, our concern in this book is the population of psychotherapy patients with chronic disorders rather than a normal population; therefore, we focus primarily on the early *maladaptive* schemas that we believe underlie personality pathology.

THE ORIGINS OF SCHEMAS

Core Emotional Needs

Our basic view is that schemas result from unmet core emotional needs in childhood. We have postulated five core emotional needs for human beings.[2]

---

[2]Our list of needs is derived from both the theories of others and our own clinical observation and has not been tested empirically. Ultimately, we hope to conduct research on this subject. We are open to revision based on research and have revised the list over time. The list of domains (see Figure 1.1 on pp. 14–17) is also open to modification based on empirical findings and clinical experience.

1. Secure attachments to others (includes safety, stability, nurturance, and acceptance)
2. Autonomy, competence, and sense of identity
3. Freedom to express valid needs and emotions
4. Spontaneity and play
5. Realistic limits and self-control

We believe that these needs are universal. Everyone has them, although some individuals have stronger needs than others. A psychologically healthy individual is one who can adaptively meet these core emotional needs.

The interaction between the child's innate temperament and early environment results in the frustration, rather than gratification, of these basic needs. The goal of schema therapy is to help patients find adaptive ways to meet their core emotional needs. All of our interventions are means to this end.

Early Life Experiences

Toxic childhood experiences are the primary origin of Early Maladaptive Schemas. The schemas that develop earliest and are the strongest typically originate in the nuclear family. To a large extent, the dynamics of a child's family are the dynamics of that child's entire early world. When patients find themselves in adult situations that activate their Early Maladaptive Schemas, what they usually are experiencing is a drama from their childhood, usually with a parent. Other influences, such as peers, school, groups in the community, and the surrounding culture, become increasingly important as the child matures and may lead to the development of schemas. However, schemas developed later are generally not as pervasive or as powerful. (Social Isolation is an example of a schema that is usually developed later in childhood or in adolescence and that may not reflect the dynamics of the nuclear family.)

We have observed four types of early life experiences that foster the acquisition of schemas. The first is *toxic frustration of needs*. This occurs when the child experiences too little of a good thing and acquires schemas such as Emotional Deprivation or Abandonment through deficits in the early environment. The child's environment is missing something important, such as stability, understanding, or love. The second type of early life experience that engenders schemas is *traumatization* or *victimization*. Here, the child is harmed or victimized and develops schemas such as Mistrust/ Abuse, Defectiveness/Shame, or Vulnerability to Harm. In the third type, the child experiences too much of a good thing: The parents provide the child with too much of something that, in moderation, is healthy for a child. With schemas such as Dependence/Incompetence or Entitlement/ Grandiosity, for example, the child is rarely mistreated. Rather, the child is coddled or indulged. The child's core emotional needs for autonomy or realistic limits are not met. Thus parents may be overly involved in the life of a child, may overprotect a child, or may give a child an excessive degree of freedom and autonomy without any limits.

The fourth type of life experience that creates schemas is *selective internalization or identification with significant others.* The child selectively identifies with and internalizes the parent's thoughts, feelings, experiences, and behaviors. For example, two patients present for treatment, both survivors of childhood abuse. As a child, the first one, Ruth, succumbed to the victim role. When her father hit her, she did not fight back. Rather, she became passive and submissive. She was the victim of her father's abusive behavior, but she did not internalize it. She experienced the feeling of being a victim, but she did not internalize the feeling of being an abuser. The second patient, Kevin, fought back against his abusive father. He identified with his father, internalized his aggressive thoughts, feelings, and behavior, and eventually became abusive himself. (This example is extreme. In reality, most children both absorb the experience of being a victim and take on some of the thoughts, feelings, or behaviors of the toxic adult.)

As another example, two patients both present with Emotional Deprivation schemas. As children, both had cold parents. Both felt lonely and unloved as children. Should we assume that, as adults, both had become emotionally cold? Not necessarily. Although both patients know what it means to be recipients of coldness, they are not necessarily cold themselves. As we discuss later in the section on coping styles, instead of identifying with their cold parents, patients might cope with their feelings of deprivation by becoming nurturing, or, alternatively, they might cope by becoming demanding and feeling entitled. Our model does not assume that children identify with and internalize everything their parents do; rather, we have observed that they *selectively* identify with and internalize certain aspects of significant others. Some of these identifications and internalizations become schemas, and some become coping styles or modes.

We believe that temperament partly determines whether an individual identifies with and internalizes the characteristics of a significant other. For example, a child with a dysthymic temperament will probably not internalize a parent's optimistic style of dealing with misfortune. The parent's behavior is so contrary to the child's disposition that the child cannot assimilate it.

Emotional Temperament

Factors other than early childhood environment also play major roles in the development of schemas. The child's emotional temperament is especially important. As most parents soon realize, each child has a unique and distinct "personality" or temperament from birth. Some children are more irritable, some are more shy, some are more aggressive. There is a great deal of research supporting the importance of the biological underpinnings of personality. For example, Kagan and his colleagues (Kagan, Reznick, & Snidman, 1988) have generated a body of research on temperamental traits present in infancy and have found them to be remarkably stable over time.

Following are some dimensions of emotional temperament that we hypothesize might be largely inborn and relatively unchangeable through psychotherapy alone.

Labile ↔ Nonreactive

Dysthymic ↔ Optimistic

Anxious ↔ Calm

Obsessive ↔ Distractible

Passive ↔ Aggressive

Irritable ↔ Cheerful

Shy ↔ Sociable

One might think of temperament as the individual's unique mix of points on this set of dimensions (as well as other aspects of temperament that will undoubtedly be identified in the future).

Emotional temperament interacts with painful childhood events in the formation of schemas. Different temperaments selectively expose children to different life circumstances. For example, an aggressive child might be more likely to elicit physical abuse from a violent parent than a passive, appeasing child. In addition, different temperaments render children differentially susceptible to similar life circumstances. Given the same parental treatment, two children might react very differently. For example, consider two boys who are both rejected by their mothers. The shy child hides from the world and becomes increasingly withdrawn and dependent on his mother; the sociable one ventures forth and makes other, more positive connections. Indeed, sociability has been shown to be a prominent trait of resilient children, who thrive despite abuse or neglect.

In our observation, an extremely favorable or aversive early environment can override emotional temperament to a significant degree. For example, a safe and loving home environment might make even a shy child quite friendly in many situations; alternatively, if the early environment is rejecting enough, even a sociable child may become withdrawn. Similarly, an extreme emotional temperament can override an ordinary environment and produce psychopathology without apparent justification in the patient's history.

SCHEMA DOMAINS AND EARLY MALADAPTIVE SCHEMAS

In our model, the 18 schemas are grouped into five broad categories of unmet emotional needs that we call "schema domains." We review the empirical support for these 18 schemas later in the chapter. In this section we elaborate on the five domains and list the schemas they contain. In Figure 1.1, the five schema domains are centered, in italics, without numbers (e.g., *"Disconnection and Rejection"*); the 18 schemas are aligned to the left and numbered (e.g., "1. Abandonment/Instability").

Domain I: Disconnection and Rejection

Patients with schemas in this domain are unable to form secure, satisfying attachments to others. They believe that their needs for stability, safety, nurturance, love, and belonging will not be met. Typical families of origin are unstable (*Abandonment/Instability*), abusive (*Mistrust/Abuse*), cold (*Emotional Deprivation*), rejecting (*Defectiveness/Shame*), or isolated from the outside world (*Social Isolation/Alienation*). Patients with schemas in the Disconnection and Rejection domain (especially the first four schemas) are often the most damaged. Many had traumatic childhoods, and as adults they tend to rush headlong from one self-destructive relationship to another or to avoid close relationships altogether. The therapy relationship is often central to the treatment of these patients.

The *Abandonment/Instability* schema is the perceived instability of one's connection to significant others. Patients with this schema have the sense that important people in their life will not continue to be there because they are emotionally unpredictable, they are only present erratically, they will die, or they will leave the patient for someone better.

Patients who have the *Mistrust/Abuse* schema have the conviction that, given the opportunity, other people will use the patient for their own selfish ends. For example, they will abuse, hurt, humiliate, lie to, cheat, or manipulate the patient.

The *Emotional Deprivation* schema is the expectation that one's desire for emotional connection will not be adequately fulfilled. We identify three forms: (1) deprivation of *nurturance* (the absence of affection or caring); (2) deprivation of *empathy* (the absence of listening or understanding); and (3) deprivation of *protection* (the absence of strength or guidance from others).

The *Defectiveness/Shame* schema is the feeling that one is flawed, bad, inferior, or worthless and that one would be unlovable to others if exposed. The schema usually involves a sense of shame regarding one's perceived defects. Flaws may be private (e.g., selfishness, aggressive impulses, unacceptable sexual desires) or public (e.g., unattractive appearance, social awkwardness).

The *Social Isolation/Alienation* schema is the sense of being different from or not fitting into the larger social world outside the family. Typically, patients with this schema do not feel they belong to any group or community.

FIGURE 1.1. Early maladaptive schemas with associated schema domains.

___

Disconnection and Rejection

(The expectation that one's needs for security, safety, stability, nurturance, empathy, sharing of feelings, acceptance, and respect will not be met in a predictable manner. Typical family origin is detached, cold, rejecting, withholding, lonely, explosive, unpredictable, or abusive.)

1. Abandonment/Instability

The perceived *instability* or *unreliability* of those available for support and connection.

Involves the sense that significant others will not be able to continue providing emotional support, connection, strength, or practical protection because they are emotionally unstable and unpredictable (e.g., have angry outbursts), unreliable, or present only erratically; because they will die imminently; or because they will abandon the individual in favor of someone better.

2. Mistrust/Abuse

The expectation that others will hurt, abuse, humiliate, cheat, lie, manipulate, or take advantage. Usually involves the perception that the harm is intentional or the result of unjustified and extreme negligence. May include the sense that one always ends up being cheated relative to others or "getting the short end of the stick."

3. Emotional Deprivation

The expectation that one's desire for a normal degree of emotional support will not be adequately met by others. The three major forms of deprivation are:

  A. ***Deprivation of Nurturance:*** Absence of attention, affection, warmth, or companionship.
  B. ***Deprivation of Empathy:*** Absence of understanding, listening, self-disclosure, or mutual sharing of feelings from others.
  C. ***Deprivation of Protection:*** Absence of strength, direction, or guidance from others.

4. Defectiveness/Shame

The feeling that one is defective, bad, unwanted, inferior, or invalid in important respects or that one would be unlovable to significant others if exposed. May involve hypersensitivity to criticism, rejection, and blame; self-consciousness, comparisons, and insecurity around others; or a sense of shame regarding one's perceived flaws. These flaws may be **private** (e.g., selfishness, angry impulses, unacceptable sexual desires) or **public** (e.g., undesirable physical appearance, social awkwardness).

5. Social Isolation/Alienation

The feeling that one is isolated from the rest of the world, different from other people, and/or not part of any group or community.

Impaired Autonomy and Performance

(Expectations about oneself and the environment that interfere with one's perceived ability to separate, survive, function independently, or perform successfully. Typical family origin is enmeshed, undermining of child's confidence, overprotective, or failing to reinforce child for performing competently outside the family.)

(cont.)

FIGURE 1.1. *(cont.)*

---

6. Dependence/Incompetence

Belief that one is unable to handle one's *everyday responsibilities* in a competent manner, without considerable help from others (e.g., take care of oneself, solve daily problems, exercise good judgment, tackle new tasks, make good decisions). Often presents as helplessness.

7. Vulnerability to Harm or Illness

Exaggerated fear that *imminent* catastrophe will strike at any time and that one will be unable to prevent it. Fears focus on one or more of the following: (A) *Medical catastrophes* (e.g., heart attacks, AIDS); (B) *Emotional catastrophes* (e.g., going crazy); (C) *External catastrophes* (e.g., elevators collapsing, victimization by criminals, airplane crashes, earthquakes).

8. Enmeshment/Undeveloped Self

Excessive emotional involvement and closeness with one or more significant others (often parents) at the expense of full individuation or normal social development. Often involves the belief that at least one of the enmeshed individuals cannot survive or be happy without the constant support of the other. May also include feelings of being smothered by or fused with others or insufficient individual identity. Often experienced as a feeling of emptiness and foundering, having no direction, or in extreme cases questioning one's existence.

9. Failure

The belief that one has failed, will inevitably fail, or is fundamentally inadequate relative to one's peers in areas of *achievement* (school, career, sports, etc.). Often involves beliefs that one is stupid, inept, untalented, lower in status, less successful than others, and so forth.

Impaired Limits

(Deficiency in internal limits, responsibility to others, or long-term goal orientation. Leads to difficulty respecting the rights of others, cooperating with others, making commitments, or setting and meeting realistic personal goals. Typical family origin is characterized by permissiveness, overindulgence, lack of direction, or a sense of superiority rather than appropriate confrontation, discipline, and limits in relation to taking responsibility, cooperating in a reciprocal manner, and setting goals. In some cases, the child may not have been pushed to tolerate normal levels of discomfort or may not have been given adequate supervision, direction, or guidance.)

10. Entitlement/Grandiosity

The belief that one is superior to other people; entitled to special rights and privileges; or not bound by the rules of reciprocity that guide normal social interaction. Often involves insistence that one should be able to do or have whatever one wants, regardless of what is realistic, what others consider reasonable, or the cost to others; or an exaggerated focus on superiority (e.g., being among the most successful, famous, wealthy) in order to achieve *power* or *control* (not primarily for attention or approval). Sometimes includes excessive competitiveness toward or domination of others: asserting one's power, forcing one's point of view, or controlling the behavior of others in line with one's own desires without empathy or concern for others' needs or feelings.

11. Insufficient Self-Control/Self-Discipline

Pervasive difficulty or refusal to exercise sufficient self-control and frustration tolerance to achieve one's personal goals or to restrain the excessive expression of one's emotions

(cont.)

FIGURE 1.1. *(cont.)*

and impulses. In its milder form, the patient presents with an exaggerated emphasis on *discomfort avoidance:* avoiding pain, conflict, confrontation, responsibility, or overexertion at the expense of personal fulfillment, commitment, or integrity.

Other-Directedness

(An excessive focus on the desires, feelings, and responses of others, at the expense of one's own needs in order to gain love and approval, maintain one's sense of connection, or avoid retaliation. Usually involves suppression and lack of awareness regarding one's own anger and natural inclinations. Typical family origin is based on conditional acceptance: Children must suppress important aspects of themselves in order to gain love, attention, and approval. In many such families, the parents' emotional needs and desires—or social acceptance and status—are valued more than the unique needs and feelings of each child.)

12. Subjugation

Excessive surrendering of control to others because one feels *coerced*—submitting in order to avoid anger, retaliation, or abandonment. The two major forms of subjugation are:

A. ***Subjugation of needs:*** Suppression of one's preferences, decisions, and desires.
B. ***Subjugation of emotions:*** Suppression of emotions, especially anger.

Usually involves the perception that one's own desires, opinions, and feelings are not valid or important to others. Frequently presents as excessive compliance, combined with hypersensitivity to feeling trapped. Generally leads to a buildup of anger, manifested in maladaptive symptoms (e.g., passive–aggressive behavior, uncontrolled outbursts of temper, psychosomatic symptoms, withdrawal of affection, "acting out," substance abuse).

13. Self-Sacrifice

Excessive focus on *voluntarily* meeting the needs of others in daily situations at the expense of one's own gratification. The most common reasons are: to prevent causing pain to others; to avoid guilt from feeling selfish; or to maintain the connection with others perceived as needy. Often results from an acute sensitivity to the pain of others. Sometimes leads to a sense that one's own needs are not being adequately met and to resentment of those who are taken care of. (Overlaps with concept of codependency.)

14. Approval-Seeking/Recognition-Seeking

Excessive emphasis on gaining approval, recognition, or attention from other people or on fitting in at the expense of developing a secure and true sense of self. One's sense of esteem is dependent primarily on the reactions of others rather than on one's own natural inclinations. Sometimes includes an overemphasis on status, appearance, social acceptance, money, or achievement as means of gaining *approval, admiration,* or *attention* (not primarily for power or control). Frequently results in major life decisions that are inauthentic or unsatisfying or in hypersensitivity to rejection.

Overvigilance and Inhibition

(Excessive emphasis on suppressing one's spontaneous feelings, impulses, and choices or on meeting rigid, internalized rules and expectations about performance and ethical behavior, often at the expense of happiness, self-expression, relaxation, close

(cont.)

FIGURE 1.1. *(cont.)*

relationships, or health. Typical family origin is grim, demanding, and sometimes punitive: performance, duty, perfectionism, following rules, hiding emotions, and avoiding mistakes predominate over pleasure, joy, and relaxation. There is usually an undercurrent of pessimism and worry that things could fall apart if one fails to be vigilant and careful at all times.)

15. Negativity/Pessimism

A pervasive, lifelong focus on the negative aspects of life (pain, death, loss, disappointment, conflict, guilt, resentment, unsolved problems, potential mistakes, betrayal, things that could go wrong, etc.) while minimizing or neglecting the positive or optimistic aspects. Usually includes an exaggerated expectation—in a wide range of work, financial, or interpersonal situations—that things will eventually go seriously wrong or that aspects of one's life that seem to be going well will ultimately fall apart. Usually involves an inordinate fear of making mistakes that might lead to financial collapse, loss, humiliation, or being trapped in a bad situation. Because they exaggerate potential negative outcomes, these individuals are frequently characterized by chronic worry, vigilance, complaining, or indecision.

16. Emotional Inhibition

The excessive inhibition of spontaneous action, feeling, or communication, usually to avoid disapproval by others, feelings of shame, or losing control of one's impulses. The most common areas of inhibition involve: (a) inhibition of *anger* and aggression; (b) inhibition of *positive impulses* (e.g., joy, affection, sexual excitement, play); (c) difficulty expressing *vulnerability* or *communicating* freely about one's feelings, needs, and so forth; or (d) excessive emphasis on *rationality* while disregarding emotions.

17. Unrelenting Standards/Hypercriticalness

The underlying belief that one must strive to meet very high *internalized standards* of behavior and performance, usually to avoid criticism. Typically results in feelings of pressure or difficulty slowing down and in hypercriticalness toward oneself and others. Must involve significant impairment in pleasure, relaxation, health, self-esteem, sense of accomplishment, or satisfying relationships.

Unrelenting standards typically present as (a) **perfectionism,** inordinate attention to detail, or an underestimate of how good one's own performance is relative to the norm; (b) **rigid rules** and "shoulds" in many areas of life, including unrealistically high moral, ethical, cultural, or religious precepts; or (c) preoccupation with **time and efficiency,** the need to accomplish more.

18. Punitiveness

The belief that people should be harshly punished for making mistakes. Involves the tendency to be angry, intolerant, punitive, and impatient with those people (including oneself) who do not meet one's expectations or standards. Usually includes difficulty forgiving mistakes in oneself or others because of a reluctance to consider extenuating circumstances, allow for human imperfection, or empathize with feelings.

Domain II: Impaired Autonomy and Performance

Autonomy is the ability to separate from one's family and to function independently comparable to people one's own age. Patients with schemas in this domain have expectations about themselves and the world that interfere with their ability to differentiate themselves from parent figures and function independently. When these patients were children, typically their parents did everything for them and overprotected them; or, at the opposite (much more rare) extreme, hardly ever cared for or watched over them. (Both extremes lead to problems in the autonomy realm.) Often their parents undermined their self-confidence and failed to reinforce them for performing competently outside the home. Consequently, these patients are not able to forge their own identities and create their own lives. They are not able to set personal goals and master the requisite skills. With respect to competence, they remain children well into their adult lives.

Patients with the *Dependence/Incompetence* schema feel unable to handle their everyday responsibilities without substantial help from others. For example, they feel unable to manage money, solve practical problems, use good judgment, undertake new tasks, or make good decisions. The schema often presents as pervasive passivity or helplessness.

Vulnerability to Harm or Illness is the exaggerated fear that catastrophe will strike at any moment and that one will be unable to cope. Fears focus on the following types of catastrophes: (1) *medical* (e.g., heart attacks, diseases such as AIDS); (2) *emotional* (e.g., going crazy, losing control); and (3) *external* (e.g., accidents, crime, natural catastrophes).

Patients with the *Enmeshment/Undeveloped Self* schema are often overly involved with one or more significant others (often parents) to the detriment of their full individuation and social development. These patients frequently believe that at least one of the enmeshed individuals could not function without the other. The schema may include feelings of being smothered by or fused with others or lacking a clear sense of identity and direction.

The *Failure* schema is the belief that one will inevitably fail in areas of achievement (e.g., school, sports, career) and that, in terms of achievement, one is fundamentally inadequate relative to one's peers. The schema often involves beliefs that one is unintelligent, inept, untalented, or unsuccessful.

Domain III: Impaired Limits

Patients with schemas in this domain have not developed adequate internal limits in regard to reciprocity or self-discipline. They may have difficulty respecting the rights of others, cooperating, keeping commitments, or meeting long-term goals. These patients often present as selfish, spoiled, irresponsible, or narcissistic. They typically grew up in families that were overly permissive and indulgent. (Entitlement can sometimes be a form of overcompensation for another schema, such as Emotional Deprivation; in these cases, overindulgence is usually not the primary origin, as we discuss in Chapter 10.) As children, these patients were not required to follow the rules that apply to everyone else, to consider others, or to develop self-control. As adults they lack the capacity to restrain their impulses and to delay gratification for the sake of future benefits.

The *Entitlement/Grandiosity* schema is the assumption that one is superior to other people, and therefore entitled to special rights and privileges. Patients with this schema do not feel bound by the rules of reciprocity that guide normal social interaction. They often insist that they should be able to do whatever they want, regardless of the cost to others. They may maintain an exaggerated focus on superiority (e.g., being among the most successful, famous, wealthy) in order to achieve power. These patients are often overly demanding or dominating, and lack empathy.

Patients with the *Insufficient Self-Control/Self-Discipline* schema either cannot or will not exercise sufficient self-control and frustration tolerance to achieve their personal goals. These patients do not regulate the expression of their emotions and impulses. In the milder form of this schema, patients present with an exaggerated emphasis on discomfort avoidance. For example, they avoid most conflict or responsibility.

Domain IV: Other-Directedness

The patients in this domain place an excessive emphasis on meeting the needs of others rather than their own needs. They do this in order to gain approval, maintain emotional connection, or avoid retaliation. When interacting with others, they tend to focus almost exclusively on the responses of the other person rather than on their own needs, and often lack awareness of their own anger and preferences. As children, they were not free to follow their natural inclinations. As adults, rather than being directed internally, they are directed externally and follow the desires of others. The typical family origin is based on conditional acceptance: Children must restrain important aspects of themselves in order to obtain love or approval. In many such families, the parents value their own emotional needs or social "appearances" more than they value the unique needs of the child.

The *Subjugation* schema is an excessive surrendering of control to others because one feels coerced. The function of subjugation is usually to avoid anger, retaliation, or abandonment. The two major forms are: (1) *subjugation of needs:* suppressing one's preferences or desires; and (2) *subjugation of emotions:* suppressing one's emotional responses, especially anger. The schema usually involves the perception that one's own needs and feelings are not valid or important. It frequently presents as excessive compliance and eagerness to please, combined with hypersensitivity to feeling trapped. Subjugation generally leads to a buildup of anger, manifested in maladaptive symptoms (e.g., passive–aggressive behavior, uncontrolled tempter outbursts, psychosomatic symptoms, or withdrawal of affection).

Patients with the *Self-Sacrifice* schema voluntarily meet the needs of others at the expense of their own gratification. They do this in order to spare others pain, avoid guilt, gain self-esteem, or maintain an emotional connection with someone they see as needy. The schema often results from an acute sensitivity to the suffering of others. It involves the sense that one's own needs are not being adequately met and may lead to feelings of resentment. This schema overlaps with the 12-step concept of "co-dependency."

Patients with the *Approval-Seeking/Recognition-Seeking* schema value gaining approval or recognition from other people over developing a secure and genuine sense of self. Their self-esteem is dependent on the reactions of others rather than on their own reactions. The schema often includes an excessive preoccupation with social status, appearance, money, or success as a means of gaining approval or recognition. It frequently results in major life decisions that are inauthentic and unsatisfying.

Domain V: Overvigilance and Inhibition

Patients in this domain suppress their spontaneous feelings and impulses. They often strive to meet rigid, internalized rules about their own performance at the expense of happiness, self-expression, relaxation, close relationships, or good health. The typical origin is a childhood that was grim, repressed, and strict and in which self-control and self-denial predominated over spontaneity and pleasure. As children, these patients were not encouraged to play and pursue happiness. Rather, they learned to be hypervigilant to negative life events and to regard life as bleak. These patients usually convey a sense of pessimism and worry, fearing that their lives could fall apart if they fail to be alert and careful at all times.

The *Negativity/Pessimism* schema is a pervasive, lifelong focus on the negative aspects of life (e.g., pain, death, loss, disappointment, conflict, betrayal) while minimizing the positive aspects. The schema usually includes an exaggerated expectation that things will eventually go seriously wrong in a wide range of work, financial, or interpersonal situations. These patients have an inordinate fear of making mistakes that might lead to financial collapse, loss, humiliation, or being trapped in a bad situation. Because these patients exaggerate potential negative outcomes, they are frequently characterized by worry, apprehensiveness, hypervigilance, complaining, and indecision.

Patients with *Emotional Inhibition* constrain their spontaneous actions, feelings, and communication. They usually do this to prevent being criticized or losing control of their impulses. The most common areas of inhibition involve: (1) inhibition of *anger*; (2) inhibition of *positive impulses* (e.g., joy, affection, sexual excitement, playfulness); (3) difficulty expressing *vulnerability*; and (4) emphasis on *rationality* while disregarding emotions. These patients often present as flat, constricted, withdrawn, or cold.

The *Unrelenting Standards/Hypercriticalness* schema is the sense that one must strive to meet very high internalized standards, usually in order to avoid disapproval or shame. The schema typically results in feelings of constant pressure and hypercriticalness toward oneself and others. To be considered an Early Maladaptive Schema, there must be significant impairment in the patient's health, self-esteem, relationships, or experience of pleasure. The schema typically presents as: (1) *perfectionism* (e.g., the need to do things "right," inordinate attention to detail, or underestimating one's level of performance); (2) *rigid rules* and "shoulds" in many areas of life, including unrealistically high moral, cultural, or religious standards; or (3) preoccupation with *time and efficiency*.

The *Punitiveness* schema is the conviction that people should be harshly punished for making mistakes. The schema involves the tendency to be angry and intolerant with those people (including oneself) who do not meet one's standards. It usually includes difficulty forgiving mistakes because one is reluctant to consider extenuating circumstances, to allow for human imperfection, or to take a person's intentions into account.

Case Illustration

Let us consider a brief case vignette that illustrates the schema concept. A young woman named Natalie comes for treatment. Natalie has an Emotional Deprivation schema: Her predominant experience of intimate relationships is that her emotional needs are not met. This has been true since early childhood. Natalie was an only child with emotionally cold parents. Although they met all of her physical needs, they did not nurture her or give her sufficient attention or affection. They did not try to understand who she was. In her family, Natalie felt alone.

Natalie's presenting problem is chronic depression. She tells her therapist that she has been depressed her whole life. Although she has been in and out of therapy for years, her depression persists. Natalie has generally been attracted to emotionally depriving men. Her husband, Paul, fits this pattern. When Natalie goes to Paul for holding or sympathy, he becomes irritated and pushes her away. This triggers her Emotional Deprivation schema, and she becomes angry. Her anger is partially justified but also partially an overreaction to a husband who loves her but does not know how to show it.

Natalie's anger further alienates her husband, and he distances himself from her even more, thus perpetuating her schema of deprivation. The marriage is caught in a vicious cycle, driven by her schema. In her marriage, Natalie continues to live out her childhood deprivation. Before marrying, Natalie had dated a more emotionally demonstrative man, but she was not sexually attracted to him and felt "suffocated" by normal expressions of tenderness. This tendency to be most attracted to partners who trigger a core schema is one we commonly observe in our patients ("schema chemistry").

This example illustrates how early childhood deprivation leads to the development of a schema, which is then unwittingly played out and perpetuated in later life, leading to dysfunctional relationships and chronic Axis I symptoms.

Conditional versus Unconditional Schemas

We originally believed that the main difference between Early Maladaptive Schemas and Beck's underlying assumptions (Beck, Rush, Shaw, & Emery, 1979) was that schemas are unconditional, whereas underlying assumptions are conditional. We now view some schemas as conditional and others as unconditional. Generally, the schemas that are developed earliest and are most at the core are unconditional beliefs about the self and others, whereas the schemas that are developed later are conditional.

Unconditional schemas hold out no hope to the patient. No matter what the individual does, the outcome will be the same. The individual will be incompetent, fused, unlovable, a misfit, endangered, bad—and nothing can change it. The schema encapsulates what was done to the child, without the child having had any choice in the matter. The schema simply *is*. In contrast, conditional schemas hold out the possibility of hope. The individual might change the outcome. The individual can subjugate, self-sacrifice, seek approval, inhibit emotions, or strive to meet high standards and, in so doing, perhaps avert the negative outcome, at least temporarily.

Unconditional schemas	*Conditional schemas*
Abandonment/Instability	Subjugation
Mistrust/Abuse	Self-Sacrifice
Emotional Deprivation	Approval-Seeking/Recognition-
Defectiveness	Seeking
Social Isolation	Emotional Inhibition
Dependence/Incompetence	Unrelenting Standards/
Vulnerability to Harm or Illness	Hypercriticalness
Enmeshment/Undeveloped Self	
Failure	
Negativity/Pessimism	
Punitiveness	
Entitlement/Grandiosity	
Insufficient Self-Control/Self-	
Discipline	

Conditional schemas often develop as attempts to get relief from the unconditional schemas. In this sense, conditional schemas are "secondary." Here are some examples:

> *Unrelenting Standards in response to Defectiveness.* The individual believes, "If I can be perfect, then I will be worthy of love."
> *Subjugation in response to Abandonment.* The individual believes, "If I do whatever the other person wants and never get angry about it, then the person will stay with me."
> *Self-Sacrifice in response to Defectiveness.* "If I meet all of this individual's needs and ignore my own, then the individual will accept me despite my flaws, and I will not feel so unlovable."

It is usually impossible to meet the demands of conditional schemas all of the time. For example, it is hard to subjugate oneself totally and never get angry. It is hard to be demanding enough to get all of one's needs met or self-sacrificing enough to meet all of the other individual's needs. At most the conditional schemas can forestall the core schemas. The individual is bound to fall short and thus have to face the truth of the core schema once again. (Not all conditional schemas can be linked to earlier ones. These schemas are conditional only in the sense that, if the child does what is expected, feared consequences can often be avoided.)

How Schemas Interfere with Traditional Cognitive-Behavioral Therapy

Many Early Maladaptive Schemas have the potential to sabotage traditional cognitive-behavioral therapy. Schemas make it difficult for patients to meet many of the assumptions of traditional cognitive-behavioral therapy noted previously in this chapter. For example, in regard to the assumption that patients can form a positive therapeutic alliance fairly quickly, patients who have schemas in the Disconnection and Rejection domain (Abandonment, Mistrust/Abuse, Emotional Deprivation, Defectiveness/Shame) may not be able to establish this kind of uncomplicated positive bond in a short period of time. Similarly, in terms of the presumption that patients have a strong sense of identity and clear life goals to guide the selection of treatment objectives, patients with schemas in the Impaired Autonomy and Performance domain (Dependence, Vulnerability, Enmeshment/Undeveloped Self, Failure) may not know who they are and what they want and thus may be unable to set specific treatment goals.

Cognitive-behavioral therapy assumes that patients can access cognitions and emotions and verbalize them in therapy. Patients with schemas in the Other-Directedness domain (Subjugation, Self-Sacrifice, Approval-

Seeking) may be too focused on ascertaining what the therapist wants to look within themselves or to speak about their own thoughts and feelings. Finally, cognitive-behavior therapy assumes that patients can comply with treatment procedures. Patients with schemas in the Impaired Limits domain (Entitlement, Insufficient Self-Control/Self-Discipline) may be too unmotivated or undisciplined to do so.

EMPIRICAL SUPPORT FOR EARLY MALADAPTIVE SCHEMAS

A considerable amount of research has been done on Young's Early Maladaptive Schemas. Most research conducted thus far has been done using the long form of the Young Schema Questionnaire (Young & Brown, 1990), although studies with the short form are in progress. The Young Schema Questionnaire has been translated into many languages, including French, Spanish, Dutch, Turkish, Japanese, Finnish, and Norwegian.

The first comprehensive investigation of its psychometric properties was conducted by Schmidt, Joiner, Young, and Telch (1995). Results from this study produced alpha coefficients for each Early Maladaptive Schema that ranged from .83 (Enmeshment/Undeveloped Self) to .96 (Defectiveness/Shame) and test–retest coefficients from .50 to .82 in a nonclinical population. The primary subscales demonstrated high test–retest reliability and internal consistency. The questionnaire also demonstrated good convergent and discriminant validity on measures of psychological distress, self-esteem, cognitive vulnerability to depression, and personality disorder symptomatology.

The investigators conducted a factor analysis using both clinical and nonclinical samples. The samples revealed similar sets of primary factors that closely matched Young's clinically developed schemas and their hypothesized hierarchical relationships. Within one sample of undergraduate college students, 17 factors emerged, including 15 of the 16 originally proposed by Young (1990). One original schema, Social Undesirability, did not emerge, whereas two other unaccounted factors did. In an effort to cross-validate this factor structure, Schmidt et al. (1995) gave the Young Schema Questionnaire to a second sample of undergraduates taken from the same population. Using the same factor-analytic technique, the investigators found that, of the 17 factors produced in the first analysis, 13 were clearly replicated in the second sample. The investigators also found three distinct higher order factors. Within a sample of patients, 15 factors emerged, including 15 of the 16 originally proposed by Young (1990). These 15 factors accounted for 54% of the total variance (Schmidt et al., 1995).

In this study, the Young Schema Questionnaire demonstrated convergent validity with a test of personality disorder symptomatology (Personality Diagnostic Questionnaire—Revised; Hyler, Rieder, Spitzer, & Williams,

1987). It also demonstrated discriminant validity with measures of depression (Beck Depression Inventory; Beck, Ward, Mendelson, Mock, & Erbaugh, 1961) and self-esteem (Rosenberg Self-Esteem Questionnaire; Rosenberg, 1965) in a nonclinical undergraduate population.

This study was replicated by Lee, Taylor, and Dunn (1999) using an Australian clinical population. The investigators conducted a factor analysis. In accord with previous findings, 16 factors emerged as primary components, including 15 of the 16 originally proposed by Young. Only the Social Undesirability scale was not supported. (We have since eliminated Social Undesirability as a separate schema and merged it with Defectiveness.) In addition, a higher order factor analysis closely fit some of the schema domains proposed by Young. Overall, this study shows that the Young Schema Questionnaire possesses very good internal consistency and that its primary factor structure is stable across clinical samples from two different countries and for different diagnoses.

Lee and his colleagues (1999) discuss some reasons that the two studies produced somewhat different factor structures depending on whether a clinical or normal population was used. They conclude that the student samples probably had range effects, as it was unlikely that many of the students were suffering from extreme forms of psychopathology. The authors state that factor structure replication depends on the assumption that the schemas underlying psychopathology in clinical populations are also present in a random sample of college students. Young suggests that Early Maladaptive Schemas are indeed present in normal populations but that they become exaggerated and extreme in clinical populations.

Other studies have examined the validity of the individual schemas and how well they support Young's model. Freeman (1999) explored the use of Young's schema theory as an explanatory model for nonrational cognitive processing. Using normal participants, Freeman found that weaker endorsement of Early Maladaptive Schemas was predictive of greater interpersonal adjustment. This finding is consistent with Young's tenet that Early Maladaptive Schemas are by definition negative and dysfunctional.

Rittenmeyer (1997) examined the convergent validity of Young's schema domains with the Maslach Burnout Inventory (Maslach & Jackson, 1986), a self-report inventory designed to assess the negative impact of stressful life events. In a sample of California schoolteachers, Rittenmeyer (1997) found that two schema domains, Overconnection and Exaggerated Standards, correlated strongly with the Emotional Exhaustion scale of the Maslach Burnout Inventory. The Overconnection schema domain also correlated, although not as strongly, with two other inventory scales, Depersonalization and Personal Accomplishment.

Carine (1997) investigated the utility of Young's schema theory in the treatment of personality disorders by using Early Maladaptive

Schemas as predictor variables in a discriminant function analysis. Specifically, Carine looked at whether the presence of Young's schemas discriminated patients with DSM-IV Axis II psychopathology from patients with other types of psychopathology. Carine found that group membership in the Axis II cluster was predicted correctly 83% of the time. In support of Young's theory, Carine also found that affect appears to be an intrinsic part of schemas.

Although the Young Schema Questionnaire was not designed to measure specific DSM-IV personality disorders, significant associations appear between Early Maladaptive Schemas and personality disorder symptoms (Schmidt et al., 1995). The total score correlates highly with the total score on the Personality Diagnostic Questionnaire—Revised (Hyler et al., 1987), a self-report measure of DSM-III-R personality pathology. In this study, the schemas of Insufficient Self-Control/Self-Discipline and Defectiveness had the strongest associations with personality disorder symptoms. Individual schemas have been found to be significantly associated with theoretically relevant personality disorders. For example, Mistrust/Abuse is highly associated with paranoid personality disorder; Dependence is associated with dependent personality disorder; Insufficient Self-Control/Self-Discipline is associated with borderline personality disorder; and Unrelenting Standards is associated with obsessive–compulsive personality disorder (Schmidt et al., 1995).

THE BIOLOGY OF EARLY MALADAPTIVE SCHEMAS

In this section we propose a biological view of schemas based on recent research on emotion and the biology of the brain (LeDoux, 1996). We stress that this section advances *hypotheses* about possible mechanisms of schema development and change. Research has not yet been undertaken to establish whether these hypotheses are valid.

Recent research suggests that there is not one emotional system in the brain but several. Different emotions are involved with different survival functions—responding to danger, finding food, having sex and finding mates, caring for offspring, social bonding—and each seems to be mediated by its own brain network. We focus on the brain network associated with fear conditioning and trauma.

Brain Systems Involved with Fear Conditioning and Trauma

Studies on the biology of the brain indicate locations at which schema triggering based on traumatic childhood events such as abandonment or abuse might occur in the brain. In his summary of the research on the biology of traumatic memories, LeDoux (1996) writes:

During a traumatic learning situation, conscious memories are laid down by a system involving the hippocampus and related cortical areas, and unconscious memories established by fear conditioning mechanisms operating through an amygdala–based system. These two systems operate in parallel and store different kinds of information relevant to the experience. And when stimuli that were present during the initial trauma are later encountered, each system can potentially retrieve its memories. In the case of the amygdala system, retrieval results in expression of bodily responses that prepare for danger, and in the case of the hippocampal system, conscious remembrances occur. (p. 239)

Thus, according to LeDoux, the brain mechanisms that register, store, and retrieve memories of the emotional significance of a traumatic event are different from the mechanisms that process conscious memories and cognitions about the same event. The amygdala stores the emotional memory, and the hippocampus and neocortex store the cognitive memory. Emotional responses can occur without the participation of the higher processing systems of the brain—those involved in thinking, reasoning, and consciousness.

Characteristics of the Amygdala System

According to LeDoux, the amygdala system has a number of attributes that distinguish it from the hippocampal system and higher cortexes.

• *The amygdala system is unconscious.* Emotional reactions can be formed in the amygdala without any conscious registration of the stimuli. As Zajonc (1984) claimed over a decade ago, emotions can exist without cognitions.[3]

• *The amygdala system is faster.* A danger signal goes via the thalamus to both the amygdala and the cortex. However, the signal reaches the amygdala more rapidly than it reaches the cortex. By the time the cortex has recognized the danger signal, the amygdala has already started responding to the danger. As Zajonc (1984) also claimed, emotions can exist before cognitions.

• *The amygdala system is automatic.* Once the amygdala system makes an appraisal of danger, the emotions and bodily responses occur automatically. In contrast, systems involved in cognitive processing are not so closely tied to automatic responses. The distinguishing feature of cognitive processing is flexibility of responding. Once we have cognition, we have choice.

---

[3]In contrast to some cognitive scientists, we define the term "cognition" in this section as *conscious* thoughts or images, not as "implicit" cognitions or simple sensory perceptions.

• *Emotional memories in the amygdala system appear to be permanent.* LeDoux writes: "Unconscious fear memories established through the amygdala appear to be indelibly burned into the brain. They are probably with us for life" (p. 252). There is survival value in never forgetting dangerous stimuli. These memories are resistant to extinction. Under stress, even fears that appear to be extinguished often spontaneously recur. Extinction prevents the expression of conditioned fear responses but does not erase the memories that underlie the responses. "Extinction . . . involves the cortical control over the amygdala's output rather than a wiping clean of the amygdala's memory slate" (p. 250). (Thus we say that schemas can probably not be completely healed.)

• *The amygdala system does not make fine discriminations.* The amygdala system is biased toward evoking conditioned fear responses to traumatic stimuli. Once an emotional memory is stored in the amygdala, later exposure to stimuli that even slightly resemble those present during the trauma will unleash the fear reaction. The amygdala system provides a crude image of the external world, whereas the cortex provides more detailed and accurate representations. It is the cortex that is responsible for suppressing responses based on cognitive appraisals. The amygdala evokes responses; it does not inhibit them.

• *The amygdala system is evolutionarily prior to the higher cortexes.* When an individual confronts a threat, the amygdala fires a fear response that has changed very little through the eons and that is shared across the animal kingdom and perhaps even in lower species. The hippocampus is also part of the evolutionarily older part of the brain but is connected to the neocortex, which contains the later developing higher cortexes.

Implications for the Schema Model

Let us consider some possible implications of this research for schema theory. As we have noted, we define an Early Maladaptive Schema as a set of memories, emotions, bodily sensations, and cognitions that revolve around a childhood theme, such as abandonment, abuse, neglect, or rejection. We might conceptualize the brain biology of a schema as follows: Emotions and bodily sensations stored in the amygdala system bear all the attributes previously listed. When an individual encounters stimuli reminiscent of the childhood events that led to the development of the schema, the emotions and bodily sensations associated with the event are activated by the amygdala system unconsciously; or, if the individual is conscious of them, the emotions and bodily sensations are activated more rapidly than the cognitions. This activation of emotions and bodily sensations is automatic and is likely to be a permanent feature of the individual's life, although the degree of activation might lessen with schema healing. In contrast, conscious memories and cognitions associated with the trauma are stored in the hippocampal system and higher cortexes.

The fact that the emotional and cognitive aspects of traumatic experience are located in different brain systems may explain why schemas are not changeable by simple cognitive methods. In a related point, the cognitive components of a schema often develop later, after the emotions and bodily sensations are already stored in the amygdala system. Many schemas develop in a preverbal stage: They originate before the child has acquired language. Preverbal schemas come into being when the child is so young that all that is stored are the memories, emotions, and bodily sensations. The cognitions are added later, as the child begins to think and speak in words. (This is one of the therapist's roles: to help the patient attach words to the experience of the schema.) Thus emotions have primacy over cognitions in working with many schemas.

When an Early Maladaptive Schema is triggered, the individual is flooded with emotions and bodily sensations. The individual may or may not consciously connect this experience to the original memory. (This is another of the therapist's roles: to help patients connect the emotions and bodily sensations to childhood memories.) The memories are at the heart of a schema, but they are usually not clearly in awareness, even in the form of images. The therapist provides emotional support as the patient struggles to reconstruct these images.

Implications for Schema Therapy

The first goal of schema therapy is psychological awareness. The therapist helps patients identify their schemas and become aware of the childhood memories, emotions, bodily sensations, cognitions, and coping styles associated with them. Once patients understand their schemas and coping styles, they can then begin to exert some control over their responses. They can increase the exercise of their free will in regard to their schemas. LeDoux says:

> Therapy is just another way of creating synaptic potentiation in brain pathways that control the amygdala. The amygdala's emotional memories, as we've seen, are indelibly burned into its circuits. The best we can hope to do is to regulate their expression. And the way we do this is by getting the cortex to control the amygdala. (p. 265)

In this light, the goal of treatment is to increase conscious control over schemas, working to weaken the memories, emotions, bodily sensations, cognitions, and behaviors associated with them.

Early childhood trauma affects other parts of the body. Primates separated from their mothers experience elevated plasma cortisol levels. If the separations are repeated, these changes become permanent (Coe, Mendoza, Smotherman, & Levine, 1978; Coe, Glass, Wiener, & Levine, 1983). Other long-lasting neurobiological changes that result from early separation from the mother include changes in adrenal gland catecholamine synthesizing enzymes (Coe et al., 1978, 1983); and hypothalamic serotonin secretion (Coe, Wiener, Rosenberg, & Levine, 1985). Primate research also suggests that the opioid system is involved in the regulation of separation anxiety and that social isolation affects the sensitivity and number of brain opiate receptors (van der Kolk, 1987). Evidently, early separation experiences result in physical changes that affect psychological functioning and that might well be lifelong.

SCHEMA OPERATIONS

The two fundamental schema operations are schema perpetuation and schema healing. Every thought, feeling, behavior, and life experience relevant to a schema can be said to either *perpetuate* the schema—elaborating and reinforcing it—or *heal* the schema—thus weakening it.

Schema Perpetuation

Schema perpetuation refers to everything the patient does (internally and behaviorally) that keeps the schema going. Perpetuation includes all the thoughts, feelings, and behaviors that end up reinforcing rather than healing the schema—all the individual's self-fulfilling prophecies. Schemas are perpetuated through three primary mechanisms: cognitive distortions, self-defeating life patterns, and schema coping styles (which are discussed in detail in the following section). Through cognitive distortions, the individual misperceives situations in such a manner that the schema is reinforced, accentuating information that confirms the schema and minimizing or denying information that contradicts the schema. Affectively, an individual may block the emotions connected to a schema. When affect is blocked, the schema does not reach the level of conscious awareness, so the individual cannot take steps to change or heal the schema. Behaviorally, the individual engages in self-defeating patterns, unconsciously selecting and remaining in situations and relationships that trigger and perpetuate the schema, while avoiding relationships that are likely to heal the schema. Interpersonally, patients relate in ways that prompt others to respond negatively, thus reinforcing the schema.

Case Illustration

Martine has a Defectiveness schema, stemming mostly from her childhood relationship with her mother. "There was nothing my mother loved about me," she tells her therapist, "and there was nothing I could do about it. I wasn't pretty, I wasn't outgoing and popular, I didn't have a lot of personality, I didn't know how to dress with a lot of style. The one thing I had, which was that I was smart, didn't mean anything to my mother."

Now Martine is 31 years old. She has few female friends. Recently her boyfriend, Johnny, introduced her to the women who were dating his friends. Martine likes these women very much, but, although they have been welcoming toward her, she feels unable to establish friendships with them. "I don't think they like me," she explains to her therapist. "I get really nervous when I'm with them. I can't settle down and relate normally."

Cognitively, affectively, behaviorally, and interpersonally, Martine acts to perpetuate her schema with these women. Cognitively, she distorts information so that it upholds the schema. She discounts the many gestures of friendliness the women have made toward her ("They're only being nice because of Johnny. They don't really like me.") and falsely interprets things they do and say as evidence of their dislike. For example, when one of the women, Robin, did not ask Martine to be a bridesmaid in her upcoming wedding, Martine jumped to the conclusion that Robin "hated" her, even though she had known Robin for too short a time to be a likely candidate for bridesmaid. Affectively, Martine has strong emotional responses to events that even slightly resemble her childhood schema triggers; she feels intensely upset at any perceived rejection, no matter how slight. When Robin did not ask her to be a bridesmaid, for example, Martine felt utterly worthless and ashamed. "I hate myself," she told her therapist.

Martine gravitates toward relationships that are likely to repeat her childhood relationship with her mother. In the group of women, Martine has most actively sought the friendship of the one who is most hard to please and critical, and, just as she did with her mother as a child, Martine behaves deferentially and apologetically toward her.

Almost all patients who have characterological disorders repeat negative patterns from their childhoods in self-defeating ways. Chronically and pervasively, they engage in thoughts, emotions, behaviors, and means of relating that perpetuate their schemas. In so doing, they unwittingly keep recreating in their adult lives the conditions that most damaged them in childhood.

Schema Healing

Schema healing is the ultimate goal of schema therapy. Because a schema is a set of memories, emotions, bodily sensations, and cognitions, schema healing involves diminishing all of these: the intensity of the memories connected to the schema, the schema's emotional charge, the strength of the bodily sensations, and the maladaptive cognitions. Schema healing also involves behavior change, as patients learn to replace maladaptive coping styles with adaptive patterns of behavior. Treatment thus includes cognitive, affective, and behavioral interventions. As a schema heals, it becomes increasingly more difficult to activate. When it *is* activated, the experience is less overwhelming, and the patient recovers more quickly.

The course of schema healing is often arduous and long. Schemas are hard to change. They are deeply entrenched beliefs about the self and the world, learned at a very young age. They are often all the patient knows. Destructive though they might be, schemas provide patients with feelings of security and predictability. Patients resist giving up schemas because the schemas are central to their sense of identity. It is disrupting to give up a schema. The whole world tilts. In this light, resistance to therapy is a form of self-preservation, an attempt to hold onto a sense of control and inner coherence. To give up a schema is to relinquish knowledge of who one is and what the world is like.

Schema healing requires willingness to face the schema and do battle with it. It demands discipline and frequent practice. Patients must systematically observe the schema and work every day to change. Unless it is corrected, the schema will perpetuate itself. Therapy is like waging war on the schema. The therapist and patient form an alliance in order to defeat the schema, with the goal of vanquishing it. This goal is usually an unrealizable ideal, however: Most schemas never completely heal, because we cannot eradicate the memories associated with them.

Schemas never disappear altogether. Rather, when they heal, they become activated less frequently, and the associated affect becomes less intense and does not last as long. Patients respond to the triggering of their schemas in a healthy manner. They select more loving partners and friends, and they view themselves in more positive ways. We give an overview of how we go about healing schemas in a later section of this chapter.

MALADAPTIVE COPING STYLES AND RESPONSES

Patients develop maladaptive coping styles and responses early in life in order to adapt to schemas, so that they do not have to experience the intense, overwhelming emotions that schemas usually engender. It is important to remember, however, that, although coping styles sometimes help the patient to avoid a schema, they do not heal it. Thus all maladaptive coping styles still serve as elements in the schema perpetuation process.

Schema therapy differentiates between the schema itself and the strategies an individual utilizes to cope with the schema. Thus, in our model, the schema itself contains memories, emotions, bodily sensations, and cognitions, but not the individual's behavioral responses. *Behavior is not part of the schema; it is part of the coping response.* The schema drives the behavior. Although the majority of coping responses are behavioral, patients also cope through cognitive and emotive strategies. Whether the coping style is manifested through cognition, affect, or behavior, it is not part of the schema itself.

The reason that we differentiate schemas from coping styles is that each patient utilizes different coping styles in different situations at different stages of their lives to cope with the same schema. Thus the coping styles for a given schema do not necessarily remain stable for an individual over time, whereas the schema itself does. Furthermore, different patients use widely varying, even opposite, behaviors to cope with the same schema.

For example, consider three patients who typically cope with their Defectiveness schemas through different mechanisms. Although all three feel flawed, one seeks out critical partners and friends, one avoids getting close to anyone, and one adopts a critical and superior attitude toward others. Thus the coping behavior is not intrinsic to the schema.

Three Maladaptive Coping Styles

All organisms have three basic responses to threat: fight, flight, and freeze. These correspond to the three schema coping styles of *overcompensation, avoidance,* and *surrender.* In very broad terms, fight is overcompensation, flight is avoidance, and freeze is surrender.

In the context of childhood, an Early Maladaptive Schema represents the presence of a threat. The threat is the frustration of one of the child's core emotional needs (for secure attachment, autonomy, free self-expression, spontaneity and play, or realistic limits). The threat may also include the fear of the intense emotions the schema unleashes. Faced with the threat, the child can respond through some combination of these three coping responses: the child can surrender, avoid, or overcompensate. All three coping styles generally operate out of awareness—that is, unconsciously. In any given situation, the child will probably utilize only one of them, but the child can exhibit different coping styles in different situations or with different schemas. (We provide examples of these three styles below.)

Thus the triggering of a schema is a threat—the frustration of a core emotional need and the concomitant emotions—to which the individual responds with a coping style. These coping styles are usually adaptive in childhood and can be viewed as healthy survival mechanisms. But they become maladaptive as the child grows older because the coping styles continue to perpetuate the schema, even when conditions change and the individual has more promising options. Maladaptive coping styles ultimately keep patients imprisoned in their schemas.

Schema Surrender

When patients surrender to a schema, they yield to it. They do not try to avoid it or fight it. They accept that the schema is true. They feel the emotional pain of the schema directly. They act in ways that confirm the schema. Without realizing what they are doing, they repeat schema-driven patterns so that, as adults, they continue to relive the childhood experiences that created the schema. When they encounter schema triggers, their emotional responses are disproportionate, and they experience their emotions fully and consciously. Behaviorally, they choose partners who are most likely to treat them as the "offending parent" did—as Natalie, the depressed patient we described earlier, chose her emotionally depriving husband Paul. They then frequently relate to these partners in passive, compliant ways that perpetuate the schema. In the therapy relationship, these patients also may play out the schema with themselves in the "child" role and the therapist in the role of the "offending parent."

Schema Avoidance

When patients utilize avoidance as a coping style, they try to arrange their lives so that the schema is never activated. They attempt to live without awareness, as though the schema does not exist. They avoid thinking about the schema. They block thoughts and images that are likely to trigger it: When such thoughts or images loom, they distract themselves or put them out of their minds. They avoid feeling the schema. When feelings surface, they reflexively push them back down. They may drink excessively, take drugs, have promiscuous sex, overeat, compulsively clean, seek stimulation, or become workaholics. When they interact with others, they may appear perfectly normal. They usually avoid situations that might trigger the schema, such as intimate relationships or work challenges. Many patients shun whole areas of life in which they feel vulnerable. Often they avoid engaging in therapy; for example, these patients might "forget" to complete homework assignments, refrain from expressing affect, raise only superficial issues, come late to sessions, or terminate prematurely.

Schema Overcompensation

When patients overcompensate, they fight the schema by thinking, feeling, behaving, and relating as though the opposite of the schema were true. They endeavor to be as different as possible from the children they were when the schema was acquired. If they felt worthless as children, then as adults they try to be perfect. If they were subjugated as children, then as adults they defy everyone. If they were controlled as children, as adults they control others or reject all forms of influence. If abused, they abuse others. Faced with the schema, they counterattack. On the surface, they are self-confident and assured, but underneath they feel the press of the schema threatening to erupt.

Overcompensation can be viewed as a partially healthy attempt to fight back against the schema that unfortunately overshoots the mark, so that the schema is perpetuated rather than healed. Many "overcompensators" appear healthy. In fact, some of the most admired people in society—media stars, political leaders, business tycoons—are often overcompensators. It is healthy to fight back against a schema so long as the behavior is proportionate to the situation, takes into account the feelings of others, and can reasonably be expected to lead to a desirable outcome. But overcompensators typically get locked into counterattacking. Their behavior is usually excessive, insensitive, or unproductive.

For example, it is healthy for subjugated patients to exert more control in their lives; but, when they overcompensate, they become *too* controlling and domineering and end up driving others away. An overcompensated patient with subjugation cannot allow others to take the lead, even when it would be healthy to do so. Similarly, it is healthy for an emotionally deprived patient to ask others for emotional support, but an overcompensated patient with emotional deprivation goes too far and becomes demanding and feels entitled.

Overcompensation develops because it offers an alternative to the pain of the schema. It is a means of escape from the sense of helplessness and vulnerability that the patient felt growing up. For example, narcissistic overcompensations typically serve to help patients cope with core feelings of emotional deprivation and defectiveness. Rather than feeling ignored and inferior, these patients can feel special and superior. However, though they may be successful in the outside world, narcissistic patients are usually not at peace within themselves. Their overcompensation isolates them and ultimately brings them unhappiness. They continue to overcompensate, no matter how much it drives away other people. In so doing, they lose the ability to connect deeply with others. They are so invested in appearing to be perfect that they forfeit true intimacy. Further, no matter how perfect they try to be, they are bound to fail at something eventually, and they rarely know how to handle defeat constructively. They are unable to take responsibility for their failures or acknowledge their limitations and therefore have trouble learning from their mistakes. When they experience sufficiently powerful setbacks, their ability to overcompensate collapses, and they often decompensate by becoming clinically depressed. When overcompensation fails, the underlying schemas reassert themselves with enormous emotional strength.

We hypothesize that temperament is one of the main factors in determining why individuals develop certain coping styles rather than others. In fact, temperament probably plays a greater role in determining patients' coping styles than it does in determining their schemas. For example, individuals who have passive temperaments are probably more likely to surrender or avoid, whereas individuals who have aggressive temperaments are more likely to overcompensate. Another factor in explaining why patients adopt a given coping style is selective internalization, or modeling. Children often model the coping behavior of a parent with whom they identify.

We elaborate further on these coping styles in Chapter 5.

Coping Responses

Coping *responses* are the *specific* behaviors or strategies through which the three broad coping styles are expressed. They include all the responses to threat in the individual's behavioral repertoire—all the unique, idiosyncratic ways in which patients manifest overcompensation, avoidance, and surrender. When the individual habitually adopts certain coping responses, then coping responses adhere into "coping styles." Thus a coping style is a trait, whereas a coping response is a state. A coping style is a collection of coping responses that an individual characteristically utilizes to avoid, surrender, or overcompensate. A coping response is the specific behavior (or strategy) that the individual is exhibiting at a given point in time. For example, consider a male patient who uses some form of avoidance in almost any situation in which his schema of abandonment is triggered. When his girlfriend threatened to break up with him, he went back to his apartment and drank beer until he passed out. In this example, avoidance is the patient's coping *style* for abandonment; drinking beer was his coping *response* in this one situation with his girlfriend. (We discuss this distinction further in the following section on schema modes.)

Table 1.1 lists some examples of maladaptive coping responses for each schema. Most patients use a combination of coping responses and styles. Sometimes they surrender, sometimes they avoid, and sometimes they overcompensate.

Schemas, Coping Responses, and Axis II Diagnoses

We believe that the Axis II diagnostic system in DSM-IV is seriously flawed. Elsewhere (Young & Gluhoski, 1996) we have reviewed its many limitations, including low reliability and validity for many categories and the unacceptable level of overlap among the categories. In this chapter, however, we emphasize what we see as more fundamental conceptual flaws in the Axis II system. We believe that in an attempt to establish criteria based on observable behaviors, the developers have lost the essence of both what distinguishes Axis I from Axis II disorders and what makes chronic disorders hard to treat.

According to our model, internal schemas lie at the core of personality disorders and the behavioral patterns in DSM-IV are primarily responses to the core schemas. As we have stressed, healing schemas should be the central goal in working with patients at a characterological level. Eliminating maladaptive coping responses permanently is almost impossible without changing the schemas that drive them. Also, because the coping behaviors are not as stable as schemas—they change depending on the schema, the life situation, and the patient's stage of life—the patient's symptoms (and diagnosis) will appear to be shifting as one tries to change them.

For most DSM-IV categories, the coping behaviors *are* the personality disorders. Many diagnostic criteria are lists of coping responses. In contrast, the schema model accounts for chronic, pervasive characterological patterns in terms of both schemas and coping responses; it relates the schemas and coping responses to their origins in early childhood; and it provides direct and clear implications for treatment. Furthermore, each patient is viewed as having a unique profile, including several schemas and coping responses, each present at different levels of strength (dimensional) rather than as one single Axis II category.

SCHEMA MODES

The concept of a schema mode is probably the most difficult part of schema theory to explain, because it encompasses many elements. Schema modes are the moment-to-moment emotional states and coping responses—adaptive and maladaptive—that we all experience. Often our schema modes are triggered by life situations to which we are oversensitive (our "emotional buttons"). Unlike most other schema constructs, we are actively interested in working with both adaptive and maladaptive modes. In fact, we try to help patients flip from a dysfunctional mode to a healthy mode as part of the schema healing process.

At any given point in time, some of our schemas or schema operations (including our coping responses) are inactive, or dormant, while others have become activated by life events and predominate in our current moods and behavior. The predominant state that we are in at a given point in time is called our "schema mode." We use the term "flip" to refer to the switching of modes. As we have said, this state may be adaptive or maladaptive. All of us flip from mode to mode over time. A mode, therefore, answers the question, "At this moment in time, what set of schemas or schema operations is the patient manifesting?"

Our revised definition of a schema mode is: "those schemas or schema operations—adaptive or maladaptive—that are currently active for an individual." A *dysfunctional* schema mode is activated when specific maladaptive schemas or coping responses have erupted into distressing emo-

TABLE 1.1. Examples of Maladaptive Coping Responses

Early Maladaptive Schema	Examples of surrender	Examples of avoidance	Examples of overcompensation
Abandonment/ Instability	Selects partners who cannot make a commitment and remains in the relationships	Avoids intimate relationships; drinks a lot when alone	Clings to and "smothers" the partner to point of pushing partner away; vehemently attacks partner for even minor separations
Mistrust/Abuse	Selects abusive partners and permits abuse	Avoids becoming vulnerable and trusting anyone; keeps secrets	Uses and abuses others ("get others before they get you")
Emotional Deprivation	Selects emotionally depriving partners and does not ask them to meet needs	Avoids intimate relationships altogether	Acts emotionally demanding with partners and close friends
Defectiveness/ Shame	Selects critical and rejecting friends; puts self down	Avoids expressing true thoughts and feelings and letting others get close	Criticizes and rejects others while seeming to be perfect.
Social Isolation/ Alienation	At social gatherings, focuses exclusively on differences from others rather than similarities	Avoids social situations and groups	Becomes a chameleon to fit into groups
Dependence/ Incompetence	Asks significant others (parents, spouse) to make all his or her financial decisions	Avoids taking on new challenges, such as learning to drive	Becomes so self-reliant that he or she does not ask anyone for anything ("counterdependent")
Vulnerability to Harm or Illness	Obsessively reads about catastrophes in newspapers and anticipates them in everyday situations	Avoids going places that do not seem totally "safe"	Acts recklessly, without regard to danger ("counterphobic")
Enmeshment/ Undeveloped Self	Tells mother everything, even as an adult; lives through partner	Avoids intimacy; stays independent	Tries to become the opposite of significant others in all ways
Failure	Does tasks in a halfhearted or haphazard manner	Avoids work challenges completely; procrastinates on tasks	Becomes an "overachiever" by ceaselessly driving him- or herself

(cont.)

TABLE 1.1. (cont.)

Early Maladaptive Schema	Examples of surrender	Examples of avoidance	Examples of overcompensation
Entitlement/ Grandiosity	Bullies others into getting own way, brags about own accomplishments	Avoids situations in which he or she is average, not superior	Attends excessively to the needs of others
Insufficient Self-Control/Self-Discipline	Gives up easily on routine tasks	Avoids employment or accepting responsibility	Becomes overly self-controlled or self-disciplined
Subjugation	Lets other individuals control situations and make choices	Avoids situations that might involve conflict with another individual	Rebels against authority
Self-Sacrifice	Gives a lot to others and asks for nothing in return	Avoids situations involving giving or taking	Gives as little to others as possible
Approval-Seeking/ Recognition-Seeking	Acts to impress others	Avoids interacting with those whose approval is coveted	Goes out of the way to provoke the disapproval of others; stays in the background
Negativity/ Pessimism	Focuses on the negative; ignores the positive; worries constantly; goes to great lengths to avoid any possible negative outcome	Drinks to blot out pessimistic feelings and unhappiness	Is overly optimistic ("Pollyanna"-ish); denies unpleasant realities
Emotional Inhibition	Maintains a calm, emotionally flat demeanor	Avoids situations in which people discuss or express feelings	Awkwardly tries to be the "life of the party," even though it feels forced and unnatural
Unrelenting Standards/ Hypercriticalness	Spends inordinate amounts of time trying to be perfect	Avoids or procrastinates in situations and tasks in which performance will be judged	Does not care about standards at all—does tasks in a hasty, careless manner
Punitiveness	Treats self and others in harsh, punitive manner	Avoids others for fear of punishment	Behaves in overly forgiving way

tions, avoidance responses, or self-defeating behaviors that take over and control an individual's functioning. An individual may shift from one dysfunctional schema mode into another; as that shift occurs, different schemas or coping responses, previously dormant, become active.

Dysfunctional Schema Modes as Dissociated States

Viewed in a different way, a dysfunctional schema mode is a facet of the self involving specific schemas or schema operations that has not been fully integrated with other facets. According to this perspective, schema modes can be characterized by the degree to which a particular schema-driven state has become dissociated, or cut off, from an individual's other modes. A dysfunctional schema mode, therefore, is a part of the self that is cut off to some degree from other aspects of the self.

A dysfunctional schema mode can be described in terms of the point on a *spectrum* of dissociation at which this particular mode lies. To the degree that an individual is simultaneously able to experience or blend more than one mode, the level of dissociation is lower. We typically refer to this mild form of a schema mode as a normal mood shift, such as a lonely mood or an angry mood. At the highest level of dissociation is a patient with dissociative identity disorder (or multiple personality disorder). In these instances, a patient in one mode may not even know that another mode exists; and, in extreme cases, a patient with dissociative identity disorder (DID) may even have a different name for each mode. We discuss this concept of modes as dissociative states in more depth later.

We have currently identified 10 schema modes, although more modes will undoubtedly be identified in the future. The modes are grouped into four general categories: Child modes, Dysfunctional Coping modes, Dysfunctional Parent modes, and the Healthy Adult mode. Some modes are healthy for an individual, whereas others are maladaptive. We elaborate further on these 10 modes in a subsequent section.

One important goal of schema therapy is to teach patients how to strengthen their Healthy Adult modes, so that they can learn to navigate, negotiate with, nurture, or neutralize dysfunctional modes.

The Development of the Mode Concept

The concept of schema modes originated from our work with patients with borderline personality disorder (BPD), although now we apply it to many other diagnostic categories as well. One of the problems we were having applying the schema model to patients with BPD was that the number of schemas and coping responses they had was overwhelming for both the patient and the therapist to deal with all at one time. For example, we find that, when we give patients with BPD the Young Schema Question-naire, it is not unusual for them to score high on almost all of the 16 schemas assessed. We found that we needed a different unit of analysis, one that would group schemas together and make them more manageable.

Patients with BPD were also problematic for the original schema model because they continually shift from one extreme affective state or coping response to another: One moment they are angry; the next they may be sad, detached, avoidant, robotic, terrified, impulsive, or filled with self-hatred. Our original model, because it focused primarily on trait con-structs—a schema or a coping style—did not seem sufficient to account for the phenomenon of shifting states.

Let us elaborate further on this state–trait distinction as it relates to schema theory. When we say that an individual has a schema, we are not saying that at every moment the schema is activated. Rather, the schema is a trait that may or may not be activated at a given moment. Similarly, indi-viduals have characteristic coping styles, which they may or may not be utilizing at a given moment. Thus our original trait model tells us about the functioning of the patient over time, but it does not tell us about the patient's current state. Because patients with BPD are so labile, we decided to move away from a trait model and toward a state model in treating them, with the schema mode as the primary conceptual construct.

When we look carefully at individual patients, we observe that their schemas and coping responses tend to group together into parts of the self. Certain clusters of schemas or coping responses are triggered to-gether. For example, in the Vulnerable Child mode, the affect is that of a helpless child—fragile, frightened, and sad. When a patient is in this mode, schemas of Emotional Deprivation, Abandonment, and Vulnera-bility may be simultaneously activated. The Angry Child mode often presents with the affect of an enraged child having a temper tantrum. The Detached Protector mode is characterized by the absence of emo-tion, combined with high levels of avoidance. Thus some of the modes are composed primarily of schemas, whereas others primarily represent coping responses.

Each individual patient exhibits certain characteristic schema modes, by which we mean characteristic groupings of schemas or coping responses. Similarly, some Axis II diagnoses can be described in terms of their typical modes. For example, the patient with BPD usually exhibits four schema modes and shifts rapidly from one to the other. One moment the patient is in the Abandoned Child mode, experiencing the pain of her schemas; the next moment she may flip into the Angry Child mode, expressing rage; she may then shift into the Punitive Parent mode, punishing the Abandoned Child; and finally she may retreat into the Detached Protector, blocking her emo-tions and detaching from people to protect herself.

Modes as Dissociated States

We mentioned briefly that our concept of a schema mode relates to a spectrum of dissociation. Although we realize that the diagnosis has become controversial, we view the different personalities of patients with DID as extreme forms of dysfunctional modes. Different parts of the self have split off into separate personalities that are often unaware of each other and that may have different names, ages, genders, personality traits, memories, and functions. The dissociative identities of these patients usually consist of either a child at a specific age who has experienced severe trauma; an internalized parent tormenting, criticizing, or persecuting the child; or an adult-like coping mode that in some way protects or blocks out the child modes. We believe that the dissociative identities in DID differ from the modes of patients with BPD mainly in degree and number. Both multiple personalities and borderline modes are parts of the self that have been split off, but the borderline modes have not been split off to nearly the same degree. Furthermore, patients with DID usually have more modes than patients with BPD because they frequently have more than one mode of each type (e.g., three Vulnerable Child modes, each a different age).

A psychologically healthy individual still has recognizable modes, but the sense of a unified identify remains intact. A healthy individual might shift into a detached, angry, or sad mood in response to changing circumstances, but these modes will differ from borderline modes in several important respects. First, as we have said, normal modes are less dissociated than borderline modes. Healthy individuals can experience more than one mode simultaneously. For example, they can be both sad and happy about an event, thus producing the sensation of "bittersweet." In contrast, when we talk about a borderline mode, we are referring to one part of the self that is split off from the other parts in a pure and intense form. The individual is overwhelmingly frightened or completely enraged. Second, normal modes are less rigid and more flexible and open to change than the modes of patients with serious characterological problems. In Piagetian terms, they are more open to accommodation in response to reality (Piaget, 1962).

To summarize, modes vary from one individual to another along several dimensions:

Dissociated ↔ Integrated
Unacknowledged ↔ Acknowledged
Maladaptive ↔ Adaptive
Extreme ↔ Mild
Rigid ↔ Flexible
Pure ↔ Blended

Another difference between healthy and more impaired individuals lies in the strength and effectiveness of the Healthy Adult mode. Although we all have a Healthy Adult mode, the mode is stronger and more frequently activated in psychologically healthy people. The Healthy Adult mode can moderate and heal dysfunctional modes. For example, when psychologically healthy people become angry, they have a Healthy Adult mode that can usually keep angry emotions and behaviors from going out of control. In contrast, patients with BPD typically have a very weak Healthy Adult mode, so that when the Angry Child mode is triggered, there is no strong counterbalancing force. The anger almost completely takes over the patient's personality.

10 Schema Modes

We have identified 10 schema modes that can be grouped into four broad categories: Child modes, Dysfunctional Coping modes, Dysfunctional Parent modes, and the Healthy Adult mode.

We believe that the Child modes are innate and universal. All children are born with the potential to manifest them. We have identified four: the Vulnerable Child, the Angry Child, the Impulsive/Undisciplined Child, and the Happy Child modes. (These labels are general terms. In actual therapy we individualize the names of modes collaboratively with patients. For example, we might refer to the Vulnerable Child mode as Little Ann, or Abandoned Carol.)

The Vulnerable Child is the mode that usually experiences most of the core schemas: It is the Abandoned Child, the Abused Child, the Deprived Child, or the Rejected Child. The Angry Child is the part that is enraged about unmet emotional needs and that acts in anger without regard to consequences. The Impulsive/Undisciplined Child expresses emotions, acts on desires, and follows natural inclinations from moment to moment in a reckless manner, without regard to possible consequences for the self or others. The Happy Child is one whose core emotional needs are currently met.

We have identified three dysfunctional coping modes: the Compliant Surrenderer, the Detached Protector, and the Overcompensator. These three modes correspond to the three coping styles of surrender, avoidance, and overcompensation. (Again, we tailor the name of the mode so that it fits the feelings and behaviors of the individual patient.) The Compliant Surrenderer submits to the schema, becoming once again the passive, helpless child who must give in to others. The Detached Protector withdraws psychologically from the pain of the schema by emotionally detaching, abusing substances, self-stimulating, avoiding people, or utilizing other forms of escape. The Overcompensator fights back either by mistreating others or by behaving in extreme ways in an attempt to disprove the schema in a manner that ultimately proves dysfunctional (see the previous discussion of overcompensation for examples). All three maladaptive coping modes ultimately perpetuate schemas.

We have identified two dysfunctional parent modes thus far: the Punitive Parent and the Demanding Parent. In these modes, the patient becomes like the parent who has been internalized. The Punitive Parent punishes one of the child modes for being "bad," and the Demanding Parent continually pushes and pressures the child to meet excessively high standards.

The 10th mode, as described earlier, is the Healthy Adult. This is the mode we try to strengthen in therapy by teaching the patient to moderate, nurture, or heal the other modes.

SCHEMA ASSESSMENT AND CHANGE

This brief overview of the treatment process presents the steps in assessing and changing schemas. Each of these procedures is described in detail in later chapters. The two phases of treatment are the Assessment and Education Phase and the Change Phase.

Assessment and Education Phase

In this first phase, the schema therapist helps patients to identify their schemas and to understand the origins of the schemas in childhood and adolescence. In the course of the assessment, the therapist educates the patient about the schema model. Patients learn to recognize their maladaptive coping styles (surrender, avoidance, and overcompensation) and to see how their coping responses serve to perpetuate their schemas. We also teach more severely impaired patients about their primary schema modes and help them observe how they flip from one mode to another. We want patients both to understand their schema operations intellectually and to experience these processes emotionally.

The assessment is multifaceted, including a life history interview, several schema questionnaires, self-monitoring assignments, and imagery exercises that trigger schemas emotionally and help patients make emotional links between current problems and related childhood experiences. By the end of this phase, the therapist and patient have developed a complete schema case conceptualization and have agreed on a schema-focused treatment plan that encompasses cognitive, experiential, and behavioral strategies, as well as the healing components of the therapist–patient relationship.

Change Phase

Throughout the Change Phase, the therapist blends cognitive, experiential, behavioral, and interpersonal strategies in a flexible manner, depending on the needs of the patient week by week. The schema therapist does not adhere to a rigid protocol or set of procedures.

Cognitive Techniques

As long as patients believe that their schemas are valid, they will not be able to change; they will continue to maintain distorted views of themselves and others. Patients learn to build a case against the schema. They disprove the validity of the schema on a rational level. Patients list all the evidence supporting and refuting the schema throughout their lives, and the therapist and patient evaluate the evidence.

In most cases, the evidence will show that the schema is false. The patient is not inherently defective, incompetent, or a failure. Rather, through a process of indoctrination, the schema was taught to the patient in childhood, much as propaganda is taught to the populace. But sometimes the evidence alone is not sufficient to disprove the schema. For example, patients might in fact be failures at work or at school. As a result of procrastination and avoidance, they have not developed the relevant work skills. If there is not enough existing evidence to challenge the schema, then patients evaluate what they can do to change this aspect of their lives. For example, the therapist can guide them to fight expectations of failure so they can learn effective work skills.

After this exercise, the therapist and patient summarize the case against the schema on a flash card that they compose together. Patients carry these flash cards with them and read them frequently, especially when they are facing schema triggers.

Experiential Techniques

Patients fight the schema on an emotional level. Using such experiential techniques as imagery and dialogues, they express anger and sadness about what happened to them as children. In imagery, they stand up to the parent and other significant childhood figures, and they protect and comfort the vulnerable child. Patients talk about what they needed but did not receive from the parents when they were children. They link childhood images with images of upsetting situations in their current lives. They confront the schema and its message directly, opposing the schema and fighting back. Patients practice talking back to significant people in their current lives through imagery and role-playing. This empowers patients to break the schema perpetuation cycle at an emotional level.

Behavioral Pattern-Breaking

The therapist helps the patient design behavioral homework assignments in order to replace maladaptive coping responses with new, more adaptive patterns of behavior. The patient comes to see how certain partner choices or life decisions perpetuate the schema, and begins to make healthier choices that break old self-defeating life patterns.

The therapist helps the patient plan and prepare for homework assignments by rehearsing new behaviors in imagery and role-playing in the session. The therapist uses flash cards and imagery techniques to help the patient overcome obstacles to behavioral change. After carrying out assignments, the patient discusses the results with the therapist, evaluating what was learned. The patient gradually gives up maladaptive coping styles in favor of more adaptive patterns.

Most of these dysfunctional behaviors are, in fact, coping responses to schemas, and they are often the main obstacles to schema healing. Patients must be willing to give up their maladaptive coping styles in order to change. For example, patients who continue surrendering to the schema—by remaining in destructive relationships or by not setting limits in their personal or work lives –perpetuate the schema and are not able to make significant progress in therapy. Overcompensators may fail to make progress in treatment because, rather than acknowledging their schemas and taking responsibility for their problems, they blame others. Or they may be too preoccupied with overcompensating—by working harder, improving themselves, impressing others—to clearly identify their schemas and apply themselves to changing.

Avoiders may fail to progress because they keep escaping from the pain of their schemas. They do not allow themselves to focus on their problems, their pasts, their families, or their life patterns. They cut off their emotions or dull them. It takes motivation to overcome avoidance as a coping style. Because avoidance is rewarding in the short run, patients must be willing to endure discomfort and to continually confront themselves with the long-term negative consequences.

The Therapist–Patient Relationship

The therapist assesses and treats schemas, coping styles, and modes as they arise in the therapeutic relationship. The therapist–patient relationship serves as a partial antidote to the patient's schemas. The patient internalizes the therapist as a "Healthy Adult" who fights against schemas and pursues an emotionally fulfilling life.

Two features of the therapy relationship are especially important elements of schema therapy: the therapeutic stance of *empathic confrontation* and the use of *limited reparenting*. Empathic confrontation involves showing empathy for the patients' schemas when they arise toward the therapist, while showing patients that their reactions to the therapist are often distorted or dysfunctional in ways that reflect their schemas and coping styles. Limited reparenting involves supplying, within the appropriate bounds of the therapeutic relationship, what patients needed but did not receive from their parents in childhood. We discuss these concepts at greater length later.

COMPARISON BETWEEN SCHEMA THERAPY AND OTHER MODELS

In the development of a conceptual and treatment approach, schema therapists adopt a philosophy of openness and inclusion. They cast a wide net, searching for solutions with little concern about whether their work will be classified as cognitive-behavioral, psychodynamic, or Gestalt. The primary focus is on whether patients are changing in significant ways. This attitude has contributed to a sense of freedom for both patients and therapists concerning what they discuss in sessions, which interventions they use, and how they implement these interventions. Moreover, the model readily incorporates the therapist's personal style.

Schema therapy is not, however, an eclectic therapy in the sense of proceeding by trial and error. It is based on a unifying theory. The theory and strategies are tightly woven into a structured, systematic model.

As a result of this inclusive philosophy, the schema model overlaps with many other models of psychopathology and psychotherapy, including cognitive-behavioral, constructivist, psychodynamic, object relations, and Gestalt approaches. Although aspects of schema therapy overlap with these other models, the schema model also differs in important respects. Although schema theory contains concepts similar to those in many psychological schools, no one school overlaps with schema therapy completely.

In this section, we highlight some key similarities and differences between schema therapy and Beck's recent formulations of cognitive therapy. We also touch briefly on some other therapy approaches that overlap in important ways with schema therapy.

Beck's "Reformulated" Model

Beck and his associates (Beck et al., 1990; Alford & Beck, 1997) have revised cognitive therapy to treat personality disorders. Personality is defined as "specific patterns of social, motivational and cognitive-affective processes" (Alford & Beck, 1997, p. 25). Personality includes behaviors, thought processes, emotional responses, and motivational needs.

Personality is determined by the "idiosyncratic structures," or schemas, that constitute the basic elements of personality. Alford and Beck (1997) propose that the schema concept may "provide a common language to facilitate the integration of certain psychotherapeutic approaches" (p. 25). According to Beck's model, a "core belief" represents the meaning, or cognitive content, of a schema.

Beck has also elaborated his own concept of a *mode* (Beck, 1996). A mode is an integrated network of cognitive, affective, motivational, and behavioral components. A mode may comprise many cognitive schemas. These modes mobilize individuals in intense psychological reactions, and are oriented toward achieving particular aims. Like schemas, modes are primarily automatic and also require activation. Individuals with a cognitive vulnerability who are exposed to relevant stressors may develop symptoms related to the mode.

According to Beck's view (Alford & Beck, 1997), modes consist of schemas, which contain memories, problem-solving strategies, images, and language. Modes activate "programmed strategies for carrying out basic categories of survival skills, such as defense from predators" (p. 27). The activation of a specific mode is derived from an individual's genetic makeup and cultural and social beliefs.

Beck (1996, p. 9) further explains that a corresponding mode is not necessarily activated when a schema is triggered. Even though the cognitive component of a schema has been triggered, we may not see any corresponding affective, motivational, or behavioral components.

In treatment, a patient learns to utilize the conscious control system to deactivate modes by reinterpreting trigger events in a manner inconsistent with the mode. Furthermore, modes can be modified.

After an extensive review of the cognitive therapy literature, we conclude that Beck has not elaborated—except in very general terms—on how the techniques for changing schemas and modes are different from those prescribed in standard cognitive therapy. Alford and Beck (1997) acknowledge that the therapeutic relationship is a valid mechanism for change and even that structured imagery work can alter cognitive structures by communicating "directly with the experiential (automatic system) [in its own medium, mainly fantasy]" (p. 70). But we cannot find detailed and distinctive change strategies for schemas or modes.

Finally, Beck et al. (1990) discuss patients' cognitive and behavioral *strategies*. These strategies seem equivalent to the schema therapy notion of coping styles. Psychologically healthy individuals cope with life situations with adaptive cognitive and behavioral strategies, whereas psychologically impaired people utilize inflexible, maladaptive responses within their vulnerable areas.

Conceptually, Beck's revised cognitive model and Young's latest statement of his schema model presented in this chapter have many points of similarity. Both emphasize two broad central structures—schemas and modes—in understanding personality. Both theories include cognition, motivation, emotion, genetic makeup, coping mechanisms, and cultural influences as important aspects of personality. Both models acknowledge the need to focus on both conscious and unconscious aspects of personality.

The differences between the two theoretical models are subtle and often reflect differences in emphasis, not fundamental areas of disagreements. Young's concept of an Early Maladaptive Schema incorporates elements of both schemas and modes, as defined by Beck (1996). Young defines schema activation as incorporating affective, motivational, and behavioral components. Both the structure and content of schemas that Beck discusses are incorporated into Young's definition of schemas.

Mode activation is very similar to Young's concept of schema activation. It is unclear why Beck (1996) needs to differentiate schemas from modes, based on his definitions of these terms. In our opinion, his mode concept could easily be broadened to encompass the elements of a schema (or vice versa). Perhaps Beck wants to differentiate schemas from modes to emphasize that modes are evolutionary mechanisms for survival. The concept of a schema, in Beck's revised model, remains closer to his original cognitive model (Beck, 1976) and as such is more closely related to other cognitive constructs such as automatic thoughts and core beliefs.

Young's concept of a schema mode is only marginally related to Beck's use of the term "mode." Beck (1996) developed his mode construct to account for intense psychological reactions that are survival related and goal oriented. Young developed his mode concept to differentiate between schemas and coping styles as *traits* (enduring, consistent patterns) and schemas and coping styles as *states* (shifting patterns of activation and deactivation). In this sense, Young's concept of a schema mode is more related to concepts of dissociation and "ego states" than to Beck's mode concept.

Another important conceptual difference is the relative emphasis placed on coping styles. Although Beck et al. (1990) refer to maladaptive coping strategies, Beck did not include them as major constructs in his reformulation (Beck, 1996; Alford & Beck, 1997). Young's model, in contrast, assigns a central role to coping styles in perpetuating schemas. This emphasis and elaboration on schema surrender, avoidance, and overcompensation is in sharp contrast with Beck's limited discussion.

Another major difference is the greater importance placed on core needs and developmental processes in schema therapy than in cognitive therapy. Although Beck and his associates agree in general that motivational needs and childhood influences play an important role in personality, they do not expand on what the core needs are or on how specific childhood experiences lead to the development of schemas and modes.

Not surprisingly, as Young's primary influence prior to developing schema therapy was Beck's cognitive approach, there are many areas of overlap in the treatments. Both encourage a high degree of collaboration between patient and therapist and advocate that the therapist play an active role in directing sessions and the course of treatment. Young and Beck agree that empiricism plays an important role in cognitive change; therefore, both treatments encourage patients to modify their cognitions—including schemas—to be more in line with "reality," or empirical evidence from the patient's life. The two approaches similarly share many cognitive and behavioral-change techniques, such as keeping track of cognitions and behavioral rehearsal. In both approaches, patients are taught strategies for altering automatic thoughts, underlying assumptions, cognitive distortions, and core beliefs.

Cognitive and schema therapies both emphasize the importance of educating the patient about the respective therapy models. Thus the patient is brought into the therapeutic process as an equal participant. The therapist shares the case conceptualization with the patient and encourages the patient to read self-help material elaborating on each approach. Homework and self-help assignments play a central role in both therapies as a mechanism for assisting patients in generalizing what they learn in the session into their lives outside. Also, to facilitate this transfer of learning, schema and cognitive therapists both teach practical strategies for handling concrete life events outside the session in an adaptive manner, rather than relying on patients to figure out for themselves how to apply general cognitive-behavioral principles.

Despite these similarities, there are also major differences in treatment approach between schema and cognitive therapies. Many of these differences flow from the fact that the treatment techniques of cognitive therapy were originally developed to reduce symptoms of Axis I disorders, whereas schema therapy strategies focused, from the beginning, on personality disorders and lifelong chronic problems. It has been our experience that there are fundamental differences in effective change techniques for symptom reduction compared with personality change.

First, schema therapy begins from the "bottom up" rather than "top down." In other words, schema therapists begin at the core level—schemas—and gradually link these schemas to more accessible cognitions, such as automatic thoughts and cognitive distortions. In contrast, cognitive therapists begin with surface-level cognitions such as automatic thoughts and address core beliefs later, if the patient remains in treatment once the symptoms have been alleviated.

In schema therapy, this bottom-up approach leads to a dramatic shift in focus early in treatment from present issues to lifelong patterns. Furthermore, in schema therapy, the majority of time is devoted to schemas, coping styles, and modes, whereas these are usually secondary in cognitive therapy. This shift in focus also leads schema therapists to impose less structure and a less formal agenda on sessions. The schema therapist needs the freedom to move fluidly between past and present, from one schema to another, within a session and between sessions. In cognitive therapy, by contrast, clearly identified current problems or sets of symptoms are pursued consistently by the therapist until they have remitted.

Furthermore, because schemas and coping styles are most central to the model, Young has elaborated 18 specific early schemas and three broad coping styles that form the basis for much of the treatment. These schemas and coping mechanisms are assessed and are further refined later in therapy to better fit each individual patient. Thus the schema therapist has valuable tools to help identify schemas and coping behaviors that might otherwise be missed through normal cognitive assessment techniques. An excellent example is the Emotional Deprivation schema, which is relatively easy to uncover using schema-focused imagery, but very difficult to recognize by asking for automatic thoughts or exploring underlying assumptions.

Another important difference is in the emphasis placed on childhood origins and parenting styles in schema therapy. Cognitive therapy lacks specificity about the origins of cognitions, including core beliefs. In contrast, schema therapists have identified the most common origins for each of the 18 schemas, and an instrument has been developed to assess them. The therapist explains these origins to patients to educate them about the normal needs of a child and to explain what happens when these needs are not met and links childhood origins with whichever schemas from the list of 18 are relevant for the patient. In addition to assessing and educating patients about the origins of their schemas, schema therapists guide patients through a variety of experiential exercises related to upsetting childhood experiences. These exercises help patients overcome maladaptive emotions, cognitions, and coping behaviors. In contrast, cognitive therapists generally deal with childhood experiences in a peripheral manner.

A crucial difference between the two approaches is in the importance of experiential work, such as imagery and dialogues. Although a small minority of cognitive therapists have begun to incorporate experiential work (Smucker & Dancu, 1999), the majority do not see this as central to treatment and use imagery primarily for behavioral rehearsal. In contrast, schema therapists view experiential techniques as one of four equal components of treatment and devote considerable time in therapy to these strategies. It is difficult to understand the reluctance of most cognitive therapists to incorporate these strategies more widely, as it is generally accepted in the cognitive literature that "hot cognitions" (when the patient is experiencing strong affect) can be changed more readily than "cold cognitions" (when the patient's affect is flat). Experiential techniques can sometimes be the only way to stimulate hot cognitions in the session.

Another primary difference is in the role of the therapy relationship. Both therapies acknowledge the importance of the relationship for effective therapy, yet they utilize it in very different ways. Cognitive therapists view the therapy relationship primarily as a vehicle to motivate the patient to comply with the treatment (e.g., completing homework assignments). They recommend that the therapist focus on cognitions related to the therapy relationship when the relationship appears to be impeding progress. However, the relationship is not generally considered to be a primary vehicle of change but rather a medium that allows change to take place. To use a medical analogy, cognitive techniques are viewed as the "active ingredients" for change, and the therapy relationship is considered the "base" or "vehicle" through which the change agent is delivered.

In schema therapy, the therapy relationship is one of the four primary components of change. As mentioned earlier in the chapter, schema therapists utilize the relationship in two ways. The first involves observing schemas as they are activated in the session and then using a variety of procedures to assess and modify these schemas within the therapy relationship. The second function involves limited reparenting. This process involves utilizing the therapy relationship as a "corrective emotional experience" (Alexander & French, 1946). Within the appropriate limits of therapy, the therapist acts toward the patient in ways that serve as an antidote to early deficits in the patient's parenting.

In terms of style, the schema therapist utilizes empathic confrontation more than collaborative empiricism. Cognitive therapists use guided discovery to help patients see how their cognitions are distorted. It has been our experience that characterological patients cannot typically see a realistic, healthy alternative to their schemas without direct instruction from the therapist. Schemas are so deeply ingrained and implicit that questioning and empirical investigation alone are not enough to allow these patients to see their own cognitive distortions. Thus the schema therapist teaches the healthy perspective by empathizing with the schema view while confronting the patient with the reality that the schema view is not working and is not in line with reality as others see it. The schema therapist must constantly confront the patient in this way or the patient slips back into the unhealthy schema perspective. As we tell patients, "the schema fights for survival." This concept of doing battle with the schema is not central to cognitive therapy.

Because schemas are far more resistant to change than are other levels of cognition, the course of treatment utilizing schema therapy for Axis II disorders is significantly longer than brief treatment that uses cognitive therapy for Axis I disorders. It is unclear, however, whether cognitive therapy and schema therapy differ in duration for Axis II problems.

Both in conceptualizing a case and in implementing change strategies, schema therapists are more concerned with changing long-term dysfunctional life patterns than with altering discrete dysfunctional behaviors in the current life situation (although both are necessary). Cognitive therapists, because they are focused on rapid symptom reduction, are much less likely to inquire about such long-term problems as dysfunctional partner choices, subtle problems with intimacy, avoidance of important life changes, or core unmet needs, such as nurturance and validation. Along the same lines, cognitive therapists generally do not place central importance on identifying and changing lifelong coping styles, such as schema avoidance, surrender, and overcompensation. Yet, in our experience, it is exactly these coping mechanisms—not simply the rigid core beliefs or schemas—that often make patients with personality disorders so difficult to treat.

We alluded earlier in this section to the concept of modes. Although cognitive and schema therapies both incorporate the concept of a mode, cognitive therapists have not yet elaborated techniques for altering them. Schema therapists have already identified 10 common schema mode states (based on Young's definition noted earlier in the chapter) and have developed a full range of treatment strategies, such as mode dialogues, to treat each individual mode. Mode work forms the basis of schema therapy for patients with borderline and narcissistic personality disorders.

Psychodynamic Approaches

Schema therapy has many parallels to psychodynamic models of therapy. Two major elements shared by both approaches are the exploration of the childhood origins of current problems and the focus on the therapy relationship. In terms of the therapy relationship, the modern psychodynamic shift toward expressing empathy and establishing a genuine relationship (cf., Kohut, 1984; Shane, Shane, & Gales, 1997) is compatible with our notions of limited reparenting and empathic confrontation. Both psychodynamic and schema approaches value intellectual insight. Both stress the need for the emotional processing of traumatic material. Both alert therapists to transference and countertransference issues. Both affirm the importance of personality structure, asserting that the kind of personality structure the patient presents holds the key to effective therapy.

There are also essential differences between schema therapy and psychodynamic models. One key difference is that psychoanalysts have traditionally attempted to remain relatively neutral, whereas schema therapists endeavor to be active and directive. In contrast to most psychodynamic approaches, schema therapists provide limited reparenting, partially meeting the patient's unmet emotional needs in order to heal schemas.

Another major difference is that, unlike classical analytic theories, the schema model is not a drive theory. Instead of focusing on instinctual sexual and aggressive impulses, schema theory emphasizes core emotional needs. Schema theory rests on the principle of cognitive consistency. People are motivated to maintain a consistent view of themselves and the world and tend to interpret situations as confirming their schemas. In this sense, the schema approach is more a cognitive than a psychodynamic model. Where psychoanalysts see defense mechanisms against instinctual wishes, schema therapists see styles of coping with schemas and unmet needs. The schema model views the emotional needs the patient is trying to fulfill as inherently normal and healthy.

Finally, psychodynamic therapists tend to be less integrative than schema therapists. Psychodynamically oriented therapists rarely assign homework, nor are they likely to utilize imagery or role-playing techniques.

Bowlby's Attachment Theory

Attachment theory, based on the work of Bowlby and Ainsworth (Ainsworth & Bowlby, 1991), had a significant impact on schema therapy, especially on the development of the Abandonment schema and on our conception of borderline personality disorder. Bowlby formulated attachment theory by drawing on ethology, systems, and psychoanalytic models. The main tenet is that human beings (and other animals) have an attachment instinct that aims at establishing a stable relationship with the mother (or other attachment figure). Bowlby (1969) conducted empirical studies of children separated from their mothers and noted universal responses. Ainsworth (1968) elaborated the idea of the mother as a secure base from which the infant explores the world and demonstrated the importance of maternal sensitivity to infant signals.

We have incorporated the idea of the mother as a secure base into our notion of limited reparenting. For patients with BPD (and with other, more severe disorders), limited reparenting provides a partial antidote to the patient's Abandonment schema: The therapist becomes the secure emotional base the patient never had, within the appropriate limits of a therapy relationship. To some extent, almost all patients with schemas in the Disconnection and Rejection domain (with the exception of the Social Isolation schema) require the therapist to become a secure base.

In the schema model, echoing Bowlby, childhood emotional development proceeds from attachment to autonomy and individuation. Bowlby (1969, 1973, 1980) argues that a stable attachment to mother (or other main attachment figure) is a basic emotional need that precedes and promotes independence. According to Bowlby, a well-loved child is likely to protest separation from parents but later develops more self-reliance. Excessive separation anxiety is a consequence of aversive family experiences, such as loss of a parent or repeated threats of abandonment by a parent. Bowlby also pointed out that, in some cases, separation anxiety can be too low, creating a false impression of maturity. An inability to form deep relationships with others may ensue when the replacement of attachment figures is too frequent.

Bowlby (1973) proposed that human beings are motivated to maintain a dynamic balance between preserving familiarity and seeking novelty. In Piagetian (Piaget, 1962) terms, the individual is motivated to maintain a balance between assimilation (integrating new input into existing cognitive structures) and accommodation (changing existing cognitive structures to fit new input). Early Maladaptive Schemas interfere with this balance. Individuals in the grip of their schemas misinterpret new information that would correct the distortions that stem from these schemas. Instead, they *assimilate* new information that could disprove their schemas, distorting and discounting new evidence so that their schemas remain intact. Assimilation, therefore, overlaps with our concept of schema perpetuation. The function of therapy is to help patients *accommodate* new experiences that disprove their schemas, thereby promoting schema healing.

Bowlby's (1973) notion of internal working models overlaps with our notion of Early Maladaptive Schemas. Like schemas, an individual's internal working model is largely based on patterns of interaction between the infant and the mother (or other main attachment figure). If the mother acknowledges the infant's need for protection, while simultaneously respecting the infant's need for independence, the child is likely to develop an internal working model of the self as worthy and competent. If the mother frequently spurns the infant's attempts to elicit protection or independence, then the child will construct an internal working model of the self as unworthy or incompetent

Utilizing their working models, children predict the behaviors of attachment figures and prepare their own responses. The kinds of working models they construct are thus very significant. In this light, Early Maladaptive Schemas are dysfunctional internal working models, and children's characteristic responses to attachment figures are their coping styles. Like schemas, working models direct attention and information processing. Defensive distortions of working models occur when the individual blocks information from awareness, impeding modification in response to change. In a process similar to schema perpetuation, internal working models tend to become more rigid over time. Patterns of interacting become habitual and automatic. In time, working models become less available to consciousness and more resistant to change as a result of reciprocal expectancies.

Bowlby (1988) addressed the application of attachment theory to psychotherapy. He noted that a large number of psychotherapy patients display patterns of insecure or disorganized attachment. One primary goal of psychotherapy is the reappraisal of inadequate, obsolete internal working models of relationships with attachment figures. Patients are likely to impose rigid working models of attachment relationships onto interactions with the therapist. The therapist and patient focus first on understanding the origin of the patient's dysfunctional internal working models; then the therapist serves as a secure base from which the patient explores the world and reworks internal working models. Schema therapists incorporate this same principle into their work with many patients.

Ryle's Cognitive-Analytic Therapy

Anthony Ryle (1991) has developed "cognitive-analytic therapy," a brief, intensive therapy that integrates the active, educational aspects of cognitive-behavioral therapy with psychoanalytic approaches, especially object relations. Ryle proposes a conceptual framework that systematically combines the theories and techniques derived from these approaches. As such, cognitive-analytic therapy overlaps considerably with schema therapy.

Ryle's (1991) formulation is called the "procedural sequence model." He uses "aim-directed activity" rather than schemas as his core conceptual construct. Ryle considers neurosis to be the persistent use of and failure to modify procedures that are ineffective or harmful. Three categories of procedures account for most neurotic repetition: traps, dilemmas, and snags. A number of the patterns Ryle describes overlap with schemas and coping styles.

In terms of treatment strategies, Ryle encourages an active and collaborative therapeutic relationship that includes a comprehensive and depth-oriented conceptualization of the patient's problems, just as schema therapy does. The therapist shares the conceptualization with the patient, including an understanding of how the patient's past led to current problems and a listing of the various maladaptive procedures the patient uses to cope with these problems. In cognitive-analytic therapy, the main treatment strategies are transference work to clarify themes and diary-keeping about maladaptive procedures. Schema therapy includes both of these components but adds many other treatment strategies.

Cognitive-analytic therapy utilizes a threefold change method: new understanding, new experience, and new acts. However, new understanding is Ryle's main focus, what he considers the most powerful agent of change. In cognitive-analytic therapy, the Change Phase primarily involves helping patients become aware of negative patterns in their lives. Ryle's emphasis is on insight: "In CAT the therapeutic emphasis is put most strongly on strengthening the higher levels (of cognition), in particular through reformulation, which modifies appraisal processes and promotes active self-observation" (Ryle, 1991, p. 200).

In schema therapy, insight is a necessary, but not sufficient, component of change. As we move toward treatment of more severe pathology, such as occurs in patients with borderline and narcissistic disorders, we find that insight becomes less important relative to the new experience provided by experiential and behavioral approaches. Ryle (1991) views new understanding as the main vehicle for change with patients with BPD. His focus is on what he calls "sequential diagrammatic reformulations." These are written diagrams summarizing the case conceptualization. The therapist places the diagrams on the floor in front of the patient and refers to them frequently. Sequential diagrammatic reformulations are intended to help patients with BPD develop an "observing eye."

Schema therapy diverges from cognitive-analytic therapy in several ways. Schema therapy places more emphasis on the elicitation of affect and on limited reparenting, especially with patients who have severe characterological disorders. Schema therapy thus does more to facilitate change on an emotional level. Ryle (1991) acknowledges that procedures for activating affect, such as Gestalt techniques or psychodrama, may be appropriate in some cases to help patients move beyond intellectual insight. In contrast, Young views experiential techniques, such as imagery and dialogues, as useful for nearly all patients.

In Ryle's (1991) approach, the therapist interacts primarily with the adult side of the patient, the Healthy Adult mode, and only indirectly with the child side of the patient, the Vulnerable Child mode. According to the schema approach, patients with BPD are like very young children and need to attach securely to the therapist before separating and individuating.

Horowitz's Person Schemas Therapy

Horowitz has developed a framework that integrates psychodynamic, cognitive-behavioral, interpersonal, and family systems approaches. His model emphasizes roles and beliefs based on "person schemas theory"

(Horowitz, 1991; Horowitz, Stinson, & Milbrath, 1996) A person schema is a template, usually unconscious, comprising one's views of self and others, and it is formed from memory residues of childhood experiences (Horowitz, 1997). This definition is virtually identical to our notion of an Early Maladaptive Schema. Horowitz focuses on the general structure of all schemas, whereas Young delineates specific schemas underlying most negative life patterns.

Horowitz (1997) elaborates on what he terms "role relationship models." Horowitz associates each role relationship with (1) an underlying wish or need (the "desired role relationship model"); (2) a core fear (the "dreaded role relationship model"); and (3) role relationship models that defend against the dreaded role relationship model. In terms of schema theory, these correspond loosely to core emotional needs, Early Maladaptive Schemas, and coping styles. Horowitz (1997) explains that a role relationship includes scripts for transactions, intentions, emotional expressions, actions, and critical evaluations of actions and intentions. As such, a role relationship contains aspects of both schemas and coping styles. The schema model conceptualizes schemas and coping responses separately, as schemas are not directly linked to specific actions. Different individuals handle the same schema with distinctive coping styles, depending on innate temperament and other factors.

Horowitz (1997) also defines "states of mind," which are similar to our concept of modes. A state of mind is "a pattern of conscious experiences and interpersonal expressions. The elements that combine to form the pattern that is recognized as a state include verbal and nonverbal expression of ideas and emotions" (Horowitz, 1997, p. 31). Horowitz does not present these states of mind as lying along a continuum of dissociation. In the schema model, more severely disturbed patients, such as those with narcissistic and borderline personality disorders, flip into states of mind that fully subsume the patient's sense of self. More than experiencing a state of mind, the patient experiences a different "self" or "mode." This distinction is important in that the degree of dissociation associated with a mode dictates major modifications in technique.

What Horowitz (1997) calls "defensive control processes" also resemble Young's coping styles. Horowitz identifies three major categories:

1. Defensive control processes that involve avoidance of painful topics through the content of what is expressed (e.g., shifting attention away or minimizing importance)
2. Those that involve avoidance through the manner of expression (e.g., verbal intellectualization)
3. Those that involve coping by shifting roles (e.g., abruptly shifting to a passive role or a grandiose role).

Within this typology, Horowitz (1997) covers many of the phenomena encompassed by schema avoidance, surrender, and overcompensation.

During the treatment, the therapist supports the patient, counteracts avoidance by redirecting the patient's attention, interprets dysfunctional attitudes and resistance, and helps the patient plan trials of new behavior. As in Ryle's (1991) work, insight is the most vital part of treatment. The therapist clarifies and interprets, focusing the patient's thoughts and discourse on role-relationship models and defensive control processes. The goal is for new "supraordinate" schemas to gain priority over immature and maladaptive ones.

In comparison with schema therapy, Horowitz (1997) does not provide detailed or systematic treatment strategies and does not utilize experiential techniques or limited reparenting. Schema therapy places more emphasis on activating affect than does Horowitz's approach. The schema therapist accesses what Horowitz (1997) terms "regressive states"—and what we term the patient's Vulnerable Child mode.

Emotionally Focused Therapy

Emotionally focused therapy, developed by Leslie Greenberg and his colleagues (Greenberg, Rice, & Elliott, 1993; Greenberg & Paivio, 1997) draws on experiential, constructivist, and cognitive models. Like schema therapy, emotionally focused therapy is strongly informed by attachment theory and therapy process research.

Emotionally focused therapy places emphasis on the integration of emotion with cognition, motivation, and behavior. The therapist activates emotion in order to repair it. Much weight is placed on identifying and repairing emotion schemes, which Greenberg (Greenberg & Paivio, 1997) defines as sets of organizing principles, idiosyncratic in content, that tie together emotions, goals, memories, thoughts, and behavioral tendencies. Emotion schemes emerge through an interplay of the individual's early learning history and innate temperament. When activated, they serve as powerful organizing forces in the interpretation of and response to events in one's life. Similar to the schema model, the ultimate aim of emotionally focused therapy is to change these emotion schemes. Therapy brings into the patient's awareness "inaccessible internal experience . . . in order to construct new schemes" (Greenberg & Paivio, 1997, p. 83).

Like schema therapy, emotionally focused therapy relies heavily on the therapeutic working alliance. Emotionally focused therapy utilizes this alliance to develop an emotionally focused "empathic dialogue" that stimulates, focuses, and attends to the patient's emotional concerns. To be able to engage in this dialogue, therapists must first create a sense of safety and trust. Once this sense is securely established, therapists engage in a delicate dialectic balance of "following" and "leading," accepting and facilitating change. This process is similar to the schema model ideal of empathic confrontation.

Like schema therapy, emotionally focused therapy recognizes that the mere activation of emotion is not sufficient to engender change. In emotionally focused therapy, change requires a gradual process of emotional activation through the use of experiential techniques, overcoming avoidance, interrupting negative behaviors, and facilitating emotional repair. The therapist helps patients recognize and express their primary feelings, verbalize them, and then access internal resources (e.g., adaptive coping responses). In addition, emotionally focused therapy prescribes different interventions for different emotions.

Despite considerable similarities, several theoretical and practical differences distinguish emotionally focused therapy from the schema model. One difference is the primacy emotionally focused therapy gives to affect within emotion schemes compared with the schema model's more egalitarian view of the roles played by affect, cognition, and behavior. Additionally, Greenberg maintains that there are an "infinite amount of unique emotional schemes" (Greenberg & Paivio, 1997, p. 3), whereas the schema model defines a finite set of schemas and coping styles and provides appropriate interventions for each one.

The emotionally focused therapy model organizes schemes in a complex, hierarchical organization, distinguishing between primary, secondary, and instrumental emotions, and breaking these further into adaptive, maladaptive, complex, and socially constructed emotions. The type of emotion scheme suggests specific intervention goals, taking into account whether the emotion is internally or externally focused (e.g., sadness vs. anger) and whether it is currently overcontrolled or undercontrolled. Compared with the more parsimonious schema model, emotionally focused therapy places a considerable burden on the therapist to analyze emotions accurately and to intervene with them in very specific ways.

The assessment process in emotionally focused therapy relies primarily on moment-by-moment experiences in the therapy room. Greenberg and Paivio (1997) contrast these techniques with approaches that rely on initial case formulations or those that rely on behavioral assessments. Although the schema model utilizes in-session information, it is more multifaceted, including structured imagery sessions, schema inventories, and attunement to the therapy relationship.

SUMMARY

Young (1990) originally developed schema therapy to treat patients who had failed to respond adequately to traditional cognitive-behavioral treatment, especially patients with personality disorders and significant characterological issues underlying their Axis I disorders. These patients violate several assumptions of cognitive-behavioral therapy and thus are difficult to treat successfully with this method. More recent revisions of cognitive therapy for personality disorders by Beck and his colleagues (Beck et al., 1990; Alford & Beck, 1997) are more consistent with schema therapy formulations. However, there are still significant differences between these approaches, especially in terms of conceptual emphasis and the range of treatment strategies.

Schema therapy is a broad, integrative model. As such, it has considerable overlap with many other systems of psychotherapy, including psychodynamic models. However, most of these approaches are narrower than schema therapy, either in terms of the conceptual model or the range of treatment strategies. There are also significant differences in the therapy relationship, the general style and stance of the therapist, and the degree of therapist activity and directiveness.

Early Maladaptive Schemas are broad, pervasive themes or patterns regarding oneself and one's relationships with others that are dysfunctional to a significant degree. Schemas comprise memories, emotions, cognitions, and bodily sensations. They develop during childhood or adolescence and are elaborated throughout one's lifetime. Schemas begin as adaptive and relatively accurate representations of the child's environment, but they become maladaptive and inaccurate as the child grows up. As part of the human drive for consistency, schemas fight for survival. They play a major role in how individuals think, feel, act, and relate to others. Schemas are triggered when individuals encounter environments reminiscent of the childhood environments that produced them. When this happens, the individual is flooded with intense negative affect. LeDoux's (1996) research on the brain systems involved with fear conditioning and trauma suggests a model for the biological underpinnings of schemas.

Early Maladaptive Schemas are the result of unmet core emotional needs. Aversive childhood experiences are their primary origin. Other factors play a role in their development, such as emotional temperament and cultural influences. We have defined 18 Early Maladaptive Schemas in five domains. A great deal of empirical support exists for these schemas and some of the domains.

We define two fundamental schema operations: schema perpetuation and schema healing. Schema healing is the goal of schema therapy. Maladaptive coping styles are the mechanisms patients develop early in life to adapt to schemas, and they result in schema perpetuation. We have identified three maladaptive coping styles: surrender, avoidance, and overcompensation. Coping responses are the specific behaviors through which these three broad coping styles are expressed. There are common coping responses for each schema. Modes are states, or facets of the self, involving specific schemas or schema operations. We have developed four main categories of modes: Child modes, Dysfunctional Coping modes, Dysfunctional Parent modes, and the Healthy Adult mode.

Schema Therapy has two phases: the Assessment and Education Phase and the Change Phase. In the first phase, the therapist helps patients identify their schemas, understand the origins of their schemas in childhood or adolescence, and relate their schemas to their current problems. In the Change Phase, the therapist blends cognitive, experiential, behavioral, and interpersonal strategies to heal schemas and replace maladaptive coping styles with healthier forms of behavior.

Chapter 2

SCHEMA ASSESSMENT AND EDUCATION

The Assessment and Education Phase of schema therapy has six major goals:

1. Identification of dysfunctional life patterns
2. Identification and triggering of Early Maladaptive Schemas
3. Understanding the origins of schemas in childhood and adolescence
4. Identification of coping styles and responses
5. Assessment of temperament
6. Putting it all together: the case conceptualization

Although the assessment is structured, it is not formulaic. Rather, the therapist develops hypotheses based on data and adjusts these hypotheses as more information accumulates. As the therapist assesses life patterns, schemas, coping styles, and temperament, utilizing the various assessment modalities described later, the assessment gradually coalesces into a unified schema-focused case conceptualization.

We now provide a brief overview of the steps in the assessment and education process. The therapist begins with the initial evaluation. The therapist assesses the patient's presenting problems and goals for therapy and evaluates the patient's suitability for schema therapy. Next, the therapist takes a life history, identifying dysfunctional life patterns that prevent the patient from meeting basic emotional needs. These patterns usually involve long-term, self-perpetuating cycles in relationships and at work that lead to dissatisfaction and symptomatology. The therapist explains the schema model and tells the patient that they will work together to identify the patient's schemas and coping styles. The patient completes questionnaires for homework, and the therapist and patient discuss the results in the sessions. Next, the therapist uses experiential techniques, especially imagery, to access and trigger schemas and to link schemas to their childhood origins and to the presenting problems. The therapist observes the patient's schemas and coping styles as they appear in the therapy relationship. Finally, the therapist assesses the patient's emotional temperament.

In the course of the assessment, patients come to recognize their schemas and to understand the origins of these schemas in childhood. They analyze how these self-destructive patterns have recurred throughout their lives. Patients identify the coping styles they have developed to deal with their schemas—surrender, avoidance, or overcompensation—and elucidate how their individual temperaments and early life experiences predisposed them to develop those styles. They link their schemas to their presenting problems, so that they have a sense of continuity from childhood to the present. Thus their schemas and coping styles become unifying concepts in the way they view their lives.

We have found that using multiple methods of assessment increases the accuracy of schema identification. For example, some patients will endorse a schema on the Young Parenting Inventory, but not on the Young Schema Questionnaire. It is easier for these patients to remember their parents' attitudes and behaviors than it is for them to access their own emotions. Patients may give inconsistent or contradictory information on questionnaires because of schema avoidance or overcompensation—processes that are likely to be less salient in the imagery work.

The Assessment Phase has both an intellectual and an emotional aspect. Patients identify their schemas rationally through the use of questionnaires, logical analysis, and empirical evidence, but they also feel their schemas emotionally through the use of experiential techniques such as imagery. The decision about whether a hypothesis about a schema "fits" the patient is based in large part on what "feels right" to the patient: A correctly identified schema usually resonates emotionally for the patient.

During the Assessment Phase, the therapist utilizes cognitive, experiential, and behavioral measures and observes the therapist–patient relationship. The assessment is thus a multifaceted endeavor in which the therapist and patient form and refine hypotheses as they gather additional sources of information. Core schemas emerge as these multiple methods converge on central themes in the patient's life. The assessment gradually crystallizes into a schema-focused case conceptualization.

The time required to complete the assessment is variable. Relatively straightforward cases might require as few as five assessment sessions, whereas patients who are more overcompensated or avoidant usually require more time.

SCHEMA-FOCUSED CASE CONCEPTUALIZATION

Schema therapy emphasizes individualized case conceptualization. Several cognitive therapists have provided excellent examples of case formulation from a cognitive perspective (e.g., Beck et al., 1990; Persons, 1989). Schema-focused case conceptualization is broader: It provides an integrative framework that includes self-defeating life patterns, early developmental processes, and coping styles, as well as schemas. Thus each patient has a unique conceptualization, based on both the patient's Early Maladaptive Schemas and his or her coping styles.

By the end of the Assessment Phase, the therapist completes the Schema Therapy Case Conceptualization Form (see Figure 2.1).[1] The form includes the patient's schemas, links to the presenting problems, schema triggers, hypothesized temperamental factors, developmental origins, core memories, core cognitive distortions, coping behaviors, modes, the effects of schemas on the therapeutic relationship, and change strategies.

The Importance of Accurate Identification of Schemas and Coping Styles

To develop an effective case conceptualization, the therapist must make an accurate assessment of the patient's Early Maladaptive Schemas and coping styles. The case conceptualization has a large impact on the course of treatment, providing tactical considerations and practical recommendations for choosing targets of change and implementing treatment procedures. Correct schema identification guides interventions, enhances the therapeutic alliance by helping the patient feel understood, and anticipates likely areas of difficulty during the Change Phase.

It is important that the therapist not jump to conclusions about which schemas are operating based solely on DSM-IV diagnosis, life history, or responses to a single assessment modality. The same Axis I diagnosis could be the outward manifestation of different schemas in different people. Almost all the schemas can result in depression, anxiety, substance abuse, psychosomatic symptoms, or sexual dysfunction. Even in a specific personality diagnosis such as BPD, patients may share some schemas and not others.

In addition, the therapist cannot assume the presence of a schema solely on the basis of simplistic analysis of a patient's childhood experiences: Patients might share similar painful childhood circumstances, yet end up with different schemas. For example, two female patients both

---

[1]All the forms and inventories mentioned in this book can be purchased as a packet from the Schema Therapy Institute. See the web site *www.schematherapy.com* for ordering information. These forms will be available in a forthcoming client workbook from The Guilford Press.

FIGURE 2.1. Schema Therapy Case Conceptualization Form for Annette

Background Information

Therapist's name: Rachel W. Patient's name: Annette G.* Age: 26
Marital status: Single
Children (Ages): None Occupation: Receptionist Ethnic background: Caucasian
Education: Completed High School

Relevant Schemas

1. Emotional Deprivation (of nurturance, empathy, and protection)
2. Self-Sacrifice   3. Mistrust/Abuse   4. Defectiveness/Shame
5. Entitlement/Grandiosity   6. Insufficient Self-Control/Self-Discipline

Current Problems

Problem 1: Depression
  Schema links: Emotional Deprivation, Defectiveness, Self-Sacrifice

Problem 2: Alcohol abuse
  Schema links: Coping response for Emotional Deprivation, Mistrust/
  Abuse, Defectiveness

Problem 3: Relationship problems : dates inappropriate men, has difficulty
  becoming intimate
  Schema links: Emotional Deprivation, Mistrust/Abuse, Defectiveness, Self-
  Sacrifice

Problem 4: Work problems: does not complete tasks, moves from job to job
  Schema links: Insufficient Self-Control/Self-Discipline, Entitlement/
  Grandiosity

Schema Triggers (Specify M–F if limited to men or women)

1. Choosing a boyfriend (M)   2. Trying to get close to a boyfriend (M)
3. Feeling alone   4. Thinking about her problems and her need for therapy
5. Being asked to do something boring, routine, or uninteresting

Severity of Schemas, Coping Responses, and Modes; Risk of Decompensation

Schemas are moderately strong. Coping responses and modes are very
strong. No suicidal ideation. Low risk of decompensation.

Possible Temperamental/Biological Factors

None

Developmental Origins

1. Mother was helpless and needy. Neither parent fulfilled Annette's
   emotional needs as a child.

(cont.)

FIGURE 2.1. *(cont.)*

Developmental Origins *(cont.)*

2. Father was angry and explosive. Annette was put in the role of protecting her mother from her father.
3. Annette had no limits or discipline as a child. Could do and have whatever she wanted.
4. Family members never shared feelings or discussed their problems.

Core Childhood Memories or Images
Father was very angry. Annette and her mother were frightened. Mother turned to Annette for help but did not offer any support, empathy, or protection for her.

Core Cognitive Distortions

1. No one will ever be there to take care of my needs. I have to be the strong one all the time.
2. There's something fundamentally wrong with me for having so many emotional problems and being so needy.
3. Most men are unpredictable, angry, and explosive.
4. I should be able to do and have whatever I want.
5. I shouldn't have to stick with tasks, activities, or relationships that are boring or uninteresting.

Surrender Behaviors

1. Does not ask others to nurture or protect her.
2. Takes care of her mother and asks little in return.
3. Does not talk about vulnerable feelings with other people.

Avoidance Behaviors

1. Abuses alcohol to block out painful feelings.
2. Seeks stimulation and novelty to avoid emotions.
3. Tries to avoid focusing on painful thoughts and feelings.
4. Avoids intimacy with men.

Overcompensating Behaviors

Acts tough and in control, even though she feels vulnerable and needy.

Relevant Schema Modes (in addition to the Healthy Adult)
1. Tough Annette (Detached Protector) 2. Little Annette (Lonely, Frightened Child) 3. "Spoiled Annette"

Therapy Relationship (Impact of schemas and modes on in-session behavior; personal reactions and/or countertransference)

Annette acts tough much of the time in session. She is reluctant to admit strong attachment, neediness, or vulnerability toward me, even though she seems engaged and connected. She tries to avoid imagery exercises and doesn't like to talk about painful emotions or events. She often doesn't follow through on written homework assignments because she says they're boring or upsetting to her.

Despite these problems, I find Annette engaging to work with and think we have a very good therapy relationship. I get somewhat frustrated by her lack of discipline and concern for others in the "Spoiled Annette" mode.

*See the case discussion of Annette in Chapter 8.

grew up with fathers who were rejecting. The first patient developed schemas of Abandonment and Defectiveness, both relatively severe. Her father treated her older sister with affection, but ignored her. She concluded that there was something wrong with her that made her unlovable to her father. Because she felt, from a young age, that anyone who liked her would eventually leave, she avoided romantic relationships entirely to escape future pain.

In contrast, the second patient had a father who was rejecting toward all the children in the family. Furthermore, her mother (unlike the first patient's mother) was a warm and loving parent who compensated for her father's coldness by providing affection and acceptance. The second patient attributed her father's rejection to limitations in her father's capacity to love, as he was equally cold to her and to her siblings. She came to believe that some men would not love her but that others would—she had to find the right ones. She later sought out loving men who further healed the damage done by her father. Although this patient had an Abandonment schema of low to moderate severity, she did not develop a Defectiveness schema. Thus two patients with rejecting fathers ended up with quite different schemas and coping styles as a result of more complex elements in their childhood experiences.

Other factors also influence which schemas a patient develops and the strength of those schemas. Many patients, such as the second woman just described, have other people in their lives who counteract a schema by providing what the patient needs, thereby preventing the schema from developing or weakening it. Patients might also have subsequent life experiences that modify or heal the schema. For example, patients might form healthy love relationships or establish close friendships and thereby partially heal schemas in the Disconnection and Rejection realm. Sometimes a patient's temperament works against the formation of a schema. Some people appear to be more psychologically resilient and do not develop strong Early Maladaptive Schemas, even under conditions of considerable adversity, whereas other people seem more psychologically vulnerable and develop maladaptive schemas with relatively mild levels of mistreatment.

Accurate identification of schemas is important because there are specific, individualized treatment interventions for each schema. For example, a patient repeatedly asks her therapist to give her advice about problems with her boyfriend. On the basis of these and similar statements, her therapist mistakenly concludes that the patient has a Dependence schema. Because the treatment strategy for the Dependence schema is to increase the patient's self-reliance by having her make her own decisions, the therapist declines to give her advice. In fact, however, the patient has an Emotional Deprivation schema. She has never had someone strong to whom she could go for guidance. The treatment strategy for Emotional Deprivation is to reparent the patient by providing nurturance, empathy, and guidance—to meet, in a limited way, the patient's unmet emotional needs. Viewing the patient in this way, the therapist offers direct advice. Thus correct schema identification points the way to the correct intervention.

Accurate identification of the patient's coping styles is equally important to the case conceptualization. Does the patient primarily surrender to, avoid, or overcompensate for schemas? Most patients use a mixture of coping styles. A patient with a Defectiveness schema might overcompensate in the workplace by overachieving and competing but avoid intimate relationships in his personal life and engage in solitary activities. Coping styles are not schema-specific: They generally cut across schemas and can serve as coping mechanisms for distressing emotions generated by many different schemas. For example, individuals who gamble compulsively in order to escape emotional upset might do so because they feel abandoned, abused, rejected, or subjugated. They could gamble to avoid the pain of almost any schema that produces psychological suffering for them.

It is important for the therapist to validate the early adaptive value of the patient's coping style. The patient developed the coping style for a good reason, in order to cope with a difficult childhood situation. However, the coping style is probably maladaptive in the adult world, in which the patient has more choices and is no longer at the mercy of the parents' mistreatment or neglect. If the coping style is avoidance or overcompensation, then it is likely to be problematic in the patient's therapy because it is a barrier to schema work. One purpose of these coping styles is to block the schema from awareness, and the patient has to become aware of a schema in order to fight it. The coping style is also problematic if it lowers the patient's quality of life, such as when the patient procrastinates, alienates others, is cut off emotionally, overspends, or abuses drugs.

Patients may respond to therapeutic interventions that trigger their schemas with the same coping styles that they use in their outside lives. It is important to recognize coping styles, because behavior that looks healthy might, in fact, represent a maladaptive coping style. The calm detachment of a patient with an avoidant coping style might resemble the demeanor of a healthy adult, but it actually indicates a dysfunctional approach to emotions.

Viewing problematic behaviors as coping styles helps us understand why patients persist in self-defeating behaviors. The resistance of these patients to change indicates their continued reliance on responses that have worked, at least to some degree, in the past.

THE ASSESSMENT AND EDUCATION PROCESS IN DETAIL

We now discuss the specific steps in the assessment and education process in greater detail.

The Initial Evaluation

The task of the initial evaluation is to identify the patient's presenting problems and therapy goals and to assess the suitability of the patient for schema therapy.

Assessing the Presenting Problems and Therapy Goals

It is important for the therapist to identify the presenting problems clearly and to stay focused on them as the patient moves through the assessment. Sometimes therapists become caught up in exploring the patient's schemas and forget to link the schemas back to the presenting problems. Framing the problems in schema terms and developing a treatment plan that addresses them help the patient feel focused and hopeful.

The therapist is specific in defining the presenting problems and treatment goals. For example, when stating a presenting problem, instead of saying, "The patient is having trouble choosing a career," the therapist says, "The patient negates potential career options and procrastinates looking for work"; or, instead of saying, "The patient has relationship difficulties," the therapist says, "The patient repeatedly chooses partners who are withholding and aloof." Operationalizing presenting problems in this manner helps the therapist formulate appropriate therapy goals.

Case Illustration. Marika is 45 years old. She has sought therapy for help with marital problems she is having. The following excerpts are taken from an interview with her conducted by Dr. Young. At the time of the interview, Marika had been in schema therapy with another therapist for 8 weeks.

In the first excerpt, Marika describes her relationship with her husband, James.

> "I've been married to James for 7 years. I married at age 38. We have no children. My husband and I both work. I manage an art gallery, he owns a construction company. We have two frenetic careers, two 'you can never do it quite right enough' personalities and busy careers.
>
> "I feel like when I was first married, I could bounce back from fights. He is, I think, verbally and emotionally abusive. I was going to make it right. Now I feel like I have no time and no patience, but I love him and want to save the marriage."

All the ways Marika has tried to improve her marriage have stopped working, and she cannot summon the energy to keep trying. She feels that her emotional needs are not being met and that her husband is verbally abusive. Her goal for treatment is to improve the quality of the marital relationship so that she will feel satisfied and so that she will no longer be treated in a demeaning manner. In the course of the assessment, the therapist will try to understand her marital problems in terms of her schemas and coping styles and in terms of her husband's schemas and coping styles.

Assessing the Suitability of the Patient for Schema Therapy

Schema therapy is not appropriate for all patients; for some patients it will become appropriate later in therapy, after acute crises and symptoms have improved, but not earlier. The following list gives some of the indications that schema therapy either may not be suitable or may need to be postponed.

1. The patient is in major crisis in some life area.
2. The patient is psychotic.
3. The patient has an acute, relatively severe, untreated Axis I disorder requiring immediate attention.
4. The patient is currently abusing alcohol or other drugs at a moderate to severe level.
5. The presenting problem is situational or does not seem to be related to a life pattern or schema.

If the patient is in crisis, then the therapist works to resolve the crisis before beginning schema therapy. If the patient has an acute, severe, untreated Axis I disorder, then the therapist first directs treatment to symptom relief through cognitive-behavioral therapy or psychotropic medication. For example, if the patient has severe panic attacks, major depression, insomnia, or bulimia, then the therapist addresses the acute disorder before undertaking schema work. If the patient is currently a serious substance abuser, then the therapist first directs treatment toward stopping the substance abuse. Once the patient has stopped or significantly reduced the addictive behavior, then the therapist turns to the schema work. It is rarely possible to do schema work effectively while the patient is seriously abusing substances because the drugs numb the very emotions the patient has to confront in order to progress. This is especially true when the patient is under the influence of drugs or alcohol during sessions.

We initially developed schema therapy as a treatment for personality disorders, but it is now being utilized for many chronic Axis I disorders as well, often in conjunction with other modalities. Treatment-resistant or relapsing anxiety and depression are often appropriate targets for schema therapy. When a patient seems to have no clear Axis I disorder or has been unresponsive to previous therapy for an Axis I disorder, then schema therapy is often indicated. For example, a 31-year-old male patient in cognitive-behavioral therapy for depression repeatedly fails to comply with homework assignments. The therapist frames the problem in terms of the patient's Subjugation schema. The homework assignments remind the patient of his school years, when he resented being controlled by parents and teachers and rebelled against authority. Just as he did then, the patient is overcompensating for his schema by not doing his homework. Because the patient wants to make progress, the therapist can ally with the patient in fighting the schema in order to complete the cognitive-behavioral work.

Other difficulties in therapy that might benefit from a schema approach include attendance problems and problems in the therapy relationship. When there are blocks to change, a schema approach can assist the therapist and patient in conceptualizing the block and generating potential solutions. It is often helpful to present the block to the patient as a mode and then to ally with the patient in responding to this mode in a healthy way.

Focused Life History

The therapist tries to determine whether the patient's presenting problems are situational or whether they reflect a pattern in the patient's life. For example, a 64-year-old man enters therapy following the death of his wife. He is deeply depressed and has not responded to pharmacological nor psychological treatment. Does his depression represent the workings of a schema, or is it merely the consequence of his grief? His depression could flow from either source.

The therapist takes a focused life history in order to answer this question, beginning with the current problem and moving back through time, tracking the problem as far back as possible. The therapist looks for periods of schema activation in the past, delving into them with the patient. Did the patient experience any traumatic losses in childhood? Patterns emerge as the same triggering events, cognitions, emotions, and behaviors repeat over time and across situations. Relationship histories, school or work difficulties, and periods of strong affect provide clues to schemas. For example, if a patient is having trouble managing her anger at her boss, it may well be that her boss is triggering one of her schemas. Further inquiry can shed light on the matter.

The therapist also works to identify the patient's coping styles of surrender, avoidance, and overcompensation. The therapist explores how patients have coped with their schemas in the past.

When patients surrender to a schema, they reenact it, just as it happened in childhood, with themselves in the same childhood role. They experience the same thoughts and feelings they did as children, and they behave the same way as they did then. In contrast, schema avoidance looks like flight from the schema, entailing the use of cognitive, emotional, or behavioral strategies to deny, escape, minimize, or detach from the schema. With schema overcompensation, the patient appears to be fighting back: He or she uses cognitive, emotional, or behavioral tactics to counterattack, compensate for, or externalize the schema.

The therapist introduces the idea of coping styles to patients by explaining that these are strategies they developed in childhood in order to adapt to distressing events. Their individual coping styles are the result of both their temperaments and parental modeling. Over time, these strategies have become generalized ways of dealing with the world. Coping styles are especially visible when schemas are triggered. The therapist tells patients that coping styles can prevent access to schemas and block therapy progress. In addition, some coping styles, such as substance abuse or emotional detachment, are problematic in themselves. This introduction to coping styles provides a rationale for administrating self-report questionnaires and prompts patients to volunteer information about how they coped during difficult times in the past.

The Case of Marika

In his interview with Marika (the patient first described on p. 70), Dr. Young takes a focused life history to determine whether her difficulties with James are unique to their relationship or part of a larger pattern in her life. In the following brief excerpt, Dr. Young asks about previous relationships. He starts with the present and works backward, staying with the information relevant to the presenting problem.

THERAPIST: What was your previous relationship like prior to James?

MARIKA: It's almost like a mirror image of the one with James. Both men were alcoholics. I was verbally abused in both. Where James abandons me emotionally, Chris abandoned me physically—he stayed out at night. Both men were generous with money and said they loved me a lot.

At this point a pattern appears to be emerging in Marika's romantic relationships. Both partners "verbally abused" and "abandoned" her. Both were generous materially. The therapist hypothesizes that she has schemas in the Disconnection and Rejection realm—perhaps Abuse or Abandonment—and inquires about her reactions to men who treated her well.

THERAPIST: What were you like with someone who was nice to you? What about the nice guys? There must have been some who treated you well.

MARIKA: They didn't last long. I ended it. They were just awful.

THERAPIST: Were they too nice?

MARIKA: One guy was very nice; he was solicitous and would give me presents.

THERAPIST: Was he critical?

MARIKA: No, he dripped all over my words. We had real conversations.

THERAPIST: What was wrong with that relationship?

MARIKA: He was European and was too "old world."

Marika's response supports the hypothesis that her problems with James are schema-driven rather than situational. A pattern is emerging in her history in which she has been attracted to men who treat her badly and uninterested in men who treat her well. This pattern fits well with our model: We believe that the triggering of schemas generates sexual chemistry in romantic relationships. Marika's explanation of why she was not attracted to the nice guy does not ring true as a satisfactory explanation but rather seems more like a rationalization for the absence of chemistry. In selecting men for romantic relationships, her coping style appears to be primarily one of surrendering to her schemas. Other coping styles are apparent in Marika's interactions with James. To overcompensate for her feelings of emotional deprivation, she becomes angry and demanding. This provokes arguments with James, just as it provoked negative responses from her father when she was a child. The result of overcompensating in this way is that she ends up feeling even more deprived. Her attempt to overcompensate ultimately serves to perpetuate her schema. This is almost always the case: The final outcome of schema avoidance and overcompensation is perpetuation of the schema.

While developing hypotheses about schemas and coping styles, the therapist notes whether some schemas are interrelated. Are there any schemas that seem to get triggered together? We call these "linked schemas." For example, Marika has the linked schemas of Emotional Deprivation and Defectiveness. When she feels deprived of love, she blames herself. She attributes James's neglect of her to her own flaws. She is not "good enough" to be loved unconditionally. Her feelings of deprivation are inextricably linked to her feelings of defectiveness.

SCHEMA INVENTORIES

Life History Assessment Forms

The life history assessment forms provide a comprehensive assessment of the patient's current problems, symptoms, family history, images, cognitions, relationships, biological factors, and significant memories and experiences. The inventory is lengthy and can be given as homework. Having the patient complete the inventory outside the session can save much therapy time. For example, the inventory asks the patient to list childhood memories, and these memories are clues to Early Maladaptive Schemas. (Sometimes patients who do not report abuse in the interview will do so on this questionnaire. They cannot bring themselves to tell the therapist face to face, but they are able to tell the therapist in writing when they are home.) The therapist can use the material to form hypotheses about life patterns, schemas, and coping styles.

Young Schema Questionnaire

The Young Schema Questionnaire (YSQ-L2; Young & Brown, 1990, 2001) is a self-report measure to assess schemas.[2] Patients rate themselves on how well each item describes them on a 6-point Likert scale. The therapist usually gives the YSQ to the patient to take home and complete after the first or second session.

Questionnaire items are grouped by schema. A two-letter code appears after each set of items to indicate to the therapist which schema is being measured. However, the name of the schema is not on the questionnaire itself. A key to the abbreviations appears on the scoring form.

The therapist does not usually compute the patient's total score or mean score for each schema in order to interpret the results. Rather, the therapist looks at the items for each schema separately, circling high scores (usually 5's and 6's) and drawing attention to patterns. The therapist reviews the completed questionnaire with the patient, asking questions about those items that the patient rated highly. We have observed clinically that, if a patient has three or more high scores (rated 5 or 6) on a particular schema, that schema is usually relevant to the patient and worthy of exploration.

The therapist uses the high-scoring items to prompt the patient to talk about each relevant schema by asking, "Can you tell me more about how this statement relates to your life?" Exploring two high-scoring items for each relevant schema with the patient in this way usually suffices to convey the essence of the schema. The therapist teaches the patient the name

---

[2]The questionnaire is available in both long and short forms. The long form version of the YSQ (YSQ-L2) contains 205 items and assesses the 16 Early Maladaptive Schemas we had identified at the time the questionnaire was constructed. We have added additional items for the forthcoming workbook, so that all of the current 18 schemas can be measured. The long form is preferable for clinical use, because it reveals more subtleties of each schema and thus provides more detailed information.

The short form of the YSQ contains 75 items and is composed of the five highest loading items for each schema from the long form, as determined by factor analysis (Schmidt et al., 1995). We will be adding additional items to this form as well, so that all 18 schemas can be measured. The short form is frequently utilized for research studies because it takes much less time to administer.

of each high-scoring schema and the meaning of the schema in everyday words and encourages the patient to read more about the schema in *Reinventing Your Life* (Young & Klosko, 1994).

By this point in the assessment, the therapist knows the patient's presenting problems and has explored patterns in the focused life history. The therapist has formed hypotheses about the patient's schemas. Responses on the Young Schema Questionnaire may support or refute these hypotheses, and they may contradict previous information. The therapist asks questions about inconsistencies. Sometimes patients misread questions, rewrite them, or interpret them in highly personal or idiosyncratic ways. The therapist clarifies discrepancies in order to ensure correct schema identification.

Some patients find that just filling out the questionnaire triggers their schemas. Fragile patients, such as those with BPD who have experienced severe early trauma, may experience strong emotions while answering items and therefore need to proceed slowly. The therapist can ask these patients to fill out a certain number of items each week, or the patient can work on the questionnaire with the therapist in the session. Some patients may respond to upsetting questions by avoiding the questionnaire. They leave items blank, they keep "forgetting" to fill out the questionnaire, or they rate items cursorily with low scores. They avoid the questionnaire in order to avoid facing their schemas. These kinds of responses point to a coping style of schema avoidance. If patients exhibit persistent difficulty completing the questionnaire, the therapist does not insist. Rather, the therapist explores reasons for not completing the questionnaire with the patient. If we cannot overcome these obstacles relatively quickly, we usually view this as a sign that the patient has significant avoidance problems and rely more on other facets of the assessment process to determine which schemas apply.

We generally spend one or two sessions going over the completed questionnaire with the patient, depending on the number of high-scoring schemas. Because patients are permitted to change the wording of questions, there is often a great deal the therapist and patient can discuss. Talking about questionnaire items usually leads patients to explore important material quickly. As the therapist and patient review the questionnaire, the therapist continually formulates and revises hypotheses about the patient's schemas and links schemas to the patient's presenting problems and life history.

Young Parenting Inventory

The Young Parenting Inventory (YPI; Young, 1994) is one of the primary means of identifying the childhood origins of schemas. The YPI is a 72-item questionnaire in which respondents rate their mothers and fathers separately on a variety of behaviors that we hypothesize contribute to the development of schemas. Like the YSQ, the YPI uses a 6-point Likert scale, and the items are grouped by schemas. We generally give the YPI to patients as homework a few weeks after the YSQ—typically around the fifth or sixth session when we discuss the origins of the patient's schemas.

If patients had stepparents, grandparents, or other parent substitutes at home when they were children, they can adapt the questionnaire by adding columns for additional parents or parent substitutes with whom they lived as children or adolescents. For example, one patient lived with her mother and father, then, after her father died when she was 5 years old, with her mother and stepfather. She added a column and rated the items on the YPI for her mother, father, and stepfather.

The inventory is a measure of the most common origins we have observed for each Early Maladaptive Schema. It reflects childhood environments that, from our observation, are likely to shape the development of specific schemas. However, it is possible that the patient experienced the childhood environment commonly associated with a particular schema but nevertheless did not develop the expected schema. This could happen for a number of reasons: (1) the patient's temperament prevented the schema from developing; (2) one parent or a significant other in the child's life compensated for the other; or (3) the patient, a significant person, or an event later in life healed the schema.

The therapist scores the YPI in a similar fashion to the YSQ. The therapist circles all items rated 5 or 6 for either parent. (We assume that scores of 5 or 6 have a high chance of being clinically significant as origins for a particular schema.) The only exceptions are items 1 through 5, which assess the origins of Emotional Deprivation and are scored in reverse: *low* scores signify the relevance of that origin for Emotional Deprivation. Unlike the YSQ, it is not necessary to have more than one high score on a particular schema for an item to be potentially significant. Although it is true that the more high scores there are for a given schema, the more certain we can be that the schema is relevant for the patient, any high-scoring item on the YPI can be meaningful as a schema origin. For example, if a patient indicates on a YPI item that she was sexually abused by a parent, it is very likely that the patient has a Mistrust/Abuse schema, even if the patient rated the other origins for that schema very low.

In the next session, after the therapist has reviewed the patient's scores, the patient and the therapist together discuss any high-scoring items. The therapist encourages the patient to expand on each origin by giving examples from childhood or adolescence that illustrate how the parent manifested the behavior. This discussion continues until the therapist has a full and accurate picture of how each parent contributed to the development of the patient's schemas. The therapist explains to the patient the relationship between each origin and the corresponding schema, and also how the childhood origin and schema may be linked to the patient's presenting problems.

Although the YPI was not designed to measure which schemas patients have but rather to identify likely origins for schemas that score high on the YSQ, the YPI has nevertheless proven to be a valuable *indirect* measure of schemas. If a patient strongly endorses items on the YPI that reflect the typical origins of a schema, we frequently observe that the patient has that schema, even if the patient rated the same schema low on the YSQ. The most likely explanation for this is that patients are often able to identify accurately what their parents were like even though they are out of touch with their own emotions. Thus, for patients with high schema avoidance, the YPI may sometimes prove to be a better measure for identifying schemas than the YSQ.

The therapist compares responses on the YPI to those on the YSQ. If high-scoring schemas on one questionnaire match high-scoring schemas on the other questionnaire, this adds to the likely significance of the schemas. Inconsistencies also yield important information. As with the YSQ, scores on the YPI might also be low as a result of schema avoidance or overcompensation. If a response is unexpectedly low, the therapist might say something like, "On your schema questionnaire, you say that throughout your life people have tried to control you, yet on your parenting inventory you indicate that your mother and father did not try to rule your life. Can you help me understand how these two statements fit for you?" Trying to resolve apparent inconsistencies like this proves very useful both in clarifying a patient's schemas and their origins and in helping patients face feelings and events that they have been avoiding or blocking.

Young–Rygh Avoidance Inventory

The Young–Rygh Avoidance Inventory (Young & Rygh, 1994) is a 41-item questionnaire that assesses schema avoidance. It includes such items as, "I watch a lot of television when I'm alone," "I try not to think about things that upset me," and "I get physically ill when things aren't going well for me." Individuals rate responses on a 6-point scale.

As with the other inventories, the therapist is not especially concerned with the total score but rather discusses high-scoring items with the patient. However, a high total score does indicate a general pattern of schema avoidance. The inventory is not schema-specific: An avoidant coping style is often a pervasive trait that can be utilized to avoid any schema.

Young Compensation Inventory

The Young Compensation Inventory (Young, 1995) is a 48-item questionnaire that assesses schema overcompensation. Items include such statements as, "I often blame others when things go wrong," "I agonize over decisions so I won't make a mistake," and "I dislike rules and get satisfaction from breaking them." The inventory uses a 6-point scale.

The therapist uses the overcompensation inventory as a clinical tool and discusses high-scoring items with the patient. For example, if the patient endorses blaming as a coping style, the therapist asks for an example. The therapist explores whether the blaming overcompensates for other, more painful feelings—perhaps feelings of shame. The therapist might ask, "Is it possible that blaming was a way for you to deal with your own feelings of shame in the situation?" As therapy progresses, patients self-monitor their use of the coping styles identified on these two inventories.

IMAGERY ASSESSMENT

At this point in the assessment process, the therapist has taken a focused life history and reviewed completed questionnaires with the patient. The therapist and patient are building an intellectual understanding of the patient's schemas and coping styles.

The next step is to trigger the patient's schemas in the therapy session so that both the therapist and the patient can feel them. The therapist usually accomplishes this with imagery. Imagery is a powerful assessment tool for most patients. With its frequently immediate and dramatic revelations of core material, it can often be the most effective way to identify schemas. A detailed description of how to do imagery work with patients is given in Chapter 4. Here we present a brief overview of the use of imagery for assessment.

The goals of imagery for assessment are:

1. To identify and trigger the patient's schemas
2. To understand the childhood origins of the schemas
3. To link schemas to presenting problems
4. To help the patient experience emotions associated with the schemas

We begin by providing patients with a convincing rationale for imagery work: that imagery will help them to feel their schemas, understand the childhood origins of their schemas, and connect their schemas to their current problems.

After giving patients this brief rationale, we ask them to close their eyes and let an image float to the top of their minds. We ask them not to force the image but to let it come on its own. Once patients picture an image, we ask them to describe it to us, out loud and in the present tense. We help them make it vivid and emotionally real.

The following exercise is an introduction to imagery that readers might wish to try themselves. It is based on a group training exercise we developed for therapists attending workshops on schema therapy (Young, 1995).

1. Close your eyes. Picture yourself in a safe place. Use pictures, not words or thoughts. Let the image come on its own. Notice the details. Tell me what you are picturing. What do you feel? Is there someone with you, or are you alone? Enjoy the relaxing, secure feeling in your safe place.

2. Keep your eyes closed and wipe out that image. Now picture yourself as a child with one of your parents in an upsetting situation. What do you see? Where are you? Notice the details. How old are you? What's happening in the image?

3. What do you feel? What are you thinking? What does your parent feel? What is your parent thinking?

4. Carry on a dialogue between you and your parent. What do you say? What does your parent say? (Continue until dialogue reaches a natural conclusion.)

5. Consider how you would like your parent to change or be different in the image, even if it seems impossible. For example, do you wish your parent would give you more freedom? More affection? More understanding? More acknowledgment? Less criticism? Be a better role model? Now tell your parent in the image how you would like him or her to change, in the words of a child.

6. How does your parent react? What happens next in the image? Keep the image going until the scene ends. How do you feel at the end of the scene?

7. Keep your eyes closed. Now intensify the feeling you have in this image as a child. Make the emotion stronger. Now, keeping the emotion in your body, wipe out the image of yourself as a child and picture an image of a situation in your *current* life in which you have the same or a similar feeling. Don't try to force it; let it come on its own. What's happening in the image? What are you thinking? What are you feeling? Say it out loud. If there is someone else in the image, tell that person how you would like him or her to change. How does the person react?

8. Wipe out the image and return to your safe place. Enjoy the relaxed feeling. Open your eyes.

The imagery assessment we conduct with patients is similar to this exercise. We start and end with a safe place. We ask patients to picture separate images of upsetting childhood situations with each parent and any other significant figures from their childhoods or adolescences. Then we instruct patients to speak to these people in their images, expressing what they are thinking and feeling and what they wish they could get from the other person. We then ask patients to switch to an image from their *current* lives that feels the same as the childhood situation. Once again, patients carry on a dialogue with the person from their adult life, saying aloud what they are thinking and feeling and what they want from the other. We repeat this process until we have covered all the significant others in childhood who contributed to the formation of the patient's schemas. (Chapter 4, on experiential techniques, provides an extended transcript of Dr. Young conducting this exercise with a patient.)

When doing imagery work with patients, it is important for the therapist to begin early in the session so that there is enough time to discuss what happens afterward. In this discussion, the therapist helps patients explore the images in order to identify schemas, understand their origins in childhood, and link them to the presenting problems. In addition, the therapist helps the patient integrate the imagery work with information from previous assessment modalities.

Sometimes patients are distraught after an imagery session. Starting imagery work early in the session helps ensure that there is enough time for patients to recover before they have to leave. When patients are afraid of the imagery work, the therapist attempts to set them at ease. The therapist tells them that they are in control of the imagery and, although the therapist is asking them to close their eyes to enhance their concentration, they may open their eyes if they become overwhelmed. Because of traumatic histories, feelings of mistrust, or anxiety, some patients participate in imagery exercises with downcast, rather than closed, eyes. Some request that the therapist not watch them during the exercises. The therapist makes the necessary accommodations. After the exercise, the therapist may need to ground these patients in the present moment before the session ends, using a mindfulness exercise.

Typically we start with an upsetting image from the patient's childhood and then work forward by linking this image to an upsetting image from the patient's current life. However, imagery exercises may proceed in other ways. For example, if the patient comes into the session already upset about a current situation, we can use an image of this situation as the starting place: We can ask the patient to picture an image of the current situation and then work back in time, asking him or her to picture an image from childhood that feels the same way. We can use an image of a specific symptom in the patient's body as the starting place. For example, we might say, "Can you picture an image of your back when you're in pain? What does it look like? What is the pain saying?" We can use strong emotions the patient experiences but does not understand as the starting place. Some examples follow.

Case Illustrations

Imagery of Childhood

Nadine is 25 years old. She has sought therapy for depression. Nadine works as an office manager in a large company. She has been consistently promoted at work because she is an excellent mediator of office disputes and because she frequently offers to take on tasks that others prefer to avoid. Although she functions at a high level, the therapist has determined that her depression is a sign that her work behavior is schema-driven and detrimental to her.

In her life history, Nadine described growing up in a religious family in which everyone was forbidden to express anger except her father. Nadine was the oldest of five children. Although her mother was ill and Nadine had a lot of responsibility for her younger siblings, she was not permitted to complain. It was her obligation to sacrifice for the sake of her parents and siblings, who were more needy than she was.

Doing imagery work about her childhood, Nadine recounted an incident in which she was falsely accused by her father of giving her mother the wrong medicine. Actually, it was Nadine's younger sister who had given the medicine, but Nadine felt it was wrong to implicate her sister and so took the blame herself. She stood before her irate father, suppressing her anger at her self-sacrifice. When the therapist asked her to picture an image of a current situation that felt the same way, Nadine came up with an image of taking the blame for a subordinate's mistake at work.

Nadine's Self-Sacrifice schema makes her well suited for exploitation at work. As in her family of origin, Nadine mediates disputes by absorbing blame and volunteering for unwanted tasks. She suppresses her anger, but her depression grows. Driven by her self-sacrifice, she helps ensure her emotional deprivation. (This is almost always true: Patients who have Self-Sacrifice schemas have Emotional Deprivation schemas as well, because they focus on meeting the needs of others rather than their own needs.) At home and at work, Nadine takes care of others, but no one takes care of her. Imagery helps Nadine recognize the origin of her Self-Sacrifice schema in her childhood and connect the schema to her depression.

Imagery Linked to an Emotion

Diane is a 50-year-old divorced woman who runs her own successful business. She reports a history of anxiety that has not responded to previous therapy. She arrived at her third session of schema therapy feeling anxious and stating that she was not sure why. When she reviewed the events of the week, she said that her 17-year-old daughter had been late picking her up at work the night before. Rationally, she had known there was no cause for alarm, but emotionally she had felt frightened. Her anxiety had persisted until that moment.

The therapist asked Diane to close her eyes and picture an image of the previous night, waiting for her daughter to pick her up. Once Diane had a vivid image and could recall the feeling of fear, the therapist asked her to picture an image of a time when she felt the same way as a child. Diane saw an image of herself as a child at summer camp, waiting for her parents to pick her up on the last day. Because her mother was manic–depressive and unable to care for her in a consistent manner and her father was a salesman who was frequently away from home, Diane was scared that no one would come for her. As she saw other children leaving with their parents, she began frantically pacing back and forth. Eventually she was the only child left. This image expressed Diane's Abandonment schema.

The therapist then asked Diane to continue the exercise by returning to the current image in which she was waiting for her daughter to pick her up. Now Diane understands why she was so frightened: Her Abandonment schema was triggered by her daughter's lateness. The imagery work helped her identify the schema underlying her anxiety. When patients have strong emotions they cannot understand, imagery can often help them discover the schema that is hidden underneath.

Imagery Linked to Somatic Symptoms

Somatic symptoms are frequently signs of schema avoidance. When patients have somatic symptoms, imagery can often help them overcome their cognitive and emotional avoidance in order to identify the underlying schemas. Paul is a 46-year-old physician. Altogether, he has spent more than 20 years in therapy trying to rid himself of his fear that he has a "migrating tumor" in his body. Despite his medical knowledge that tells him that this is not possible and despite years of medical tests that have failed to detect any biological abnormality, Paul persists in fearing he is terminally ill and will be killed by the tumor at any time.

In imagery, the therapist asks Paul to identify where the tumor is in his body at that moment. The therapist asks him to picture an image of the tumor and describe its size, texture, shape, and color. The therapist instructs him to talk to the tumor and ask why it is in his body and then to take the role of the tumor and answer. Speaking as the tumor, Paul says that he has not been doing his best work and is very bad. The tumor is in his body to punish him. Paul had better work more conscientiously or the tumor will strike him dead.

The therapist then asks Paul to picture an image of someone who made him feel the same way when he was a child. Paul pictures an image of himself as a child with his exacting father. His father is telling him that his school grades are unacceptable and that he must work harder. Like the tumor, the father embodies Paul's Unrelenting Standards schema. The imagery helps Paul access the schema underlying his somatic symptom and understand the origins of the schema in his childhood relationship with his father.

Overcoming Schema Avoidance

Schema avoidance is the most common obstacle to imagery assessment work. Schema avoidance may manifest itself in a number of ways. Patients might refuse to do the exercise, stating disdainfully that it will not be helpful. (This is a likely response from a narcissistic patient.) Patients might stall by asking questions or bring up unrelated topics in order to distract the therapist. Patients might keep opening their eyes or insist that they only see a "blank screen." Their images may be too vague to make out, or they may see only "stick figures."

There are many possible causes for schema avoidance. Some can be easily overcome: The patient may be self-conscious about "performing," worried about doing the exercise "right," or too nervous to concentrate. Often the therapist can resolve these difficulties simply by restating the rationale for the imagery work and reassuring the patient that the difficulties can be overcome. The therapist can also begin with less threatening material: For example, the therapist might begin with pleasant or neutral images and then gradually introduce more upsetting images.

We have several methods for overcoming schema avoidance of imagery work. We describe them more fully in the chapter on experiential techniques (Chapter 4), but we list them briefly here. They include:

1. Educate the patient about the rationale for imagery work.
2. Examine the pros and cons of doing the exercise.
3. Start with soothing imagery and gradually introduce more anxiety-provoking material.
4. Conduct a dialogue with the avoidant side of the patient (mode work).
5. Use affect regulation techniques such as mindfulness or relaxation training.
6. Initiate psychotropic medication.

Some patients have trouble visualizing themselves as children. When this happens, it can be helpful to have patients picture themselves in the present, then work backward to early adulthood, adolescence, and then finally to childhood. It can also be helpful to ask patients to picture their parents or siblings as they were when the patients were children. Sometimes patients cannot visualize themselves, but they can visualize other people and places from childhood. In addition, patients can bring in photographs of themselves as children to stimulate imagery. The therapist and patient can look at the photographs together, and the therapist can ask questions such as, "What might the child be thinking? What is the child feeling? What does the child want? What happens next in the picture?"

Another method for overcoming schema avoidance is conducting a dialogue with the avoidant side of the patient. We call this side the "Detached Protector" mode (see Chapter 8). The Detached Protector protects the patient by cutting off feelings. The therapist negotiates with the Detached Protector to gain access to the vulnerable part of the patient where the core schemas are—the Vulnerable Child mode.

However, sometimes it is not so easy for the therapist to deal with schema avoidance. Persistent schema avoidance may indicate that the patient's schemas are severe. For example, patients who have been abused may be too mistrustful to make themselves emotionally vulnerable. Very fragile patients may be too frightened to experience the affect connected to their schemas because of the possibility of decompensation. Severe schema avoiders and overcompensators have trouble with imagery because they cannot tolerate the negative affect. All of these patients may need to form a more stable and trusting bond with the therapist before attempting imagery work. Imagery work often becomes possible as the therapeutic relationship grows over time.

Some patients have great difficulty with childhood imagery because something traumatic happened to them and they are blocking it; or, at the other extreme, they experienced neglect and deprivation so great that the atmosphere was empty and flat. They have few memories of childhood. In these cases, the therapist must obtain knowledge of the schemas through other assessment methods. However, it is possible for traumatized or neglected patients to report sensations and emotions that give clues to schemas. For example, patients may feel trapped when they close their eyes, or they may report feeling alone. These sensations and emotions can help the therapist build hypotheses about the patient's schemas.

Assessing the Therapeutic Relationship

The patient's schemas also appear in the therapy relationship. (Of course, this is true of the therapist's schemas as well: The therapist's own schemas are triggered. We discuss this issue of countertransference in Chapter 6 on the therapeutic relationship.) The triggering of the patient's schemas in the therapy relationship represents an opportunity for the therapist to gather more assessment material. The therapist and patient can discuss what transpired, working to identify schemas, triggers, and associated thoughts and feelings, covering both the current circumstance and related events in the past. The therapist asks patients to remember other people who have prompted them to feel the same way.

Early Maladaptive Schemas produce characteristic behaviors in therapy. For example, a patient with a Dependence schema might repeatedly ask for help with questionnaires and homework assignments; a patient with a Self-Sacrifice schema might be overly solicitous of the therapist and frequently inquire about the therapist's health or mood; a patient with an Entitlement schema might repeatedly make requests for special treatment, such as scheduling changes or extra time; a patient with an Abandonment schema might resist relying on the therapist out of fear of being deserted; a patient with a Mistrust/Abuse schema might ask suspiciously about the therapist's note taking or adherence to confidentiality; a patient with a Defectiveness schema might avoid making eye contact or have difficulty accepting compliments; a patient with an Enmeshment schema might copy aspects of the therapist's appearance or style. The therapist can learn about the patient's schemas by observing how the patient behaves in the therapy relationship. The therapist shares this information with the patient, speaking about it empathically in schema terms.

ASSESSING EMOTIONAL TEMPERAMENT

As we noted in Chapter 1, we have identified seven hypothesized dimensions of emotional temperament, drawn from the scientific literature and from our own clinical observations:

Labile ↔ Nonreactive
Dysthymic ↔ Optimistic
Anxious ↔ Calm
Obsessive ↔ Distractible
Passive ↔ Aggressive
Irritable ↔ Cheerful
Shy ↔ Sociable

We conceptualize temperament as a set of points on these dimensions. Temperament influences the coping styles individuals adopt to handle their schemas.

There are several reasons to assess temperament. First, temperament is inborn and will always be a significant part of how the patient responds to the environment. Although each temperament poses some drawbacks, it also presents some benefits. Each person's temperament has advantages and disadvantages. Patients can learn to accept and appreciate their natures and still overcome their problems. Knowledge of one's temperament can be illuminating. People do not choose their temperaments. They do not generally choose to feel emotional, aggressive, or shy. It is neither good nor bad; it is just the way they are. For example, recognizing their intensely emotional natures can often help patients with BPD build self-esteem. They can see that they are not "bad" for having intense feelings, even if their intensity was problematic for their parents. Rather, it is their nature to be passionate human beings. Patients can also learn strategies for modulating their temperaments and can learn to behave in appropriate ways in spite of their emotional makeup.

We should note that we do not yet have adequate assessment measures to determine with certainty someone's innate temperament. The best we can do is to make an educated guess by obtaining a detailed history. For clinical purposes, however, it does not matter whether a patient's lifelong mood state is innate or a result of early life experiences. If it has been a part of them for most of their lives, it is usually extremely resistant to change through psychotherapy and thus can be addressed as though it were innate.

The therapist begins to conceptualize the patient's temperament by asking a series of questions related to affective states. Some patients can identify their baseline or prevailing moods. The therapist asks questions such as, "What do your family members say you were like (emotionally and interpersonally) as a child?"; "Are you generally a high energy or a low energy person?"; "What is your general outlook on life? Are you generally optimistic or pessimistic?"; "How do you usually feel when you're alone?"; "How often do you cry?"; "How often do you lose your temper?"; "Do you worry a lot?"

Lifelong traits are likely to be temperamental. Thus, for each of these questions, the therapist asks whether this has always been true for the patient or has been true only for certain periods in the patient's life. The more consistent and long-term the feelings are and the earlier they began, the more likely it is that they are part of the patient's innate temperament rather than a response to life events.

In addition to interviewing the patient, the therapist observes the patient's emotional reactions in therapy sessions and asks about emotional reactions in the patient's outside life. Finally, the therapist considers what it feels like to be with the patient in the sessions. The affective tone of the meetings can reveal a great deal about the patient's temperament.

OTHER ASSESSMENT METHODS

Schemas are often triggered naturally in the course of the patient's life. Current events can trigger a patient's schemas. The therapist and patient can watch for instances in which the patient has a strong emotional reaction to a current event and talk about it in the session. Group therapy is another context in which the patient's schemas may be evident. How the patient responds to other group members and to the topics discussed can provide valuable material for individual sessions. Schemas are also ap-

parent in dreams. Patients can record their dreams—especially recurring dreams and dreams involving strong affect—and discuss them with
the therapist in subsequent sessions. Dreams often portray the patient's
schemas, and they can be a starting place for imagery work. Books and
movies can trigger schemas. Therapists can assign specific books or movies to the patient for this purpose, based on the therapist's hypotheses
about the patient's schemas. The patient's reactions can support or dis-
confirm the therapist's hypotheses.

EDUCATING PATIENTS ABOUT SCHEMAS

Throughout the assessment process, the therapist educates the patient
about the schema model. Patients become educated primarily through discussion, assigned readings, and self-observation. As they learn about the
model, patients can participate more fully in the formation of their case
conceptualizations.

Reinventing Your Life

We assign *Reinventing Your Life* (Young & Klosko, 1994) to patients to help
them learn about their schemas, referred to as "lifetraps" in the book. The
book presents extensive case examples. We have found that patients relate
well to the characters in these examples and thus engage emotionally with
the material. The book explains the nature of "lifetraps" and describes the
three coping styles of surrender, avoidance, and overcompensation (called
"surrender," "escape," and "counterattack"). The book next presents chapters on each of 11 lifetraps. These chapters provide their own questionnaires, which patients can take to ascertain whether they are likely to have
that lifetrap. The chapters then describes the typical childhood origins of
the lifetrap; danger signals in potential partners (who perpetuate rather
than heal the lifetrap); how the lifetrap manifests itself in relationships,
particularly romantic ones; and specific strategies for change.

   We recommend that patients read the first five short introductory
chapters and then one or two chapters about their primary schemas. Even
if the patient has many more schemas, we work on only the primary one or
two first. We may recommend other chapters later, as the topics arise naturally in the patient's everyday life or in therapy sessions.

Self-Observation of Schemas and Coping Styles

As patients learn about their schemas, they begin to observe the activity of
their schemas in their current lives. They self-monitor their schemas and
coping styles using the Schema Diary form. We say more about the self-

monitoring of schemas and coping styles in Chapter 3. Self-observation helps patients see how automatically their schemas are triggered and how pervasive they are in their lives. Patients can observe what is happening and can often recognize that they are behaving in self-destructive ways, even if they are not yet able to change their behavior patterns.

THE COMPLETED SCHEMA-FOCUSED CASE FORMULATION

As a last step before the Change Phase begins, the therapist summarizes the case conceptualization for the patient using the Schema Therapy Case Conceptualization Form. This initial conceptualization is open to refinement as treatment unfolds (see Figure 2.1).

SUMMARY

This chapter discusses the Assessment and Education Phase of schema therapy. This phase has six major goals: (1) identification of dysfunctional life patterns; (2) identification and triggering of Early Maladaptive Schemas; (3) understanding of the origins of schemas in childhood and adolescence; (4) identification of coping styles and responses; (5) assessment of temperament; and (6) formulation of the case conceptualization.

The assessment is multifaceted, utilizing self-report, experiential, behavioral, and interpersonal measures. It begins with the initial evaluation, in which the therapist ascertains the patient's presenting problems and goals for therapy, and evaluates the patient's suitability for schema therapy. Next, the therapist takes a life history, identifying maladaptive life patterns, schemas, and coping styles. The patient gradually completes the following questionnaires as homework assignments: (1) life history assessment forms; (2) Young Schema Questionnaire; (3) Young Parenting Inventory; (4) Young–Rygh Avoidance Inventory; and (5) Young Compensation Inventory. The therapist and patient discuss the results of the questionnaires in sessions, in the course of which the therapist educates the patient about the schema model. Next, the therapist uses experiential techniques, especially imagery, to access and trigger the patient's schemas and to link schemas to their origins in childhood and to current problems. Throughout, the therapist observes the patient's schemas and coping styles as they appear in the therapy relationship. Finally, the therapist assesses the patient's emotional temperament. As the therapist and patient formulate and refine hypotheses, the assessment gradually adheres into a case conceptualization.

Schema avoidance is the most common obstacle to the imagery assessment work. We present methods for overcoming schema avoidance of imagery, including educating the patient about the rationale for imagery work; examining the advantages and disadvantages of doing the exercise; starting with soothing imagery and gradually introducing more emotionally charged material; conducting a dialogue with the avoidant side of the patient (mode work); using affect regulation techniques such as mindfulness or relaxation training; and initiating psychotropic medication.

Chapter 3

COGNITIVE STRATEGIES

After completing the Assessment and Education Phase described in the previous chapter, the therapist and patient are ready to begin the Change Phase. This phase incorporates cognitive, experiential, behavioral, and interpersonal strategies to modify schemas, coping styles, and modes. We usually begin the change process with cognitive techniques, which are the focus of this chapter.[1]

As part of the Assessment and Education Phase, the therapist has already filled out the case conceptualization form and educated the patient about the schema model. The therapist and patient have identified the patient's dysfunctional life patterns and Early Maladaptive Schemas, explored the childhood origins of the schemas, and linked the schemas to the presenting problems. They have also identified the patient's coping styles, emotional temperament, and modes.

Cognitive strategies help the patient articulate a healthy voice to dispute the schema, strengthening the patient's Healthy Adult mode. The therapist helps the patient build a logical, rational case against the schema. Usually patients have not questioned their schemas: They have accepted them as "givens" or as truths in their lives. In their internal psychological worlds, their schemas have reigned supreme. There has been no strong Healthy Adult mode to counter the schema. Cognitive strategies help patients step outside the schema and evaluate its veracity. Patients see that there is a truth outside of the schema and that they can fight the schema with a truth that is more objective and empirically sound.

---

[1]With patients with BPD, the therapist does not begin with cognitive work but focuses instead on forming a stable bond with the patient. This is discussed further in Chapter 9.

OVERVIEW OF COGNITIVE STRATEGIES

It is through the cognitive strategies that the patient first recognizes that the schema is inaccurate—either untrue or greatly exaggerated. The therapist and patient begin by agreeing to regard the schema as open to question. Rather than an absolute truth, it is a hypothesis to be tested. They then subject the schema to logical and empirical analyses. They examine the evidence supporting and refuting the schema in the patient's life; they go through the evidence the patient has used to uphold the schema, and they find alternative interpretations of these same events; they conduct debates between the "schema side" and the "healthy side"; and they list the advantages and disadvantages of the patient's current coping styles. Based on this work, the patient and therapist generate healthy responses to the schema. They write these responses on schema flash cards and read the flash cards whenever the schema is triggered. Finally, patients practice responding to schemas on their own using the Schema Diary form.

When the cognitive strategies are effective, patients gain a heightened appreciation of how distorted the schema actually is. They have gained more psychological distance from the schema and no longer view it as an absolute truth. They have some insight into how the schema twists their perceptions. They begin to wonder whether the schema really has to run— and ruin—their lives. They realize they might have a choice.

Successfully treated patients have internalized the cognitive work as part of a Healthy Adult mode that actively counters the schema with rational arguments and empirical evidence. After completing the cognitive component of schema therapy, patients are usually no longer dependent on the therapist's assistance in challenging the schema. When a schema is triggered in their lives outside of therapy, they are able to fight the schema using the cognitive techniques. Even though patients may still *feel* as though the schema is true, they know that it is not factually true. They have a heightened intellectual awareness that the schema is false.

THERAPEUTIC STYLE

We call the primary stance that the schema therapist takes throughout treatment "empathic confrontation" or "empathic reality-testing." In the cognitive stage of treatment, empathic confrontation means that the therapist empathizes with the reasons for patients having the beliefs that they do— namely, that their beliefs are based on their early childhood experiences— while simultaneously confronting the fact that their beliefs are inaccurate and lead to unhealthy life patterns that patients must change in order to improve. The therapist acknowledges to patients that their schemas seem right to them because they have lived entire lives that seem to verify their schemas and that they adopted certain coping styles because it was the only way to survive adverse childhood circumstances. Consistent with constructivist models, the therapist validates patients' schemas and coping styles as understandable conclusions based on their life histories. At the same time, the therapist reminds patients about the negative consequences of their schemas and maladaptive coping styles. Their schemas and coping styles were adaptive in early childhood but now are maladaptive. A therapeutic stance of empathic confrontation acknowledges the past while distinguishing the realities of the past from the realities of the present. It supports the patient's ability to see and to accept what is.

Empathic confrontation requires constant shifting between empathy and reality-testing. Therapists often err in one direction or the other. Either they are so empathic that they do not push patients to face reality, or they are too confrontational and cause patients to feel defensive and misunderstood. Either way, patients are unlikely to change. With empathic confrontation, the therapist strives for the optimal balance between empathy and reality-testing that will enable patients to progress. When the therapist is successful in this endeavor, patients feel truly understood and affirmed, perhaps for the first time in their lives. Feeling understood, they are more likely to accept the necessity of change, and they are more receptive to healthy alternative perspectives offered by the therapist. Further, patients experience the therapist as allying with them against the schema. Rather than viewing the schema as a core part of who they are, they begin to view it as foreign.

The therapist explains to patients that, given their life histories, it makes sense that they see things as they do and behave as they do. However, in the end, the ways in which they see and behave have only served to perpetuate their schemas. The therapist builds a case in favor of fighting their schemas with new ways of behaving rather than persisting in the same self-defeating patterns. The material gathered in the Assessment Phase enables the therapist to substantiate the destructiveness of the schemas and coping styles in their lives. The therapist encourages patients to respond to schema triggers in healthier ways. In so doing, they can eventually heal their schemas and meet their basic emotional needs. The following excerpt provides a brief example of empathic confrontation and is taken from the interview Dr. Young conducted with Marika, a patient whom we introduced in Chapter 2. Marika entered therapy to improve her marriage. Marika and her husband, James, are stuck in a repetitive, vicious cycle in which she becomes more and more aggressively demanding of attention and affection, and he becomes more and more withdrawn, indifferent, and cold. After exploring her childhood relationship with her father, Dr. Young speaks to Marika about her approach to James.

"Marika, I know it feels natural to you to try to get James upset in order to get his attention. But, even though it's the only way you think he'll give you any caring, you still need to approach him in a more vulnerable way. Let him know why you need his love and see if he responds before moving so quickly to that other style of upsetting him. I understand it was the only way that got you any attention from your father, but it might not be the only way that works with James."

Thus the therapist empathizes with Marika's reason for approaching James in such an aggressive way—because that was the only way she got anything from her father—while still presenting the negative consequences of this approach and the wisdom of approaching James in a more vulnerable way.

COGNITIVE TECHNIQUES

Cognitive techniques in schema therapy include the following:

1. Testing the validity of a schema
2. Reframing the evidence supporting a schema
3. Evaluating the advantages and disadvantages of the patient's coping styles
4. Conducting dialogues between the "schema side" and the "healthy side"
5. Constructing schema flash cards
6. Filling out Schema Diary forms

The therapist typically goes through the cognitive techniques with patients in the order we have listed them here, as the techniques build on one another.

Testing the Validity of the Schemas

The therapist and patient test the validity of a schema by examining the objective evidence for and against the schema. This process is similar to testing the validity of automatic thoughts in cognitive therapy, except that the therapist uses the patient's whole life as empirical data and not just the present circumstances. The schema is the hypothesis to be tested.

The therapist and patient make a list of evidence from the past and present supporting the schema; then they make a list of evidence refuting the schema. Patients usually find it remarkably easy to compose the first list, evidence supporting the schema, because they already believe this evidence. They have been rehearsing it all their lives. Generating evidence that supports the schema feels natural and familiar to them. In contrast, patients usually find it extremely difficult to compose the second list, evidence refuting the schema, and frequently require a good deal of input from the therapist, because they do not believe the evidence against the schema. They have spent their lives ignoring or downplaying this evidence. They do not have ready access to this evidence as a result of schema perpetuation, which has continuously induced them to accentuate information confirming the schema and negate information contradicting the schema. The discrepancy between the patient's ease at playing the schema side and difficulty playing the healthy side often proves highly instructive to the patient. The patient observes firsthand how the schema works to preserve itself.

To illustrate this technique, we examine one patient's evidence regarding her Defectiveness schema. Shari is 28 years old, married with two children, and works as a psychiatric nurse. Her Defectiveness schema originated in her childhood with her alcoholic mother. (Her father divorced her mother and left the family when Shari was 4 years old. Although he provided money, Shari rarely saw him after that.) Throughout her childhood, her mother frequently humiliated her by appearing intoxicated in public places. She once came drunk to one of Shari's school plays and disrupted the performance. Shari avoided bringing friends home out of fear of what her mother might do. Her home life was barren and chaotic.

Here is Shari's list of evidence that she is defective:

1. I'm not like everyone else. I'm different and always have been.
2. My family was different from other families.
3. My family was shameful.
4. No one ever loved me or cared for me when I was a child. I never belonged to anyone. My own father didn't care to see me.
5. I'm awkward, stilted, obsessive, afraid, and self-conscious with other people.
6. I'm inappropriate with other people. I don't know the rules.
7. I'm fawning and pandering with other people. I need acceptance and approval too much.
8. I get too angry inside.

It is important to mention that, despite Shari's critical appraisal of her social ability, she is actually highly socially skilled. Her problem is one of social anxiety, not one of social skills.

Not surprisingly, Shari found it extremely difficult to compose the second list, evidence refuting the schema. When it came to this part of the exercise, she could not think of anything to write down at all. She sat there bewildered and silent. Even though she is both personally and professionally successful and has a multitude of commendable traits, she could not think of a single positive quality to ascribe to herself. The therapist had to suggest every one.

The therapist asks leading questions designed to draw from the patient the evidence against the schema. For example, if a patient has a Defectiveness schema such as Shari does, the therapist might ask, "Has anyone ever loved you or liked you?" "Do you try to be a good person?" "Is there anything at all good about you?" "Is there anyone you care about?" "What have other people told you is good about you?" Such questions—often worded in an extreme manner—spur the patient to generate positive information. The therapist and patient gradually develop a list of the patient's good qualities. Later the patient can use this list to counter the schema.

Here is the list Shari compiled with the help of her therapist.

1. My husband and children love me.
2. My husband's family loves me. (My sister-in-law asked me to take her children if she and my brother-in-law died.)
3. My friends Jeanette and Anne Marie love me.
4. My patients like and respect me. I get really good feedback from them pretty much all the time.
5. Most of the staff at the hospital likes me and respects me. I get good evaluations.
6. I'm sensitive to other people's feelings.
7. I loved my mother, even if she cared about drinking more than she cared about me. I was the one who was there for her until the end.
8. I try to be good and do the right thing. When I get angry, it's for good reason.

It is important for the therapist to write down the evidence against the schema, because patients tend to quickly dismiss or forget it.

Shari is fortunate, because there is an abundance of evidence against her Defectiveness schema. Not all patients have such good fortune. If there is not much evidence to contradict the schema, the therapist acknowledges it, but says, "It doesn't have to be this way." For example, a male patient with a Defectiveness schema might actually have very few loving people in his life. Through surrendering to the schema (choosing significant others who are rejecting and critical), avoiding the schema (staying out of close relationships), or overcompensating for the schema (treating others arrogantly and pushing them away), the patient might look back on a whole life without love. The therapist says,

"I agree you haven't developed loving relationships in your life, but it's for a good reason. It's because of what happened to you as a child that it's been so hard for you. Because you learned very young to expect criticism and rejection, you stopped reaching out to people. But we can change this pattern. We can work together to help you choose people who are warm and accepting and let them become part of your life. You can work on gradually getting close to some of these people and letting them gradually get close to you. You could try to stop denigrating yourself and others. If you take these steps, things could be different for you. This is what we'll work on in therapy."

As therapy progresses and the patient develops a greater ability to form close relationships, the therapist and patient can add new information to the list of evidence against the schema.

As another step in this process of examining the evidence, patients look at how they discount the evidence against the schema. They write down how they negate evidence. For example, Shari listed the ways she discounts the evidence against her Defectiveness schema.

1. I tell myself that I'm fooling my husband and children, and that's why they love me. They don't know the real me.
2. I do more for my family and friends than they do for me, and then I feel like that's the only reason they care about me.
3. When people give me good feedback, I don't believe them. I think that there's some other reason they're saying it.
4. I tell myself that I'm only sensitive to people's feelings out of weakness. I'm afraid to assert myself.
5. I get down on myself for getting angry and resentful while I was taking care of my mother.

After writing down how they negate evidence, patients "reclaim" the evidence against the schema. The therapist shows how invalidating the evidence against the schema is simply another form of schema perpetuation.

Reframing the Evidence Supporting the Schema

The next step is to take the list of evidence supporting the schema and to generate alternative explanations for what happened. The therapist takes events the patient views as proving the schema and reattributes them to other causes. The goal is to discredit the evidence supporting the schema.

Evidence from the Patient's Early Childhood

The therapist discounts early childhood experiences as reflecting pathological family dynamics, including poor parenting, rather than the truth of the schema. The therapist points out any activities that occurred within the family that would not have been acceptable in healthy families. In addition, the therapist and patient consider the psychological health and character of the parents (and other family members) one by one. Did the parent truly have the patient's best interests at heart? What role did the parent assign to the patient? The therapist points out that parents often assign roles to children that do not serve the children's needs but the needs of the parents. These roles do not reflect inherent flaws in the children, but instead reflect flaws in the parents. Did the parent use the patient in any selfish way? The therapist goes on exploring in this fashion until patients shift to a more realistic perspective of their family history. They stop viewing their early childhood experiences as proof of their schemas.

For example, one item on Marika's list of evidence supporting her Defectiveness schema was, "My father didn't love me or pay attention to me." Marika attributed her father's lack of love to her inherent unlovability: He did not love her because she was unworthy of love. In her view, she was too needy. The therapist spent time exploring the patterns in Marika's family of origin. Then the therapist suggested an alternative explanation: Her father was *incapable* of loving his children. In fact, he did not love her brother, either. Her father did not show love for her because of his own psychological limitations, not because she was unlovable. Marika's father was narcissistic and incapable of genuine love. He did not have the ability to be a good father. A good father would have loved her. She was an affectionate child who wanted a close relationship with her father, but he could not have this kind of relationship.

Evidence from the Patient's Life Since Childhood

The therapist discounts experiences since childhood that support the schema by attributing them to schema perpetuation. The coping styles patients learned in childhood have carried their schemas forward into their adult lives. The therapist notes that, because of their schema-driven behaviors, patients have never given their schemas a fair test. For example, another item on Marika's list of evidence supporting her Defectiveness schema was, "All the men in my life have treated me badly." She reported that she had had three boyfriends. One of them abused her, one left her, and one frequently slept with other women.

Marika believes that her boyfriends treated her badly because she is undeserving of respect and love, and they knew it. The therapist suggests an alternative explanation: Since she started dating as an adolescent and continuing until the present day, her Defectiveness schema has caused her to keep choosing partners who were critical and rejecting and who would thus treat her badly. (Partner selection is frequently an important aspect of schema perpetuation.)

THERAPIST: Well, let's look at the type of people you chose. Did you choose partners who at the beginning you had reason to believe would be caring to you—loyal, committed, honest, loving people?

MARIKA: Well, no. Joel from the beginning was trouble. He was sleeping around.

THERAPIST: And how about Mark?

MARIKA: No, he had beaten up his previous girlfriend.

In sum, the therapist takes evidence supporting the schema and reframes it. If it is evidence from childhood, the therapist reframes it as a problem with the parents or family system. If it is evidence from the patient's life since childhood, the therapist reframes it as schema perpetuation, which has turned the schema into a self-fulfilling prophecy in the patient's life.

Evaluating the Advantages and Disadvantages of the Patient's Coping Responses

The therapist and patient study each schema and coping response individually and list its advantages and disadvantages. (The therapist and patient have already identified the patient's coping styles in the Assessment and Education Phase.) The goal is for patients to recognize the self-defeating nature of their coping styles and to discern that, if they were to replace these coping styles with healthier behaviors, they could increase the chances for happiness in their lives. The therapist also points out that their coping styles were adaptive as children but are maladaptive as adults in the wider world outside their families or adolescent peer group.

For example, a young female patient named Kim has an Abandonment schema. She copes with her schema by using an avoidant coping style. She stays away from men by turning down most requests for dates and spending her free time alone or with her girlfriends. On the rare occasions that she goes out with men whom she likes, she ends the relationship abruptly after a few dates:

THERAPIST: So, would it be OK with you if we list the advantages and disadvantages of your coping style—of all the ways you avoid getting close to men and your history of ending promising relationships?

KIM: Yes. That sounds OK.

THERAPIST: So, what are the advantages, do you think? What do you gain by avoiding men and ending relationships prematurely?

KIM: That's easy. I don't have to go through the pain of being left. I leave them so they can't leave me.

The advantage of Kim's avoidant coping style is that it provides her with an immediate sense of control over what happens in her relationships with men. In the short run, she feels less anxious. The disadvantage, however, is significant: In the long run, she is alone. (As usual, attempts at schema avoidance result in schema perpetuation.)

THERAPIST: What are the disadvantages of avoiding men and breaking up with them when things are going well? What are the disadvantages of your coping style?

KIM: Well, one disadvantage is that I lose a lot of good relationships.

THERAPIST: How do you feel about losing your last boyfriend, Jonathan?

KIM: (*pause*) Relieved. I feel relieved. I don't have to worry about it all the time anymore.

THERAPIST: Do you feel anything else about it?

KIM: Yeah, well, of course. I feel sad. I miss him. I feel sad that he's gone. We were really close for a while.

The exercise helps Kim face the reality of her situation. If she continues with her current method of coping with her Abandonment schema, she will surely end up alone. However, if she is willing to tolerate her anxiety and commit to a promising relationship, then there is a possibility that she might get what she wants most: a relationship with a man who will heal, rather than reinforce, her Abandonment schema.

Conducting Dialogues between the "Schema Side" and the "Healthy Side"

With the next cognitive technique, patients learn to conduct dialogues between their "schema side" and "healthy side." Adapting the Gestalt "empty chair" technique, the therapist instructs patients to switch chairs as they play the two sides: In one chair they play the schema side, in the other they play the healthy side.

Because patients normally have little or no experience expressing the healthy side, the therapist first plays the healthy side and the patient plays the schema. The therapist might introduce the technique by saying: "Let's have a debate between the schema side and the healthy side. I'll play the healthy side, and you play the schema side. Try as hard as you can to prove that the schema is true, and I'll try as hard as I can to prove that the schema is false." Beginning this way gives the therapist the opportunity to model the healthy side for the patient and enables the therapist to come up with answers to whatever arguments the patient raises while playing the schema side.

Eventually the patient takes over the role of the healthy side, with the therapist acting as coach. Either the therapist or patient can play the schema side; when the patient plays both sides, the patient moves back and forth between two different chairs, each chair representing one side of the debate. At first the patient needs a lot of prompting from the therapist to come up with healthy responses. The therapist gradually withdraws into the background, however, as the patient more easily generates healthy answers. The goal is for patients to learn how to play the healthy side on their own, naturally and automatically.

In the following example, Dr. Young helps a patient conduct a dialogue between his Mistrust/Abuse and Defectiveness schemas and his "healthy side." The patient is a 35-year-old man named Daniel, whom we present in greater detail in the next chapter on experiential strategies. Daniel had a traumatic childhood: His father was alcoholic, and his mother was sexually, physically, and emotionally abusive. At the time of his interview with Dr. Young, Daniel had been in traditional cognitive therapy with another therapist for about 9 months. He had sought therapy for social anxiety and anger-management problems. Daniel's ultimate goal was to meet a woman and get married, but he both mistrusted women and expected them to reject him. He thus avoided social situations in which he might meet women.

In order to prepare the patient for the dialogue, Dr. Young began the session by helping the patient build a case against the schema. Dr. Young thus provided the patient with some ammunition to use against the schema side. In the following excerpt, Daniel plays both the schema side and the healthy side.

THERAPIST: What I'd like to do now is to have what I call a dialogue between the schema side, which feels women can't be trusted and they're not going to find you attractive, and then this healthy side that you're trying to build up but which is still not as strong. Do you know what I'm saying?

DANIEL: Yes.

THERAPIST: So I'm going to ask you to go back and forth. Maybe you can start as if you're in a room at a dance about to approach a woman, but you're feeling avoidant, you want to run. First be the schema side that wants to run out and say what you're afraid of.

DANIEL: (*as the schema side*) "I'm in a very nervous state and I'm sort of hoping that the dance will not be a success, and that, contrary to what I've heard, that there's always more women than men at the dances, that the reverse will be true, and that will give me a reason to leave."

Dr. Young encourages the patient to overcome his desire to escape and stay at the dance despite his anxiety:

THERAPIST: Now imagine that you're at the dance and you actually see a woman you're attracted to. Now be the schema side.

DANIEL: (*as the schema side*) "She looks like a really nice person, but I don't think she'd go for me. I'm probably not even up to this person, on either an intellectual level or an emotional level. She's probably way ahead of me maturity-wise. And she'll probably go for one of these other guys, and they'll probably ask her before me anyway."

THERAPIST: All right, now be the healthy side that we're trying to build up and have it answer. Talk back to that side.

DANIEL: (*as the healthy side*) "Don't be so quick to judge. You have a lot of good parts to yourself that probably would be very appealing to this woman. You have a definite value system, you know boundaries, you can allow her to be her own person, you have a definite sensitivity towards female issues, and she probably would like you a lot."

Here Daniel is using his prior cognitive work against the schema. Dr. Young elicits more of the schema side:

THERAPIST: Now go back to the schema side.

DANIEL: (*as the schema side*) "But even so, when it comes down to continuing the conversation to the point of asking her for a date, you know, I don't think you should, because then you're going to have to deal with other issues, such as, maybe becoming more intimate and figuring out where to go after the date, whether you should go to bed or whether you shouldn't go to bed. It's better that you don't get involved because of that."

THERAPIST: Now be the healthy side again.

DANIEL: (*as the healthy side*) "I don't think that's the issue right now, and you wouldn't have to be worried about it for a long time."

THERAPIST: Try to answer it, though. Try to answer it even though you're right, you don't have to worry about it till later, but try to at least give some hope that there's an answer to it.

The therapist encourages Daniel to answer every argument posed by the schema.

DANIEL: (*as the healthy side*) "I think that, when it gets to that point, that I could do very well giving affection and being emotionally supportive and being sensitive when it comes time to being sexually intimate, possibly. (*Speaks hesitantly.*) I don't think that'll be a problem."

THERAPIST: (*coaching the patient as the healthy side*) "I have to be sure I trust the woman before I try to do anything sexual."

The therapist helps Daniel when he falters. Sexual intimacy is an issue he is only beginning to explore in his relationships with women.

DANIEL: (*continuing as the healthy side*) "I would have to trust. I would just have to learn how to trust the woman and feel safe."

THERAPIST: Now be the schema side that says, "You'll never do that, women can't be trusted."

The therapist tries to elicit all the counterarguments the schema utilizes to preserve itself.

DANIEL: (*as the schema side*) "Women can't be trusted, and they're very unreasonable and erratic, and it will be very difficult to figure out just what to do. And I don't think you can do it."

THERAPIST: OK, now be the other side.

DANIEL: (*as the healthy side*) "Women are people just like men are, and they can be very reasonable, and they're very nice to be with."

The therapist tries to help the patient differentiate his mother, who was the primary cause of his schemas, from other women.

THERAPIST: Try to distinguish your mother from other women in your answer.

DANIEL: (*continuing as the healthy side*) "And all woman aren't necessarily like your mother. Each woman is a unique person just like I am, and they have to be treated as individuals. And there are many women who have value systems that are probably even better than mine."

THERAPIST: Now be the schema side.

DANIEL: (*as the schema side*) "Well, that's easier said than done, because your mother really fixed it so no woman could possibly be good to you. The women here are just like all women. Women in general are like your mother, and they're just concerned about one thing, using you and abusing you. And that's just about what you're gonna wind up with. Eventually you'll be used or abused."

THERAPIST: Now be the healthy side.

DANIEL: (*as the healthy side*) "Again, all women are not like my mother, and all women are not abusive. Women are neither totally bad nor totally good. They're like every other person; they have good parts and bad parts."

The patient goes back and forth between the chairs. The therapist continues the exercise until the healthy side has the final word.

It takes most patients a long time and a lot of practice before they can play the healthy side with assurance. It takes many months of repeating the exercise to "chip away" at the schema and fortify the healthy side. The therapist asks patients to repeat the dialogues until they can play the healthy side independently. Even though they can speak the words, however, patients still say, "I don't really believe the healthy side." The therapist can answer: "Most patients feel the way you do at this point in the therapy: Rationally they understand the healthy side, but emotionally they don't believe it yet. All I'm asking you to do now is to say what you know to be *logically* true. Later we'll work on helping you take in what you're saying on a more emotional level."

Schema Flash Cards

After completing the schema restructuring process, the therapist and patient begin to write schema flash cards. Schema flash cards summarize healthy responses to specific schema triggers. Patients carry the flash cards around with them and read them when the relevant schemas are triggered. Ideally, flash cards contain the most powerful evidence and arguments against the schema and provide patients with continual rehearsals of rational responses.

We provide a Schema Therapy Flash Card template (see Figure 3.1) for the therapist to use as a guide (Young, Wattenmaker, & Wattenmaker, 1996). Using the template, the therapist collaborates with the patient in composing flash cards. The therapist plays such an active role because, at this point in therapy, the patient's healthy side is not strong enough to write a truly convincing answer to the schema. Usually the therapist dictates the flash card while the patient writes it down on an index card.

In the following excerpt, Dr. Young and Daniel create a flash card for him to read in social situations with women in which he feels anxious.

THERAPIST: There are various techniques we can use to try to help you overcome situations you tend to avoid. One is flash cards. A flash card is a card you carry around with you that basically answers a lot of the fears you have and the schemas that come up. In fact, if you want, I could dictate one to you and you could jot it down. How would that be?

DANIEL: That would be wonderful.

THERAPIST: Maybe we'll pick one based on what we've already talked about in here, as if you're at one of these dances and you're trying to meet a woman. How would that be?

DANIEL: That sounds good.

FIGURE 3.1. Schema Therapy Flash Card.

Acknowledgment of current feeling

Right now I feel _____ because _____
              (emotions)
_____.
                              (trigger situation)

Identification of schema(s)

However, I know that this is probably my _____
                                              (relevant schema)
schema(s), which I learned through _____
                                           (origin)
_____.

These schemas lead me to exaggerate the degree to which _____
                                                           (schema distortions)
_____.

Reality-testing

Even though I believe _____
                                   (negative thinking)
_____,

the reality is that _____
                                   (healthy view)

The evidence in my life supporting the healthy view includes: _____
                                                               (specific life examples)
_____.

Behavioral instruction

Therefore, even though I feel like _____
                                             (negative behavior)
_____,

I could instead _____
                             (alternative healthy behavior)
_____.

_____

THERAPIST: I'll dictate and you can just jot it down. You can revise it if it doesn't seem to fit.

THERAPIST: (*dictating*) "Right now I'm feeling nervous about approaching a woman because I'm worried she won't find me desirable." Is "desirable" the right word? Is there a better word?

DANIEL: "Attractive."

THERAPIST: "Attractive"? OK. And also, I'm trying to get at the deeper part of that, like "I won't be able to love her enough," or "I won't be able to show love to her."

DANIEL: "Able to be loving."

THERAPIST: "Able to be loving." That's good. "I also am worried that I can't trust her to be . . . "?

DANIEL: "Honest and trustworthy."

Dr. Young tries to use the patient's own words while constructing the flash card.

THERAPIST: OK. "However, I know that these are my Defectiveness and Mistrust/Abuse schemas being triggered. These are based on my feelings about my mother and have nothing to do with my value or this woman's trustworthiness. The reality is. . . ." Now we want to fill in some evidence that you have to the contrary, that you are lovable and desirable and attractive to women in different ways.

DANIEL: "The reality is I am a very affectionate person capable of being warm and loving."

THERAPIST: Maybe we'll put in parentheses a person you've shown that to.

DANIEL: "I can be an affectionate person with my son."

THERAPIST: And now, "Furthermore . . ." Now I want to say something about the woman you are with. That objectively, women are no less trustworthy than men.

DANIEL: "Women can be very reasonable and trustworthy, just as men can be."

THERAPIST: Good. Now, the end of the card would say something like, "Therefore, I must approach this woman, even though I feel nervous, because it's the only way to get my emotional needs met." How's that seem to you?

DANIEL: It seems very good.

The complete flash card reads as follows:

Right now I'm feeling nervous about approaching a woman because I'm worried that she won't find me attractive and that I won't be able to be loving. I also am worried that I can't trust her to be honest and trustworthy.

However, I know that these are my Defectiveness and Mistrust/Abuse schemas being triggered. These are based on my feelings about my mother and have nothing to do with my value or this woman's trustworthiness. The reality is that I am a very affectionate person capable of being warm and loving. (For example, I'm an affectionate person with my son.) Furthermore, women can be very reasonable and trustworthy, just as men can be.

Therefore, I must approach this woman, even though I feel nervous, because it's the only way to get my emotional needs met.

Daniel can take the flash card with him when he goes to social events and read it when he feels anxious. We expect that reading the flash card before going into the situation will help him shift into a more positive point of view, and reading the card during the event when he feels disheartened will help him interact with women in more positive ways. By repeatedly reading the flash card, Daniel can act to weaken his Defectiveness and Mistrust/Abuse schemas and strengthen his healthy side.

Some patients with BPD carry large numbers of flash cards, one for each of many schema triggers. In addition to helping these patients manage affect and behave in healthier ways, the flash cards serve as transitional objects. Patients with BPD often report that carrying flash cards feels as if they are carrying the therapist along with them. The presence of the flash card is comforting.

Schema Diary

The Schema Diary (Young, 1993) is a more advanced technique than the flash card. With the flash card, the therapist and patient construct a healthy response ahead of time for a specific schema trigger, and the patient reads the flash card as needed before and during the event. With the Schema Diary, patients construct their own healthy responses as their schemas are triggered in the course of their daily lives. The therapist therefore introduces the Schema Diary later in treatment, after the patient has become proficient at using flash cards.

The therapist instructs patients to carry copies of the Schema Diary form with them as they go about their lives. When a schema is triggered, patients fill out the form in order to work through the problem and arrive at a healthy solution. The Schema Diary asks the patient to identify trigger events, emotions, thoughts, behaviors, schemas, healthy views, realistic concerns, overreactions, and healthy behaviors.

We provide a case example. Emily is 26 years old. She recently began a job as the project director of a grant for an arts foundation. Her Subjugation schema has made it difficult for her to manage her staff effectively. She has had the greatest difficulty with a domineering and condescending subordinate named Jane. By the time Emily entered therapy, she was allowing her staff to make most of her administrative decisions. When Jane behaved in an angry way toward her, Emily apologized. "It's like she's my boss instead of my being her boss," Emily says.

With schema therapy, Emily identifies her Subjugation schema and explores the origins of her schema in childhood. She observes how her schema stops her from asserting herself, especially with Jane. Emily filled out a Schema Diary form at work (see Figure 3.2), moments after Jane requested a meeting with her later in the day.

FIGURE 3.2. Emily's Schema Diary.

Trigger: Jane said she wants to meet with me at three o'clock this afternoon.

Emotions: I feel scared and want to hide.

Thoughts: She'll tell me off and I won't know what to do. I can't stand up to her.

Actual Behaviors: I agreed to meet with her. I'm filling out this form so I can figure out what to do.

Schemas: I remember having to be available to my father and my first husband and how I had to be careful not to upset them. When they got angry, look out. Even now, I let my second husband tell me what to do, and he's nice. My Subjugation schema makes me want to give Jane whatever she wants so she won't get mad at me.

Healthy View: I don't know what Jane wants to meet about. Anyway, I don't have to give her whatever she wants. I deserve respect and can end the meeting if she turns abusive.

Realistic Concerns: Jane is very intimidating with people. She could yell at me. I'm not perfect at this job, but I'm getting better. I know she can find something I did wrong if she really wants to.

Overreactions: I jumped to two conclusions. The first one is that Jane wants to berate me and the second one is that there's nothing I can do about it. That makes me feel passive and helpless, like the best I can do is just survive the meeting. This attitude paralyzes me.

Healthy Behavior: I can meet with Jane and find out what she wants instead of stewing about this. If she's rude, I can end the meeting. On the other hand, I might not be attacked, so I won't prepare to attack back. The bottom line is I have time to prepare and I can find a solution that works for me.

SUMMARY

Cognitive strategies increase the patient's intellectual awareness that the schema is either not true or is greatly exaggerated. The therapist and patient begin by agreeing to view the schema as a hypothesis to be tested. They examine the evidence in the patient's past and present life that supports and refutes the schema. Next, the therapist and patient generate alternative explanations for the evidence supporting the schema. The therapist attributes evidence from childhood to disturbed family dynamics, and evidence since childhood to schema perpetuation. The therapist helps the patient learn to conduct dialogues between the "schema side" and the "healthy side."

Next, the therapist and patient list the advantages and disadvantages of the patient's current coping styles, and the patient commits to attempting more adaptive behaviors. The patient practices healthy behaviors, first by using flash cards and later by filling out the Schema Diary form. The steps in the cognitive work fit together sequentially and build on one another. The cognitive work prepares the patient for the experiential, behavioral, and interpersonal work that lies ahead.

The therapist and patient continue doing cognitive work throughout the treatment process. As therapy progresses, patients add to the list of evidence against their schemas. For example, as Emily made more independent decisions and behaved more proactively at work, she accumulated successes. At one point, a board member of her project wanted to talk to her about the budget. Rather than feeling helpless and procrastinating, Emily prepared for the meeting. She role-played the meeting in her therapy session. She studied all the relevant facts. At the meeting, Emily responded to all of the board member's questions and was able to suggest some new ideas. As Emily continued to progress, she amassed more evidence against her Subjugation schema. As she fought her schema and improved her coping responses, her life increasingly proved her schema wrong.

Chapter 4

EXPERIENTIAL STRATEGIES

Experiential techniques have two aims: (1) to trigger the emotions connected to Early Maladaptive Schemas and (2) to reparent the patient in order to heal these emotions and partially meet the patient's unmet childhood needs. For many of our patients, experiential techniques seem to produce the most profound change. Through experiential work, patients can make the transition from knowing intellectually that their schemas are false to believing it emotionally. Whereas the cognitive and behavioral techniques draw their power from the accumulation of small changes achieved through repetition, the experiential techniques are more dramatic. They draw their power from a few deeply convincing corrective emotional experiences. The experiential techniques capitalize on the human capacity to process information more effectively in the presence of affect.

This chapter describes the experiential techniques that we use most often in schema therapy. We present the experiential techniques for the Assessment Phase and then for the Change Phase.

IMAGERY AND DIALOGUES FOR ASSESSMENT

Our primary experiential assessment technique is imagery. This section describes how to introduce imagery work to patients and how to conduct an assessment imagery session, moving from a relaxing image to upsetting images of childhood to upsetting images from the patient's current life. We show how schema therapists utilize experiential strategies to identify schemas, understand the childhood origins of schemas, and relate schemas to the patient's presenting problems.

Introducing Imagery Work to Patients

It is best to plan to devote almost the whole therapy hour to the first imagery assessment session with a patient. We generally allot about 5 minutes to presenting the rationale and answering any questions; do imagery work for about 25 minutes; then take about 20 minutes more to process with the patient what happened during the imagery session. Later imagery assessment sessions may only require the first half of a session.

Presenting the Rationale

At this point in treatment, patients have completed a life review and have filled out and discussed the Young Schema Questionnaire and the Young Parenting Inventory. Patients are starting to build an intellectual understanding of their schemas. The therapist and patient have discussed hypotheses about the patient's core schemas and how they developed in childhood.

Imagery work is a powerful technique with which to continue this hypothesis testing because it triggers schemas in the office—often in a way that allows both the patient and the therapist to *feel* them. It is one thing for patients to see rationally that they might have certain schemas from their childhood and another thing for them to feel the schemas, to remember what it was like when they were children, and to connect this feeling to their current problems. Imagery work moves the understanding of the schema from the intellectual to the emotional realm. It turns the idea of the schema from a "cold" into a "hot" cognition. Discussing what happened during an imagery session helps to further educate patients about schemas and their own unmet needs as children.

The rationale for imagery assessment work is thus threefold:

1. To identify those schemas that are most central for the patient.
2. To enable patients to experience schemas on an affective level.
3. To help patients link emotionally the origins of their schemas in childhood and adolescence with problems in their current lives.

We generally present a brief rationale to patients for doing the imagery assessment work. Most patients do not require more. We explain that the purpose of doing imagery is to enable them to feel their schemas and to understand how their schemas began in childhood. Imagery thus deepens the intellectual understanding they derived from the cognitive work with emotional understanding.

Beginning Imagery

When doing imagery work with patients, one guiding principle is to give the least amount of instruction necessary for the patient to produce a workable image. We want the images that patients produce to be totally their own. The therapist avoids making suggestions and gives as few prompts as possible. The aim is to capture as accurately as possible the patient's experience, rather than inserting the therapist's own ideas or hypotheses. The goal is to elicit core images—those connected with such primary emotions as fear, rage, shame, and grief—that are linked to the patient's Early Maladaptive Schemas.

The therapist generally instructs the patient as follows: "Now close your eyes and let an image float to the top of your mind. Don't force the image; just let an image come into your mind and tell me what you see." The therapist asks the patient to describe the image out loud in the present tense and in the first person, as though it were happening right now. The therapist tells the patient to use pictures to make the image, not words or thoughts: "Imagery is not like thinking or free association, in which one thought leads to another; rather, imagery is like watching a movie inside your mind. But more than just watching the movie, I want you to experience it—to become part of the movie and live through all the events that unfold." With this goal in mind, the therapist helps the patient to elaborate on the image, to make it vivid, and to become absorbed in the image.

The therapist can help the patient by asking questions such as, "What are you seeing?"; "What are you hearing?"; "Can you see yourself in the image? What is the look on your face?" Once the image is distinct, the therapist explores the thoughts and emotions of all the "characters" in the image. Is the patient in the image? What is the patient thinking? What is the patient feeling? Where in the body does the patient feel these emotions? What does the patient have the impulse to do? Is anyone else in the image? What is that person thinking and feeling? What does that person want to do? The therapist tells the patient to speak out loud and have the characters tell one another what they are feeling. How do the characters feel about each other? What do they wish they could get from one another? Could they say it out loud?

The therapist ends the imagery session by asking patients to open their eyes and then asking such questions as, "What was the experience like for you?"; "What did the images mean to you?"; "What were the themes?"; "What schemas are related to those themes?"

In addition to helping patients feel their schemas more intensely, the therapist's goal is to experience the image with the patient in order to understand it on an emotional level. This kind of empathic experiencing of the patient's imagery is a powerful way to diagnose schemas.

Imagery of a Safe Place

Initially, we start and end imagery sessions with an image of a safe place. This is especially important for fragile patients and traumatized patients. Starting with a safe-place image is a simple, nonthreatening way to introduce imagery work. Starting this way also provides the patient with a chance to practice doing imagery before getting into more significant, emotionally laden material. At the end of an imagery session, returning to the safe place gives patients a refuge when the imagery material has left them upset.

In this example, the therapist and patient generate a safe-place image. Hector is 42 years old and entered therapy at the insistence of his wife, Ashley, who is threatening to divorce him. Her main complaints are that he is detached, cold, and prone to angry outbursts. As the excerpt begins, the therapist has already given Hector the rationale for doing imagery and is moving into constructing a safe-place image.

THERAPIST: Would you like to do an imagery exercise now?

HECTOR: OK.

THERAPIST: Please close your eyes and picture yourself in a safe place. Just let an image of a safe place come into your mind, and tell me what it is.

HECTOR: I see a photograph (*long pause*).

THERAPIST: What is it a photograph of?

HECTOR: It's a photograph of my brother and I looking out the window of our tree house. My uncle built it for us.

THERAPIST: Tell me what you see when you look at the photograph.

HECTOR: I see the two of us. . . . (*Opens eyes.*) This really is a photograph, I remember this photograph. (*Closes eyes.*) I see the two of us, and we're smiling.

THERAPIST: OK, keeping your eyes closed, can you see yourself?

The therapist helps the patient stay focused on the image. When he wanders, the therapist leads him back into the imagery.

HECTOR: Yeah.

THERAPIST: How old are you?

HECTOR: Oh, I'm about 7.

THERAPIST: What season is it?

HECTOR: It's fall. The leaves are changing, they're falling and blowing around.

THERAPIST: Good. Now, keeping your eyes closed, I'd like you to become the little boy in the photograph. I'd like you to look around you, from the boy's perspective, and tell me what you see.

HECTOR: OK. I'm next to my brother, looking out the window of my tree house.

THERAPIST: What else do you see?

HECTOR: I see my grandfather standing on the side of our house taking our picture. I see the street, and the trees, and my neighborhood. All the houses are the same, and they're close together, each with its little piece of lawn.

THERAPIST: What sounds do you hear?

HECTOR: (pause) I hear traffic, and people's voices. And birds chirping.

THERAPIST: Now I'd like you to turn and look around the inside of the tree house. What do you see?

HECTOR: Well, I see this little wooden room. It's built out of these uneven planks, and there are gaps where I can see out. It's in the middle of a big tree, and the branches go all the way down to the ground. It's a little dark inside. Outside it's daylight, but no one can see in. And if we're quiet, no one can tell that we're here.

THERAPIST: And what do you hear in there?

HECTOR: It's very, very quiet. I only hear the leaves rustling once in a while, and the wind whistling.

THERAPIST: And does it have a smell?

HECTOR: Yeah. It smells like pine. And like earth.

THERAPIST: And how do you feel in there?

HECTOR: Good. I feel good. I feel like it's a secret place, a special, secret place. It feels very peaceful here.

THERAPIST: How does your body feel?

HECTOR: Relaxed. My body feels relaxed.

The therapist helps Hector elaborate on the image and experience it as though it were happening in the present moment.

Certain stylistic concerns are important when doing safe-place imagery. Unlike other imagery, which has the goal of triggering negative emotions, the goal of safe-place imagery is to calm the patient. The therapist tries to soothe and relax the patient, avoiding negative elements. The therapist phrases ideas in positive terms: for example, instead of saying, "There is no danger," the therapist says, "You are safe"; instead of saying, "You are free of anxiety," the therapist says, "You feel calm." The therapist guides the patient away from psychologically charged themes, striving for images that are warm, uplifting, and comforting.

Some patients—usually those who have had traumatic experiences of being abused or neglected as children—are unable to generate safe-place images on their own. They may never have had a safe place. The therapist helps these patients construct safe-place images. Beautiful natural scenes such as beaches, mountains, meadows, or forests sometimes work well. However, even with our help, some patients cannot imagine anyplace where they feel safe. When this happens, the therapist can try using the office as the safe place: The therapist orients patients to the surroundings in the office at the beginning and end of imagery sessions. The therapist asks patients to look around and describe everything they see, hear, feel—until they report feeling calm. We sometimes have to postpone imagery until later in therapy, when the patient feels safe with the therapist and can view the office as a safe place.

Return to the Safe Place

The therapist ends the first imagery session by bringing patients back to the safe-place image and then asks them to open their eyes. In most cases, this is enough to calm and center the patient, and the therapist can move on to discussing the imagery.

In cases in which the patient is fragile or the imagery was traumatic, then more soothing is required on the part of the therapist. When patients seem intensely agitated following an imagery session, the therapist works to ground them in the present moment, where they are safe. The therapist asks them to open their eyes and to look around the office, describing what they see and hear, and talks with them about mundane matters—where they are going and what they will be doing right after the session. The therapist allows time for the affect stirred up by the images to subside. These measures help patients make the transition from upsetting imagery material back to ordinary life.

It is important to leave enough time for patients to calm down and to fully discuss imagery sessions. If it can be avoided, the therapist does not allow patients to leave the session extremely depressed, frightened, or angry as a result of imagery, because these feelings can occasionally spill over into their lives outside the session in undesirable ways. If necessary, the therapist suggests that patients sit in the waiting room until they feel ready to leave. The therapist can talk briefly with the patient between sessions. The therapist can also follow up with a phone call at night to check up on the patient's progress.

Imagery from Childhood

Overview

Now that we have provided a rationale and presented safe-place imagery to patients so that they feel comfortable, we move into childhood imagery. Our purpose is to observe the patient's affect and the themes that emerge, in order to identify schemas and understand their origins.

We generally elicit the following images from patients in the order presented (we typically work on only one image in a given session).

1. Any upsetting childhood image.
2. One upsetting image with each parent (i.e., an image with the mother and an image with the father).
3. Upsetting images of any other significant others, including peers, who may have contributed to the formation of a schema.

The therapist starts with an unstructured image, simply instructing the patient to picture an upsetting image from childhood. This gives patients the opportunity to communicate whatever they feel was most difficult about their childhoods. Moving into structured images ensures that the therapist covers all significant others who contributed to the patient's schemas.

Case Illustration

The following excerpt is taken from an imagery session Dr. Young conducted with Marika, a patient introduced in the previous chapter, who sought therapy for help with marital problems. She states that there is a lack of intimacy in the marriage and that her husband, James, is aloof, critical, and emotionally abusive.

On her questionnaires, Marika wrote that her father was "aloof" and "sarcastic" and that, with him, "crumbs would have to do." She had already practiced a safe-place image with her therapist. In this excerpt, the therapist asks Marika to picture an upsetting image of her father when she was a child.

THERAPIST: Would you like to do an exercise now?

MARIKA: Yes.

THERAPIST: Good, maybe you could close your eyes for a while.

MARIKA: OK.

THERAPIST: What I'm going to ask you to do is just keep your eyes closed, and I want you to get an image of yourself with your father when you were a child. And don't try to force it, let it come on its own.

MARIKA: OK.

THERAPIST: What are you seeing?

MARIKA: (*Suddenly starts to cry.*) It's just me, and he's sitting down, and he's reading his paper, and he has on a white shirt, and he has lots of pens in his shirt pocket. And I go up and I just tap on the paper, like, "tap, tap," and he looks at me like, you know, like, "you're bothering me." But I know he's going to let me crawl up on his lap. (*Cries quietly.*)

THERAPIST: So it's like he doesn't really want you to be there.

MARIKA: But I know he'll let me get up on his lap, you know, and then, and then I sit on his lap and he might read to me, but he always reads the stories that he wants to read, not the ones I want.

And then I start taking his pens out of his pen holder, and stuff like that, and he always makes me put them back, 'cause he wants them back. And then, if I go too far, he takes my fingers and he bends them back. And it hurts, and then I have to say "uncle," and then I go away. Or sit there and try to make nice again, so he . . . (*long pause*).

THERAPIST: So he'll like you again?

MARIKA: So he'll like me again.

THERAPIST: So it seems like you have to do everything he wants to do and it's always on his terms?

MARIKA: Yeah.

THERAPIST: And you have to take the crumbs, whatever he'll give you, even though it's not what you really want.

MARIKA: Yeah.

THERAPIST: Can you, in this image now, tell your father what you would have liked him to be like?

MARIKA: All right.

THERAPIST: And what he doesn't give you that you need. Tell him what you need, all right?

MARIKA: Well, I wouldn't have minded if we went outside and walked down the street and just got out of the house. And I wouldn't have minded if you'd laughed a little more. And, I wouldn't have minded if you could have taken my brother and me and gone somewhere and played with us. But you never wanted to play with us.

The first thing one notices about this imagery session with Marika is how quickly her affect shifts. As soon as she closes her eyes and pictures her father, she begins to cry. This rapid shifting of the patient's affect is common when doing imagery work.

The predominant emotion Marika expresses in the session is grief:

Her crying expresses grief for the emotional needs not met by her father. The core theme is Emotional Deprivation—her father is reluctant to pay attention to her and to give her physical affection, and he lacks empathy for her feelings. He seems uninterested in her. This is the essence of Emotional Deprivation: The parent is emotionally disconnected from the child. The child keeps trying to get the parent to connect, but the parent rarely does.

Two other related schemas are Subjugation and Mistrust/Abuse. Everything is on the father's terms: He deigns to let Marika climb up on his lap; they read the stories he wants to read. When she is with him, she must do what he wants to do. He is in control; she has no power to get the attention and affection she wants from him. She has to "make nice" to be accepted, even after her father bends her fingers back—she has to accept mistreatment if she wants attention from her father.

A more subtle but still important theme is Defectiveness. Most neglected children have the feeling that the reason their parent is not paying attention to them is that they are somehow unworthy. Marika's father's indifference to her is rejecting, and the theme of rejection is part of the Defectiveness schema. Marika wants to be worthy of his love, and, when faced with her father's inability to give her love, she feels that she must be the one who is to blame. She feels unlovable. (This theme emerges more clearly as the session progresses.)

Imagery Linking the Past to the Present

After exploring a significant childhood image—one that elicits negative affect related to an Early Maladaptive Schema—the therapist asks the patient to switch to an image of a current or adult situation that feels the same. In this way, the therapist forges a direct link between the childhood memory and the patient's adult life.

The following example is a continuation of the imagery session with Marika. Dr. Young asks Marika to picture an image of herself with her husband, James, that feels the same as the image with her father. The therapist then asks Marika to talk to James in the image, to tell James what she wants from him.

THERAPIST: Can you tell James what you want from him now in this image? Just say it out loud.

MARIKA: (to James) James, I want you to stop yelling at me. And I want you to ask me every single day how my day was. And to listen to me when I tell you all my silly stories. And to not look at me when I talk like you wish I would either hurry up or shut up.

And I wish we would go out and have a little bit more fun together. Like just to laugh or, even if you don't want to laugh, you could just laugh at the silly things I do or something, just so I know that you're enjoying being with me, just a little. (*Cries.*)

THERAPIST: You just want to feel that he enjoys you a little bit.

MARIKA: I know there's got to be a reason that we're married.

THERAPIST: What does he say to you when you say that? Be him now. Have him answer you.

MARIKA: Well, he just starts to tell me all the reasons why: We do a lot, and he has a very important job. And you know it takes a lot of hours. And he's very tired and, you know, "I can only do so much." And, you know, almost like, "How dare you have any demands," because he's doing the best he can.

THERAPIST: Sort of like your father, feeling that because he works hard and gives you material things, you should be happy?

MARIKA: Uh-huh.

THERAPIST: The same thing. If they're working and giving you money, you should be satisfied?

MARIKA: Yes.

Almost everything Marika says to James in this image, she might have said to her father. The themes are the same. There is the Emotional Deprivation: Marika wants James to pay attention to her, listen to her, have fun with her. There is the Subjugation: James sets the terms of the relationship. Because he works so hard, he gets to determine when he shows affection. Marika has no right to make any demands. And there is the Defectiveness: Marika wants James to find her appealing and enjoy being with her, instead of behaving in a rejecting way.

Conceptualizing Imagery in Schema Terms

The therapist helps the patient conceptualize what happened in the imagery session in schema terms. This provides an intellectual context for what happened during the session and helps the patient develop greater insight into the meaning of the imagery. In the following excerpt, the therapist and Marika discuss the implications of the imagery session for the understanding of her schemas. Conceptualizing the imagery session in schema terms helps the patient integrate what happened during the imagery session with the assessment material that preceded it.

The therapist focuses on the core schemas of Emotional Deprivation, Defectiveness, and Subjugation. He begins by describing Marika's Emotional Deprivation schema. As often happens with this schema, Marika is only dimly aware of her emotional deprivation.

THERAPIST: It's interesting that on your questionnaire that you filled out, the Schema Questionnaire, the ones that scored highest were, I think, Unrelenting Standards—let's see, I wrote them down here . . . Self-Sacrifice. . . .

MARIKA: Yeah, all the ones I don't think apply to me. (*Laughs.*)

THERAPIST: Yeah, I have a feeling that the ones that are more painful for you aren't the ones you scored highest on. But maybe sometimes you're not aware of some of the deeper things going on with you.

MARIKA: Yes.

THERAPIST: Let me tell you some of the ones that occur to me that might be your schemas, judging from what you've said here today so far. One of them I call Emotional Deprivation, which is the feeling that you're not going to get your normal needs met for emotional support—that there are not going to be people who love you, who are strong, who understand you and listen to you and take your needs into account, that there's no one to nurture you and really try to take care of you and pay attention to you. Does that feel right, that that might be one of the issues?

MARIKA: Well, certainly you have to qualify it for men, because with my women friends. . . .

THERAPIST: Yes, right. Your mother was different. Your mother was very loving. But at least as it relates to men, emotional deprivation seems like it's a very big issue. Your father wasn't very emotionally nurturing or giving.

MARIKA: Right.

THERAPIST: And neither is James, right?

MARIKA: Yeah.

THERAPIST: And yet that's what you want. That's what you ask them both for. You ask them to just give you some attention, give you some emotional caring.

The therapist points out the core theme in Marika's relationships with her father and husband. Both men reinforce her sense of emotional deprivation. The therapist continues by describing Marika's Defectiveness schema.

THERAPIST: Let's go to another one that I thought might be an issue. There's one called Defectiveness, which is the sense that you're inwardly defective in some way, or unlovable. And it seems to me that a lot of what you've described with your father would have to lead to that feeling. He would have made you feel that there's something wrong with you that makes it so that you can never get his attention, something about you that makes it so that he doesn't want to be with you, that makes him give you that disdainful look. That must create inside of you, I would think, a deeper feeling of being somehow inadequate or not up to what he needs, to his expectations. Does that feel right?

MARIKA: (*Cries.*) Yeah. Well, and it's also a woman's issue, 'cause there hasn't been one day in my life that I haven't criticized what I look like. My hair is too straight, I'm overweight, I'm not pretty enough, you know, on and on and on, since the time I can remember, because that's what my mother did.

THERAPIST: And, implicitly, that's what your father was doing, too, by not giving you attention, ignoring you, he was leading you to feel that you were not good enough—that there were flaws in you that made it so he didn't want to pay attention to you. So, between your mother being critical and your father ignoring you, you would have had the feeling that you deserve to be criticized, do you know what I mean?

MARIKA: (*Sighs deeply.*) Yeah.

The therapist points out that Marika acts to reinforce her Defectiveness schema.

THERAPIST: And I wonder if that's the feeling, the Defectiveness feeling, that you have. You keep doing it to yourself, you keep finding fault, you keep finding more evidence, your weight or your appearance, that you can use to put yourself down, to keep you feeling defective. Do you know what I'm saying?

MARIKA: Yeah. It's automatic. If I weighed 120 pounds, there's something still wrong.

THERAPIST: And that's the schema talking.

MARIKA: Yeah, I realized that, finally, when I did lose a lot of weight, my problems weren't over.

THERAPIST: The Defectiveness feeling was still there, even when the weight was low. And then, of course, again you've chosen a husband who reinforces it, who's criticizing you.

MARIKA: Yes.

THERAPIST: Who contributes to your sense of feeling defective. And then you try to fight back by defending yourself, but deep down some part of you believes him, and that's the schema.

As the therapist describes the themes that emerged during the imagery session, he relates these themes to examples from Marika's current life. In doing so, he helps Marika see the workings of her schema in her day-to-day life.

Imagery of Other Significant Figures from the Patient's Childhood

Like Marika, most patients have schemas that are connected to childhood experiences with parents, and images of parents are almost always the most significant. However, we also explore other relevant childhood images: We explore whatever images we hypothesize as most central to the development of the patient's schemas. Most often these involve parents, but sometimes they involve siblings, extended family members, peers, teachers, or even strangers. If we believe from obtaining the life history that some other individual from the patient's childhood or adolescence played a significant role in the development of a schema, then we include imagery of the patient with that person as well. For example, if we know a patient was abused by his brother as a child, we also say, "Close your eyes now and picture an image of yourself as a child with your brother"; or, if we know a patient was teased by her peers at school, we say, "Close your eyes and picture an image of yourself as a child in the school yard."

Summary of Imagery for Assessment

Doing imagery work for assessment helps both the therapist and the patient to identify and feel core schemas, to understand their origins in childhood, and to link these origins to the patient's current problems. Further, imagery work enriches both the therapist's and the patient's understanding of the patient's schemas, helping them move from recognizing the patient's schemas intellectually to experiencing them emotionally.

EXPERIENTIAL STRATEGIES FOR CHANGE

Several sessions pass between the use of experiential techniques for assessment and the use of experiential techniques for change. After conducting the imagery assessment, we move to conceptualizing the patient's schemas and then to the cognitive techniques for battling schemas described in the preceding chapter, such as examining the evidence for and against schemas and using flash cards. It is at that point that we introduce experiential techniques for change.

This section on experiential change techniques presents the following: (1) the rationale for including such techniques in treatment; (2) how to conduct imagery dialogues; (3) "reparenting" imagery work; (4) imagery of traumatic memories; (5) writing letters as homework assignments; and (6) imagery for pattern-breaking.

Rationale

The rationale for experiential work is to fight schemas affectively. At this point in treatment, the therapist and patient have already examined the evidence for and against the schema and built a rational case against it. After completing this cognitive stage, the patient often says something like, "I understand on a rational level that my schema isn't true, but I still feel the same way. I still *feel* like my schema is true." It is primarily the experiential work (in combination with limited reparenting) that helps the patient fight the schema on this emotional level.

Imagery Dialogues

Imagery dialogues are one of our primary experiential change techniques. We instruct patients to conduct dialogues in imagery, both with the people who caused their schemas in childhood and with the people who reinforce their schemas in their current lives. The imagery dialogues we describe in this section are a simplified form of mode work, which we elaborate on in a later chapter. We utilize three modes in this simplified version: the Vulnerable Child, the Healthy Adult, and the Dysfunctional Parent.

As we have noted, most often the significant childhood figures are parents, and parents are the first characters we use for imagery dialogues. We ask patients to close their eyes and to picture themselves with a parent in an upsetting situation. Often these images are the same as or similar to memories that arose in the imagery for assessment. We then focus on helping patients to express strong affect toward the parent, particularly anger. We help patients identify the needs that were not met by their parent, and we help them get angry with the parent in the image for not meeting these needs.

Why do we want the patient, the child in the image, to get angry at the parent whose behavior caused the schema? The rationale is not simply getting the patient to vent, although venting anger is in itself cathartic and of some value. Our main goals are to empower the patient to fight back against the schema and to distance the patient from the schema. It is empowering for patients to express anger and stand up for their rights with the offending parent. Anger provides emotional strength to fight the schema. The schema represents a world gone wrong, and anger sets the world right again. When patients say, "I won't let you abuse me anymore," "I won't let you criticize me," "I won't let you control me," "I needed love and you didn't give it to me," "I had a right to feel angry," or "I had a right to a separate identity," they feel revived and worthwhile. They validate their own rights as human beings. They assert that they deserved better than what happened to them as children.

What we are trying to convey to the patient is a feeling of entitlement to basic human rights. The therapist educates patients about what we believe to be the universal needs and basic rights of children. For example, we teach the patient with a Defectiveness schema that all children are entitled to be treated with respect. We teach the patient with Emotional Deprivation that all children are entitled to affection, understanding, and protection. We teach the patient with a Subjugation schema that all children are entitled to express their feelings and needs (within reasonable limits). We tell them that, as children, they were entitled to these things, too. Our hope is that, when patients leave the session and go out into the world, they will take with them some of this healthy entitlement that they did not learn as children.

Expressing anger at the parent in sessions is of foremost importance in this stage of the experiential work. Sometimes patients try to talk the therapist out of doing this work. They say they have resolved their anger already in prior therapy. They say, "I'm already past this. I've dealt with my anger. I understand my parents. I forgive them." However, we have found that when we take such claims at face value, we usually are mistaken. Later we realize that the patient has never really experienced genuine anger toward the parent. If patients have not done this part of the experiential work—if they have not gotten angry at the parent in a meaningful way, either in therapy or in their actual lives—then they have not gone through this stage. (We generally discourage patients from expressing anger directly at their parents "in real life" unless we have carefully weighed the pros and cons with the patient.) Later in treatment the therapist and patient will speak about whether or not the patient can forgive the parent. Later the therapist will help the patient see the good aspects of the parent and accept the parent's limitations. However, in order to move from being wronged to forgiveness and to make headway against the schema, most patients must first go through anger. For most patients, expressing the anger in therapy is crucial. Without it, patients still believe emotionally that the schema is true, even though they might know intellectually that it is not.

Sometimes patients say that they feel too guilty to do this exercise. They believe that it is wrong to get angry at their parents. They believe that somehow their anger will hurt the parents, that they are betraying their parents by doing the exercise, or that their parents do not deserve the anger because "they did the best they could." When this happens, we tell patients that it is only an exercise. Furthermore, we are not condemning the parents as bad people by getting angry at them in imagery; we are getting angry at particular errors in their parenting.

It is also important that patients express grief about what happened to them in childhood. Grief is almost always mixed in with the anger. Going through the process of grieving helps patients differentiate the past, when the schema was true, from the present, when it no longer has to be true. Grieving helps patients let go of unrealistic expectations that the parent will change and helps them acknowledge the parent's good qualities. It also helps them accept the fact that their childhood was painful and that they cannot undo that, but that it is possible to focus on the future and make it as gratifying as possible.

Patients often realize that, despite everything, they still love the parent. They become able to negotiate a workable relationship with the parent. When all reasonable efforts to do so have failed, however, grieving helps patients let go of the parent, leaving them more open to forming other, healthier attachments. Finally, grieving helps patients build compassion for their childhood selves, replacing their more typical attitudes of scorn or indifference toward themselves. Grieving helps patients forgive themselves.

The second purpose we mentioned for venting anger at the parent was to help the patient gain emotional distance from the schema. One reason it is so hard for patients to fight their schemas is that their schemas feel ego-syntonic. Patients have internalized the messages their parents gave them, and now they say to themselves what the parent used to say (or imply through their behavior): "Your feelings don't matter," "You deserve to be abused," "You are unlovable," "You will always be alone," "No one will ever meet your needs," "You must always do what the other person wants." The parent's voice has become the patient's own voice, and it feels right. When patients vent anger at a parent in imagery, they help reverse this process. They externalize the schema as the "parent's voice." In this way, the patients achieve a sense of distance from what feels like their own voice. Now it is the parent who criticizes, controls, deprives, or hates them—and not a core part of themselves. The schema becomes ego-dystonic. The therapist allies with the patient to fight the schema, represented by the parent.

Case Illustration

The following excerpts are from an interview Dr. Young conducted with Daniel, a patient we introduced in Chapter 3. Daniel had been in traditional cognitive therapy with another therapist for about 9 months for social anxiety and anger-management problems. He is 36 years old and is the single father of a young son. Five years ago he divorced his wife after discovering she had been secretly having affairs with other men. Except for his child, he has been alone since then. Daniel's long-term therapy goal is to establish a successful intimate relationship with a woman.

Daniel's childhood was traumatic. His father was an alcoholic who drank at neighborhood bars every night. Daniel can remember even as a small child walking through town alone at night to find his father and bring him home. While his father was out drinking, Daniel's mother stayed at home entertaining her boyfriends, drinking and having sex with them while Daniel was there. When there was no boyfriend available, Daniel's mother displayed her naked body to him in a sexually provocative way, under the guise of educating him about sex. In addition, Daniel's mother was physically and verbally abusive to him.

As one might expect from his history, Daniel's core schema—particularly in regard to intimate relationships with women—is Mistrust/Abuse. Daniel's mother sexually, physically, and verbally abused him, and both parents used him for their own purposes. As Daniel said himself, "People will use and abuse me." This is his basic belief. A number of other schemas cluster around this core. Like most abuse victims, Daniel feels defective. His mother's abuse and his father's neglect left him feeling inadequate, ashamed, worthless, and unlovable. In addition to Defectiveness, Daniel also has strong Subjugation and Emotional Inhibition schemas.

In this excerpt, Dr. Young instructs Daniel to carry on imagery dialogues with his mother and then his ex-wife. Dr. Young's purpose is to help Daniel express anger toward the people in his past who have hurt him and to assert his rights. As the excerpt begins, Daniel is describing an image of an upsetting childhood situation with his mother.

DANIEL: I'm upstairs in the house, and my mother is making herself up and dying her hair. She usually spent tons of time doing that kind of stuff. She's naked, and she has the door wide open to the bathroom, and when she sees me, she stands up and makes the remark that she can prove she's a blonde, by the color of her genital hair.

THERAPIST: What are you feeling as she's saying these things?

DANIEL: Disgust and contempt. I'm not feeling sexual at all. . . .

THERAPIST: And what does she do next?

DANIEL: She's pointing out her parts, like her breasts, and kind of bragging about things.

THERAPIST: Can you be her, her voice, and have her say that?

DANIEL: (*as his mother*) "It's all right for you to look at me, it might be good, you might learn a little bit. You need to learn a little bit about sex. And this is what it looks like."

THERAPIST: How are you feeling as she says that?

DANIEL: Kind of perplexed and disgusted. I feel like she's violated my boundaries. I feel like I don't even have a mother that I can talk to properly. I've got this crazy nut in my house.

Having determined what the mother did that was hurtful and how Daniel felt about it, the therapist moves on to exploring the patient's unmet needs. He asks Daniel what he wished he could have gotten from his mother.

THERAPIST: Can you tell her what you need from her right now? Tell her what you really need her to be like as a mother, even though you wouldn't, of course, have told her as a child. But try to imagine, in this image, that as a child you say to her what you need from her.

DANIEL: (*as a child, to his mother*) "It's wrong of you to use me in this way. It's bad enough I have to deal with Dad's problems. I have a lot of problems just like you have a lot of problems. And I really need you to, kind of, be there for me, to help me deal with my problems once in a while. Not for you to do this. I need you to be a parent, an understanding and caring parent that I feel I can turn to. And instead, you're a little girl yourself, not even a grown-up. I feel I can't even have a happy childhood."

THERAPIST: What does she say back?

DANIEL: (*as his mother*) "We all have problems, and I have more problems than you've got. You should feel lucky you have a house to live in." (*Pause.*)

Up until this point, the patient's affect has been somewhat flat. The therapist helps him vent with greater emotional intensity by exaggerating the mother's behavior. (As we demonstrate in later chapters, to do this the therapist uses mode work. He introduces the "Angry Child" mode as a character in the imagery.)

THERAPIST: I want you to keep this image, and now I want you to bring into the picture a different Daniel, the Angry Daniel, the Daniel that's infuriated with her for treating you this way. Can you get an image of Angry Daniel—that's maybe out of control and enraged at her?

DANIEL: Yes.

THERAPIST: What do you see?

DANIEL: I see myself yelling at her.

THERAPIST: Can I hear it?

DANIEL: (*Speaks loudly.*) You're nothing but a goddamn slut and a bitch! I hate you! I wish I had somebody else for a mother. I have a father that I can't even deal with, and you, I can't even deal with either.

THERAPIST: Let me be her, and I want you to keep getting angry. (*as the mother*) "Look, we've all got problems. My problems are worse than yours. You're lucky you've got a house to live in."

DANIEL: You're full of baloney! I'm the child in this house. It's your responsibility to protect me and see to it that I have what I need.

THERAPIST: (*as the mother*) "I have to think about me, your father doesn't."

DANIEL: That's all you do is think about you. You're always putting your goddamn make-up on, your smelly hair dye, and thinking about men. And I get left home alone. And I've got to see all this shit. And I'm sick and tired of it! I'm sick and tired of him and you, and, if I had a choice, I wouldn't be here.

THERAPIST: (*as the mother*) "I don't like it when you yell like that. I'm going to pull your hair and drag you around. . . . "

DANIEL: You'd better not pull my hair anymore because I'm tired of it! Go punch somebody your own size.

THERAPIST: (*as the mother*) "I try to do nice things for you, like showing you my body. Doesn't that make you feel good, if I teach you about sex?"

DANIEL: Yeah, nice things. What's the matter, the men are not enough for you? The men have to sneak in and out, it's not enough for you to have that, and now you have to have me, too? Well, I'm sick of it, I'm sick of your disgusting body. You can keep it to yourself because I don't want to see it!

The therapist, playing the part of Daniel's mother in the imagery dialogue, is deliberately being provocative and inflammatory. We often adopt this tactic when playing the part of the parent in role-plays with emotionally inhibited patients. In order to increase the patient's level of affect, we say whatever will most enrage the patient, so long as what we say is "in character," based on what we have already learned about the parent. Note that the therapist, playing the part of the patient's mother, virtually quotes verbatim what the patient himself said when he played the part of his mother earlier in the dialogue and uses information that the patient has already provided, such as the fact that his mother pulled his hair to punish him when he was a child.

The therapist moves on to Daniel's first wife, who cheated on him, and continues to help him vent anger at the people who have hurt and betrayed him in the past.

THERAPIST: Now I want you to bring your ex-wife into the image, after you found out that she'd had affairs, OK? I want you to now tell her how you feel.

DANIEL: (*Speaks sadly.*) I'm extremely hurt that you cheated on me. We were supposed to be married, husband and wife. I'm not the best husband in the world, I'm not perfect, but this is really, this is the pits. It makes me feel like garbage. Is this the only thing that's important to you? To ruin our marriage?

THERAPIST: What does she say in the image? Be her, and say what she says.

DANIEL: (*as his ex-wife*) "Well, it's no big deal. Everyone's doing it today. You don't have any control over me. I can do whatever I want, I can go where I want! Who the hell are you to tell me what to do?"

THERAPIST: Answer her back.

DANIEL: I'm your husband. And I married you, for better or for worse, for the purpose of being together. And I'm really disappointed in you, that you were unfaithful. And I don't think I'm gonna put up with it. I'm *not* gonna put up with it.

THERAPIST: How are you feeling now as you're saying this to her?

DANIEL: Well, I feel like I'm appropriately asserting my anger. It's a little bit of a relief to do this.

In encouraging Daniel to vent anger at his mother and ex-wife, the therapist helps him feel both more empowered in regard to his abusers and more distant from his childhood sense of helplessness.

Imagery Work for Reparenting

Imagery work for reparenting is especially helpful for patients with most of the schemas in the Disconnection and Rejection domain (Abandonment, Mistrust/Abuse, Emotional Deprivation, and Defectiveness). When these patients were children, their ability to relate to others and feel safe, loved, nurtured, or worthy was largely destroyed. Through reparenting in imagery work, the therapist helps patients go back into that child mode and to learn to get from the therapist, and later from themselves, some of what they missed. This approach is a form of "limited reparenting."

As with the imagery dialogues we have described thus far, the reparenting work in imagery that we describe here is a simplified form of mode work. We use the same three modes of the Vulnerable Child, Maladaptive Parent, and Healthy Adult, but now we bring the Healthy Adult into the image to defend the child against the Dysfunctional Parent and to nurture the Vulnerable Child.

The three steps in this process are as follows: (1) The therapist asks permission to enter the image and speak directly to the Vulnerable Child; (2) the therapist reparents the Vulnerable Child; and (3) later, the patient's Healthy Adult, modeled after the therapist, reparents the Vulnerable Child.

*Step 1: The Therapist Asks Permission to Enter the Image
and Speak Directly to the Vulnerable Child*

First, the therapist must access the patient's Vulnerable Child mode. To do this, the therapist asks patients to close their eyes and picture an image of their little child mode, either now or in some past situation. The therapist then carries on a dialogue with the patient's Vulnerable Child, using the patient as an intermediary. Rather than speaking directly to the child, the therapist asks the patient to relay messages.

Here is an example with Hector, the patient we described earlier who entered therapy at the insistence of his wife, who was threatening to leave him. Hector generally presented in a detached manner and had some trouble adjusting to imagery work. Even after several imagery practice sessions, he found it difficult to stay focused on negative childhood images.

Hector's mother is schizophrenic, and she was in and out of mental hospitals throughout his childhood. He and his younger brother spent time in foster homes. This image expresses his Abandonment and Mistrust/Abuse schemas.

THERAPIST: Can you get an image of yourself as a child in one of those foster homes?

HECTOR: Yes.

THERAPIST: What do you see?

HECTOR: I see me and my brother in a strange bedroom, sitting on the bed.

THERAPIST: What do you see when you look at Little Hector in the image?

HECTOR: He looks scared.

The therapist asks the patient for permission to speak directly to "Little Hector," the patient's Vulnerable Child.

THERAPIST: Can I talk to Little Hector in the image?

HECTOR: No. He's too scared of you to talk. He doesn't trust you yet.

THERAPIST: What is he doing?

HECTOR: He's crawling under the covers of the bed. He's too scared to talk to you.

The patient is protecting the Vulnerable Child from being hurt. This is understandable for patients with core schemas in the Disconnection and Rejection realm. They are detached from the affect connected to their schemas, and they have difficulty opening up to the pain involved in doing this work. Patients who were abused as children are literally afraid of the therapist.

At this point, the therapist begins a dialogue with the part of the patient that is being avoidant (the "Detached Protector" mode). The therapist tries to persuade the patient that it is safe to let the therapist talk to the Vulnerable Child.

THERAPIST: Why doesn't Little Hector trust me? What's he afraid I'm going to do?

HECTOR: He thinks you're going to hurt him.

THERAPIST: How does he think I'd hurt him?

HECTOR: He thinks you're going to be mean to him and make fun of him.

THERAPIST: Do you agree with him? Do you think that's how I would really treat him? That I would be mean to him and make fun of him?

HECTOR: (*pause*) No.

THERAPIST: Well, then, could you tell that to him? Could you tell him that I'm a good person who's been good to you and that I won't hurt him?

The therapist continues in this way until the patient grants the therapist permission to talk directly to the Vulnerable Child. With a severely damaged patient, it may take the therapist many sessions to get to this point.

Step 2: The Therapist Reparents the Vulnerable Child

Once the therapist has permission to speak directly to the patient's Vulnerable Child, the therapist enters the image and reparents the child.

THERAPIST: Can you see me now in the image? Can you see me kneeling next to the bed so I can talk to Little Hector?

HECTOR: Yes.

THERAPIST: Can you talk to me in the image as Little Hector and tell me what you're feeling?

HECTOR: I'm feeling scared. I don't like it here. I want my mother. I want to go home.

THERAPIST: What do you want from me?

HECTOR: I want you to stay with me. Maybe to hold me.

THERAPIST: How about if I sit next to you in the image and put my arm around you? How would that be?

HECTOR: Good. That's good.

THERAPIST: (*in the image*) I'll stay here with you. I'll take care of you. I won't leave you.

The therapist says to the child, "What do you want from me? What can I do to help you?" Sometimes patients say, "I just want you to play with me. Would you play a game with me?" Or they say, "I want you to hold me," or "Tell me I'm a good child." Whatever the patient wants (if it is appropriate behavior for a parent with a child, of course), we try to provide in the image. For patients who want us to play a game with them, we ask, "What game do you want to play?" For patients who want to be held, we say, "Why don't I put my arm around you in the image?" As the Healthy Adult in the image, the therapist provides the antidote to the patient's core schemas.

Step 3: The Patient's Healthy Adult, Modeled after the Therapist, Reparents the Vulnerable Child

After we reparent the Vulnerable Child, we ask patients to access a nurturing part of themselves, modeled after the therapist, that can do the same. Often we wait until a later session to do this, when the patient's healthy side is stronger.

THERAPIST: I want you to bring yourself into the image as an adult. Imagine that you are there in the image as an adult, and you see Little Hector, and you see the room, and your little brother there with you. Can you see it?

HECTOR: Uh-huh.

THERAPIST: Could you talk to Little Hector? Could you try to help him feel better?

HECTOR: (*to Little Hector*) I can see this is really hard for you. You're really scared. Do you want to talk about it? Why don't you just come over here with me, and we'll be together for awhile.

THERAPIST: And how does Little Hector feel when he hears that?

HECTOR: He feels better, like someone's there for him.

The goal is for the patient's Healthy Adult to meet the emotional needs of the Vulnerable Child in the imagery. Doing this exercise helps patients build up a part of themselves that can satisfy their unmet emotional needs and thus fight their schemas.

The reparenting imagery work also serves an important purpose for the therapy sessions that come later. Once the therapist has spoken directly to the patient's Vulnerable Child, the therapist can appeal to this mode in later sessions whenever the patient is cut off in an avoidant or compensatory mode. The therapist can reach the vulnerable part of the patient hiding behind the avoidance or compensation. Following is an example with Hector, who often came to therapy sessions in a detached mode.

THERAPIST: You seem distant and a little sad today.

HECTOR: Yeah.

THERAPIST: What's going on? Do you know why?

HECTOR: No. I don't know why.

THERAPIST: Can we do an exercise to find out? Could you close your eyes and picture Little Hector? Could you picture him here right now and tell me what you see?

HECTOR: I see him curled up into a ball. He's scared.

THERAPIST: What's he scared about?

HECTOR: He's scared Ashley's gonna leave him.

Often when patients say they do not know what they are feeling, they are out of touch with their Vulnerable Child. When the therapist asks them to close their eyes and picture their Vulnerable Child, they suddenly can recognize what it is they are feeling. The therapist then has something to work on in the session that was inaccessible a moment before.

Once the therapist has established a link with the patient's Vulnerable Child, the therapist has a strategy for the remainder of therapy for tapping in to what the patient is feeling at the core, even when the adult side of the patient does not seem to know. Whenever the patient says, "I don't know what I'm feeling right now," or "I feel scared and I don't know why," or "I feel angry and I don't know why," the therapist can say, "Close your eyes and picture your little child." Accessing the Vulnerable Child mode almost always provides us with information about what the patient is feeling and why.

Traumatic Memories

This section presents a discussion of imagery dialogues for patients dealing with traumatic memories, usually of abuse or abandonment. Imagery of traumatic memories differs from other imagery in the following ways: It is more difficult for patients to endure; the affect it generates is more extreme; the psychological damage is more severe; and the memories are more often blocked

We have two goals when conducting imagery of traumatic memories. The first goal is getting the patient to release blocked affect—the "strangulated grief" associated with the experience of trauma. The therapist helps the patient relive the trauma, feeling and expressing all of the associated emotions. Our second goal is to provide protection and comfort to the patient in the image by bringing in the Healthy Adult. As with the other imagery dialogues we have described, the dialogues we describe in this section are a form of mode work, using the three main characters of the

Vulnerable Child, the Abusive or Abandoning Parent, and the Healthy Adult.

When doing nontraumatic imagery work, typically we persuade avoidant patients to persist. We push them to work past the point at which they feel comfortable. We encourage them to vent fully the emotions connected to the image. However, when dealing with memories of abuse or other trauma—especially blocked memories—we do not push the patient. Rather, we go slowly, letting patients set their own pace. The goal of helping the patient to feel safe takes precedence over all other considerations. More often than not, imagery work with traumatic memories is terrifying for patients. The therapist tries to maximize the patient's sense of control over the work. If blocked memories of abuse are coming to the surface, then the therapist takes the admonition to go slowly even more seriously and deals with the patient's memories in small increments. The therapist gives the patient plenty of time to absorb new information and to work through all the implications before moving on.

There are many steps the therapist can take to help the patient maintain a sense of control during and after traumatic imagery sessions. The therapist can agree on a signal patients can use during the session—for example, raising their hands—whenever they want to stop the imagery. The therapist can begin and end with a safe-place image. Framing the imagery in this way can help patients contain the affect evoked by the work.

Another way in which the therapist can help patients contain affect is to discuss the imagery session thoroughly after it is over. In this discussion, the therapist gives patients the opportunity to talk through everything that happened—what they thought, felt, needed, learned. For example, the therapist might go through 15 minutes of traumatic imagery with a patient and then wait several weeks before doing related imagery again. During those weeks, the patient would spend a lot of time processing with the therapist all that took place during the previous imagery session.

During the imagery itself, we have found that it is generally best for the therapist to remain quiet. The therapist just listens, without reality-testing or confronting, gently asking open-ended questions—"What's happening now in the image?" or "What happens next?"—when the patient appears stuck. Later in therapy, once the patient has understood the full extent of the trauma and relived it fully, the therapist can intervene more actively. When the patient becomes too frightened to work on an image, the therapist can provide the child in the image with some kind of barrier or weapon against the perpetrator, hopefully allowing the patient to feel safe enough to continue working on the image. We discuss this further in Chapter 9, on borderline personality disorder. (As we explain in that chapter, we do not suggest bringing weapons into the images of patients who have a history of violence.)

One important principle is for the therapist to refrain from making any suggestions about what happened to the patient. It is not the thera-pist's place to make pronouncements about what "really happened," nor to make inferences about what happened. Rather, patients are left free to dis-cover their own stories. If the therapist suspects that the patient has been sexually abused but the patient is neither talking about it nor raising it in imagery work, the therapist does not bring it up. The therapist just waits silently and hopes the patient will eventually bring it up. Generally we have found that, if we work long enough with patients, over time they feel safe enough and they trust us enough to finally bring up abuse if it has oc-curred. Particularly in light of the current debate about false memories, we believe it is essential for therapists to err on the side of caution. Therefore we say nothing; we just schedule regular imagery sessions and we wait.

After completing traumatic imagery sessions about their childhoods, patients sometimes will deny that the image was true. They will say, "That never really happened. That was not really a memory. I made it up." We feel that the proper response to this assertion is that, in terms of the ther-apy, it does not matter whether the image is literally true. What we are ad-dressing in therapy is the theme of the image, not the accuracy. The image has an emotional truth, and the therapist and patient are working together to find that truth and to help the patient heal from it. We can work with the image without deciding about its accuracy or validity. Even though a memory may be false in the sense that certain details might be inaccurate, the theme of the image—the theme of being deprived, controlled, aban-doned, criticized, abused—is usually on target. We try not to get caught up in worrying about whether an image is accurate or not, and we do not be-have with patients as though the image is necessarily accurate. We focus on the theme of the image—the schema—and work with that.

With extremely fragile patients, particularly patients with BPD, a risk exists of their dissociating or decompensating during and after experien-tial work. We elaborate on this in Chapter 9.

Letters to Parents

Another experiential technique that we often give patients as a homework assignment is to write letters to their parents or to other significant people who hurt them when they were children or adolescents. Patients bring the letters to subsequent sessions and read them aloud to the therapist. (Pa-tients do not actually send the letters to their parents, except in rare in-stances, as we discuss shortly.)

The rationale for writing letters to parents is to summarize what the patient has learned about the parent as a result of doing the cognitive and experiential work. Patients can use the letters as opportunities to state their feelings and assert their rights. The therapist can suggest that they address certain topics: what the parent did (or did not do) that was damaging in the patient's childhood; how the patient felt about it; what the patient wished for at the time from the parent; what the patient wants from the parent now.

In most cases, we recommend to patients that they not actually send the letters. Occasionally, patients do decide to send them, but only after we have spent a lot of time going over all the possible repercussions. For example, patients might enrage their parents; parents might become depressed; patients might feel guilty later; or patients might alienate siblings and end up excluded from their families. The therapist is careful to cover all possible scenarios thoroughly before a patient actually sends a letter.

This is an example of a letter written by a patient named Kate, a 26-year-old young woman who writes copy for an advertising agency. Kate sought treatment for depression and anorexia nervosa. Her core schema is Defectiveness. Kate wrote this letter to her mother, who was critical and rejecting when she was a child.

Dear Mom,

When I was a child, you didn't love me. I always knew I wasn't what you wanted. I wasn't pretty and popular. I think you hated me. And you were always angry at me for not looking the way you wanted, for not being what you wanted. You were always criticizing me. I felt like I couldn't do anything to make you happy. I can't remember a single time I was ever able to please you.

I feel angry and cheated and hurt. I hate myself and have to live with that, for now at least. I hope that someday I won't have to live with it anymore. I hate myself for all the things you hated me for, the way I look and how unpopular I am. And I feel so sad. I feel like I have a bottomless pit of sadness.

I wish you could have loved what was good about me. You made me feel like there was nothing good about me, but it wasn't true. I was a good girl. I was sensitive to other people's feelings. I wish you could have felt love for me and shown it to me, but you never did.

I had a right to be accepted by you. I had a right to be respected for who I was. I had a right to be free of your constant putting me down. I still have a right to these things, and if you can't give them to me, I don't want to talk to you anymore about anything that really matters to me.

I can't tell you how many times I've picked up the phone and called you, excited to tell you something, and then hung up the phone after talking to you, feeling down. I want you to stop pulling the rug out from under my feet. I want you to stop hating me and being angry at me. I want you to stop putting me down. You make me feel like I'm no one and I have nothing.

I don't think you'll be able to do what I want. First of all, half the time I don't think you even know you're putting me down. You think

you're helping me. You think you do everything for me. If I send this
letter, you probably won't know what I'm talking about. You'll just get mad
at me. I wish you could understand, but, if you could, I probably wouldn't
be writing this letter in the first place.

> Your daughter,
> Kate

This letter summarizes the essential elements of the cognitive and experiential work Kate had done thus far in the treatment regarding her
mother. The letter expresses how Kate's mother hurt her as a child. It asserts Kate's right to feel and express her anger about what happened and to
expect her mother to behave appropriately from now on. Although Kate
never sent her mother the letter, writing it helped Kate fight her schemas
and clarify the issues in their relationship.

Imagery for Pattern-Breaking

We also use imagery techniques to help patients push through their coping
styles of avoidance and overcompensation to discover new ways of relating. Patients imagine behaving in healthy ways, rather than retreating into
their typical coping styles. For example, a patient with a Failure schema
imagines something he would ordinarily avoid, like asking his boss for an
important assignment; or a patient with a Defectiveness schema imagines
relating in a vulnerable way to her spouse rather than overcompensating
by adopting a superior stance. Imagery helps these patients face their
schemas and fight them directly.

The following excerpt involves Daniel, the patient described previously whose father was alcoholic and whose mother was sexually and
physically abusive. In the excerpt, he practices imagery for pattern-
breaking. Daniel's long-term therapy goal is to establish an intimate relationship with a woman. In this excerpt, the therapist asks Daniel to close
his eyes and imagine being at a dance with single women. He then instructs Daniel to carry on a dialogue between his Mistrust/Abuse and Defectiveness schemas, which are pressuring him to leave the situation, and
his Healthy Adult, which is encouraging him to stay and master the situation. Dr. Young then instructs Daniel to imagine staying at the dance and
breaking through his avoidance.

THERAPIST: Keep your eyes closed, and I want you to switch to an image of
yourself at a dance where there are single women available that you
might meet. And you're just entering the room. Can you picture yourself in a situation like that?

DANIEL: Yes. I'm at a dance, and I'm feeling very uncomfortable. I actually feel like I could make a beeline for the door at any minute. But I'm forcing myself to stay because I know it's important.

THERAPIST: I want you to be the part of yourself right now that wants to just leave, and talk to me. Why do you want to leave right now?

DANIEL: I don't feel I have too much confidence in starting up a conversation, and, you know, getting to the point where somebody might even like me enough to date me.

THERAPIST: Why won't they like you?

DANIEL: Um, because I'm, you know, just not a lovable person. I'm not lovable, and I'm not sure I can give love (*pause*).

Daniel has shifted into an avoidant mode at the dance. If this were "real life" rather than an imagery exercise, he would probably remain frozen in this mode for the remainder of the dance, or he would leave. The therapist pushes Daniel to imagine overcoming his avoidance and connecting with a woman.

THERAPIST: Try in the image to go up to them anyway, even though you want to run out because you think it's going to be a waste of time and you'll be rejected anyway. Try to imagine yourself going forward and approaching women anyway, and tell me what you see happening.

DANIEL: (*long pause*) I go over to a table and I ask a woman if I can sit down and talk, and she says, "OK." And we're talking, we're talking about the dance, talking about the music.

THERAPIST: How's it going, the conversation?

DANIEL: So far, so good.

THERAPIST: Do you feel comfortable with it yet, or do you still feel nervous?

DANIEL: I feel nervous. I feel like I can't be myself, I have to try to make more of myself than I am and try to force the conversation, that there shouldn't be any quiet spots in the conversation.

THERAPIST: Can you say this out loud to her, even though of course you wouldn't normally?

DANIEL: (*to woman in image*) I'm kind of uncomfortable being here because it's kind of a scary thing. I haven't been out to a dance in a long time, and I really don't know what to say or what to do. But I like being here, and I like being here sitting talking with you.

THERAPIST: Tell her how you feel, that you can't be yourself.

DANIEL: I feel a little uncomfortable because I feel I can't be real, that if I'm real you might not like me.

THERAPIST: What does she say to you?

DANIEL: (*pause*) She tells me she's feeling that way, too.

THERAPIST: About herself?

DANIEL: Yes.

THERAPIST: And how do you feel when she says that?

DANIEL: It makes me feel a little more relaxed.

THERAPIST: Tell her the things that you're ashamed of or afraid she's going to find out, that you can't show her.

DANIEL: (*to woman in image*) I feel uncomfortable saying this, but, even though I want to be emotionally supportive and loving towards a woman, I'm not sure if I can, and I'm afraid that you're going to sense this.

THERAPIST: Tell her about your anger toward women.

DANIEL: And because of some of the things that happened in my childhood with my mother, I have a lot of rage toward women.

THERAPIST: How does she react?

DANIEL: (*pause*) She tells me she has some rage towards men because of some of the things that have happened to her.

THERAPIST: How do you feel when she says that?

DANIEL: A little more relaxed. A little more at ease, because she's being honest with me.

Note that the therapist is not asking Daniel to rehearse what he would actually say to a woman at a dance. Rather, the therapist is asking Daniel to fight his schemas and avoidant coping style. Rather than shutting down emotionally and withdrawing into himself as he would normally do—thus perpetuating his Mistrust/Abuse and Defectiveness schemas—the therapist helps Daniel imagine approaching women and speaking in a more genuine and vulnerable way. The assumption of a more open attitude toward women opposes his schemas and leads to a better outcome. The exercise helps Daniel build up the part of himself that is able to behave constructively in social situations with women. The imagery also helps Daniel see that his fears about women are not realistic but are schema-driven. This reduces some of his shame and thus his avoidance.

Having given a voice to Daniel's Defectiveness schema, the therapist moves on to his Mistrust/Abuse schema.

THERAPIST: Is there some question whether you can trust her? Are you trying to figure out if you can trust her?

DANIEL: Well, as we're trying to be more real with each other, that seems to be diminishing, that feeling, but there is a feeling there.

THERAPIST: Be the part of yourself that's suspicious of her, and I want to hear what that side is saying.

DANIEL: (*pause*) I'm afraid you're going to just use me. If we decided to go out on a date, you'll get me to wine and dine you, and then I won't hear from you again, or you'll reject me. I'm suspicious that maybe you'll use me to just fill in some of your dating time until you get something better. I'm afraid you're going to use me.

THERAPIST: What does she say?

DANIEL: She says, "Don't be silly. I like you."

THERAPIST: When she says that, do you feel at all reassured, or are you still suspicious of her?

DANIEL: I feel a little bit reassured.

The therapist discusses the imagery exercise with the patient.

THERAPIST: Why don't you open your eyes?

DANIEL: (*Opens eyes.*)

THERAPIST: How did it feel, during that?

DANIEL: I felt it was a good exercise, putting me into a social situation.

THERAPIST: Are those the feelings that you think are coming up in those situations, that are blocking you from getting close?

DANIEL: I think so. And also the idea about being more honest, and more vulnerable, I have started to realize that's one of the important things I have to work on.

THERAPIST: And there's so much anger and fear, that you tend not to do that, because you're worried that you're going to be either rejected or used.

DANIEL: Yes.

THERAPIST: So instead you have to hide yourself, protect yourself.

DANIEL: Yes.

Once again, the therapist's aim was not for Daniel to practice what he actually would say in a social situation with a woman. Rather, his aim was for Daniel to fight his schemas by recognizing that his schema-driven fears are unrealistic.

OVERCOMING OBSTACLES TO EXPERIENTIAL WORK: SCHEMA AVOIDANCE

Most patients quickly take to imagery. They easily produce clear images and carry on dialogues, become involved with them on an affective level, and require minimal prompting and assistance. However, a significant minority of patients needs more assistance: Their images are vague, sparse, or nonexistent, or they seem emotionally detached from their images.

Schema avoidance is the central obstacle to doing experiential work. Imagery work is painful, and many patients act automatically and unconsciously to avoid that pain. They close their eyes and say, "I don't see anything," "I only see a blank screen," "I see an image but it's vague and I can't make it out." The therapist can use several strategies to overcome schema avoidance.

Educating the Patient about the Rationale

Imagery work evokes painful affect, and the patient needs a good reason to endure it. When patients avoid doing experiential work, we first make sure that they understand the rationale. We present all the advantages. We contrast intellectual understanding with emotional understanding and tell patients that experiential work is most potent in fighting the schema on an emotional level. We explain that schemas change more quickly when patients relive their childhood experiences in imagery. We tell them that, until they do the experiential work, they will still believe that the schema is true. We empathize with the fact that experiential work is difficult, but we point out the costs and benefits just the same.

Wait and Give Permission

The next option the therapist has is to wait.

THERAPIST: Close your eyes and let an image from your childhood float to the top of your mind.

PATIENT: I'm trying, but I don't see anything.

THERAPIST: Don't worry, just keep your eyes closed. Something will come (*long pause*).

PATIENT: I still don't see anything.

THERAPIST: It's okay to take your time. Take five minutes if necessary, and let's see what comes. Even if nothing comes, it's OK.

The therapist can also give the patient permission to generate any image at all.

THERAPIST: It doesn't matter what kind of image it is. It doesn't have to be real. It can be a fantasy. It can be colors, shapes, lights.

Sometimes the combination of the therapist's permission and a few minutes of time is enough, and the patient finally produces an image. However, when this does not work, there are other options.

Relaxation Imagery with Gradually Increasing Affective Strength

Another way to counter schema avoidance is to begin with a safe-place or other relaxing image and then gradually introduce elements that are slightly more threatening. This is a kind of graduated exposure which contains a hierarchy of characters and situations, and the therapist introduces increasingly more threatening characters and situations as the imagery progresses.

For example, the therapist might start the patient with a safe-place image, then bring one of the patient's close friends into the image, then bring in the slightly more problematic lover, and finally bring in the even more problematic father. The therapist might take several sessions to do this, exploring each step fully with the patient before moving on to the next one.

Medication

Sometimes patients are too depressed or labile to handle the imagery work: The imagery work activates powerful emotions, and it is hard for the patient to shake free of these emotions after they leave the session. Their emotions feel scary and unmanageable to them. This often happens to traumatized patients. Sometimes medication can help contain the affect so these patients can continue with the work.

One danger is that the medication can diminish the affect so much that the patient becomes numb and cannot do the exercises. The goal with medication is to reach an optimal level of arousal at which patients can still feel emotion but not so strongly that they feel unable to cope. If patients are too highly aroused, they feel too overwhelmed by the experiential techniques; if they are not sufficiently aroused, they are unable to generate enough affect to benefit from the techniques.

Body Work

When patients have difficulty feeling or expressing emotion, the therapist can sometimes help by focusing them on their bodies. The therapist can add sounds or motions to the feeling. For example, the therapist can tell patients to speak more loudly or to hit a pillow while attempting to express anger; or the therapist can instruct patients to assume certain positions, such as a fetal position, an open position, or a trapped position.

For example, in the preceding illustration with the patient Daniel, when the therapist encouraged Daniel to express his anger at his sexually abusive mother, the therapist could have instructed him to pound a pillow or the couch with his fist as he spoke to her.

Dialogue with the Detached Protector

Another option is for the therapist to open a dialogue with the part of the patient that is avoiding. We call this part of the patient the Detached Protector mode. We elaborate on this mode in greater detail in Chapter 8. However, here we briefly illustrate this technique as a means of overcoming schema avoidance. The therapist speaks directly to the part of the patient that is avoiding feeling or expressing the emotions connected to the imagery, the Detached Protector. Until we speak directly to the Detached Protector, we usually do not know why the patient is avoiding, and we therefore have difficulty finding a way to overcome the avoidance. Once we speak to the Detached Protector, we can usually find out why the patient is avoiding, and then devise a plan to overcome it.

Here is an example with Hector, the 42-year-old patient we described previously whose mother was schizophrenic throughout his childhood. Hector is doing an imagery exercise in which he is visualizing himself as a child with his mother. In the image, his mother is sitting next to him on a bus, loudly talking about "traitors." The therapist is trying to get the child to vent anger at his mother for embarrassing him in the image, and Hector is resisting. The therapist initiates a dialogue with the Detached Protector.

THERAPIST: Little Hector is so angry and he wants to express it. Why won't you let him express his anger? Be the side of you that wants to stop him from showing anger.

HECTOR: (*as Detached Protector*) "Well, what if Little Hector feels it, what can he do about it anyway? There's nothing he can do anyway, so what good is it for him to feel it?"

THERAPIST: Well, the value is that now we're here to help him, and we can protect him, and it's safe for him to express his anger. He has a right to feel his anger. He has a right to express his anger.

HECTOR: What if he goes out of control? What if he goes out of control and hurts someone?

THERAPIST: Has he ever done that? Has he ever gone out of control and hurt someone?

HECTOR: No. Never. I mean, not more than to yell at someone.

THERAPIST: How about if we try an experiment? How about if you try letting him express a little bit of anger and see how that feels? See if he feels better.

HECTOR: (*pause*) OK.

Until we understand why the patient's Detached Protector mode is interfering, we do not know how to respond. Once we give the Detached Protector a voice, we can learn why the patient cannot feel or express the emotion. We then are able to reason and negotiate with the Detached Protector.

We discuss this type of mode work further in this book. However, this example shows one way in which mode work can be helpful. By taking an avoidant coping style and making it into a mode, we give it a voice to which we can speak and with which we can negotiate.

If, after all this work, patients still insist that they cannot do imagery, we try one last technique. We tell patients that an overwhelming percentage of patients who say they cannot do imagery actually are able to. We then ask them to try an experiment: to look at the therapist for a full minute, then close their eyes and try to picture the therapist in an image. Almost all patients say they can see the therapist. This experiment illustrates that most patients are capable of seeing images. It is the Detached Protector who is stopping the patient from seeing them.

SUMMARY

Experiential techniques help the therapist and patient first identify and then fight the patient's schemas on an affective level.

The purpose of experiential assessment techniques is to identify the patient's core schemas, understand their origins in childhood, and link them to the presenting problem. We described how to conduct an imagery assessment session, moving from a safe-place image to disturbing images from the patient's childhood to images of the patient's current life problems.

The therapist introduces experiential change strategies following the cognitive change techniques. The goal is to help patients bolster rational understanding of their schemas with emotional understanding. Many experiential change techniques represent a simplified version of mode work, using imagery dialogues with the three main characters of the Vulnerable Child, the Dysfunctional Parent, and the Healthy Adult. The therapist brings the Healthy Adult into the patient's images of childhood to reparent the Vulnerable Child. The aim is for the patient to develop an internalized

Healthy Adult mode, modeled after the therapist. We also discussed other experiential change techniques, such as letters to parents and imagery for behavioral pattern-breaking.

Finally, we discussed overcoming obstacles to experiential work, primarily schema avoidance. The solutions we proposed included educating the patient about the rationale, giving the patient permission to take several minutes to generate an image, using relaxation imagery with gradually increasing affective strength, medication, body work, and conducting dialogues with the Detached Protector mode.

In the next chapter, we describe the behavioral component of schema therapy—what we call "behavioral pattern-breaking."

Chapter 5

BEHAVIORAL PATTERN-BREAKING

In the behavioral pattern-breaking stage of treatment, patients attempt to replace their schema-driven patterns of behavior with healthier coping styles. Behavioral pattern-breaking is the longest and, in some ways, the most crucial part of schema therapy. Without it, relapse is likely. Even if patients have insight into their Early Maladaptive Schemas, and even if they have done the cognitive and experiential work, their schemas will reassert themselves if patients do not change their behavioral patterns. The progress they have made will erode, and eventually they will fall back under the sway of their schemas. For patients to achieve and maintain full gains, it is essential that they change their behavioral patterns.

Of the four main change components in schema therapy, behavioral pattern-breaking is usually the final one that the therapist focuses on. If the patient has not progressed adequately through the cognitive and experiential stages, the patient is unlikely to achieve lasting changes in schema-driven behavior. The other parts of treatment prepare the patient for the task of behavioral change. They give the patient psychological distance from the schema, helping him or her to view the schema as an intruder rather than as a core truth about the self. The cognitive and experiential stages strengthen the healthy side of the patient, especially the ability of the healthy side to fight the patient's schemas. Once the behavioral part of treatment is underway, they help the patient overcome blocks to behavioral change.

Thus the behavioral stage of treatment takes place within the framework of the schema model and incorporates the other schema strategies, such as flash cards, imagery, and dialogues. Where relevant, the therapist also uses traditional behavioral techniques, such as relaxation training, assertiveness training, anger management, self-control strategies (i.e., self-monitoring, goal-setting, self-reinforcement) and graduated exposure to feared situations. (We assume that readers are familiar with these standard techniques from behavior therapy, so we will not elaborate on them in this book.)

COPING STYLES

Behavioral pattern-breaking targets coping styles: The behaviors that are the focus of change are the ones patients use in surrendering to, avoiding, and overcompensating for their Early Maladaptive Schemas. These are the self-defeating behaviors patients employ to cope when their schemas are triggered: the unfounded jealous accusations of the patient with an Abandonment schema, the self-deprecatory comments of the patient with a Defectiveness schema, the advice-soliciting of the patient with a Dependence schema, the obedience of the subjugated patient; the phobic avoidance of the patient who has a Vulnerability to Harm or Illness schema. These surrender, avoidance, and overcompensatory behaviors ultimately serve to perpetuate schemas. Patients must change their coping styles in order to heal their schemas and thereby fill the unmet needs that brought them into therapy.

Case Illustration

A young woman named Ivy comes for schema therapy. She is feeling frustrated and unhappy in many life areas. The pattern is the same: in her family, in her love life, at work, with her friends, she assumes a caretaking role while asking virtually nothing for herself. As she puts it, "I take care of everybody, but nobody takes care of me." She is depressed, overwhelmed, exhausted, and resentful. In the Assessment Phase, Ivy and the therapist agree that she has a Self-Sacrifice schema. Her main coping style is surrendering to the schema. She takes care of others but does not allow others to take care of her.

Ivy meets her best friend Adam for dinner every few weeks. The dinners follow the same pattern: Adam asks Ivy about her life, and Ivy gives short, positive answers, basically conveying, "Everything's fine," and then asks Adam about his life. Adam answers by raising a troubling issue in his own life, and the two spend the rest of dinner discussing the issue he has raised. Why does Ivy not share anything of importance about herself with her friend? The answer is that her friend's questions trigger her Self-Sacrifice schema. Ivy feels guilty and selfish talking about herself. She copes with the triggering of her schema by giving quick nonanswers and shifting the focus back to Adam. Ivy ends up feeling emotionally deprived

(almost all patients with Self-Sacrifice schemas have linked Emotional De-privation schemas.)

In the behavioral part of treatment, Ivy decides to bring greater balance into her intimate relationships. She decides to begin with her relationship with Adam. To prepare her, the therapist asks her to close her eyes and picture an image of herself sitting at dinner with Adam and telling him about her life. In imagery, Ivy conducts a dialogue between her Self-Sacrifice schema, which tells her to switch the focus back to Adam, and her healthy side, which promulgates the wisdom of sharing a problem with her friend. Next, switching chairs between the "schema" and the "healthy side," Ivy gets angry at her schema, asserting her right to be taken care of by others. In imagery she connects the situation to her childhood with her fragile, needy mother. She tells her mother, "It cost me too much to take care of you. It cost me my sense of self."

Next, in imagery, she visualizes sharing a problem with Adam, dealing with all the obstacles that arise.

THERAPIST: So what do you want to tell Adam?

IVY: I want to tell him what it's like to have my mother getting sick and needing so much from me.

THERAPIST: OK, so could you imagine telling him about that in the image? About your mother getting sick, and your feelings about it?

IVY: I want to tell him, but I feel scared.

THERAPIST: And what is the scared side saying?

IVY: It's saying, "It's not supposed to be this way. Adam's not supposed to be taking care of me, I'm supposed to be taking care of him."

THERAPIST: What are you afraid will happen if you let Adam take care of you?

IVY: I'm afraid he won't like me anymore.

THERAPIST: Are you afraid of anything else?

IVY: I'm afraid I'll start crying, or something.

THERAPIST: And what would be so bad about that?

IVY: I'd be really embarrassed.

THERAPIST: Well, that's your Self-Sacrifice schema talking, everything you've been saying: "You're not supposed to let anyone take care of you. People won't like you if you show your own vulnerability. You're not supposed to cry." What does the healthy side say to that? Could you answer as the healthy side in the image?

IVY: Well, yeah, the healthy side is saying, "It's all right to let my friends take care of me. They'll still like me. It's okay to cry with a close friend."

Finally, as a behavioral homework assignment, Ivy practices responding more authentically to her friend when he asks about her life. The next
time they meet for dinner, she shares an issue concerning her love relationship. Adam responds warmly and supportively, countering Ivy's Self-
Sacrifice (and Emotional Deprivation) schemas.

Maladaptive Coping Styles Associated with Specific Schemas

Each schema is associated with certain dysfunctional behavior patterns
that tend to characterize the patient's approach to partners and significant
others (including the therapist). Table 5.1 gives an example of each coping
style for each schema.

As Table 5.1 shows, behavioral pattern-breaking refers not only to
how one behaves in specific situations but also to the types of situations
one generally selects: whom one marries; the career one chooses; one's cir-
cle of friends. Behavioral pattern-breaking involves major life decisions, as
well as everyday behaviors. Patients maintain their Early Maladaptive
Schemas by making major life decisions that perpetuate their schemas.

Patients can often change discrete, situation-specific behaviors with
standard cognitive-behavioral techniques, but lifelong behavioral patterns driven by Early Maladaptive Schemas require an integrative approach. Assertiveness training might help a patient who has difficulty
setting limits with his girlfriend, but assertiveness training alone will
probably not be sufficient to change a broader life pattern of subjugation
to significant others. Patients subjugate because they fear punishment,
abandonment, or criticism, and they must work through these underlying issues in order to overcome the pattern. The linked schemas tied to
these underlying issues—Punitiveness, Abandonment, Defectiveness—
block progress. If the patient has a Mistrust/Abuse schema, he is going
to be afraid that, if he asserts himself, his girlfriend will become abusive.
If the patient has an Abandonment schema, he is going to be afraid that
his girlfriend will leave him if he asserts himself. If the patient has a Defectiveness schema, he is not going to feel he has the right to be assertive with his girlfriend, even if he knows the steps necessary for self-
assertion. Skills training is frequently not the primary intervention. The
schema has cognitive and emotional aspects that the treatment must address beforehand.

It is often easier for patients to change their cognitions and emotions
than it is to break lifelong patterns of behavior. For this reason, the therapist must be patient but persistent throughout the behavioral stage, employing the rule of empathic confrontation. The therapist expresses empathy for how hard it is to change deeply instilled patterns of behavior yet
continually confronts the necessity for that change.

TABLE 5.1. Examples of Coping Styles Associated with Specific Schemas

Schema	Surrender	Avoidance	Overcompensation
Abandonment/ Instability	Selects partners and significant others who are unavailable or unpredictable.	Avoids intimate relationships altogether out of fear of abandonment.	Pushes partners and significant others away with clinging, possessive, or controlling behaviors.
Mistrust/Abuse	Chooses untrustworthy partners and significant others; is overvigilant and suspicious of others.	Avoids close involvement with others in personal and business life; does not confide or self-disclose.	Mistreats or exploits others; acts in an overly trusting manner.
Emotional Deprivation	Chooses cold, detached partners and significant others; discourages others from giving emotionally.	Withdraws and isolates; avoids close relationships.	Makes unrealistic demands that others meet all of his or her needs.
Defectiveness/ Shame	Chooses critical partners and significant others; puts him- or herself down.	Avoids sharing "shameful" thoughts and feelings with partners and significant others due to fear of rejection.	Behaves in a critical or superior way toward others; tries to come across as "perfect."
Social Isolation/ Alienation	Becomes part of a group but stays on the periphery; does not fully join in.	Avoids socializing; spends most of his or her time alone.	Puts on a false "persona" to join a group, but still feels different and alienated.
Dependence/ Incompetence	Asks for an excessive amount of help; checks decisions with others; chooses overprotective partners who do everything for him or her.	Procrastinates on decisions; avoids acting independently or taking on normal adult responsibilities.	Demonstrates excessive self-reliance, even when turning to others would be normal and healthy.
Vulnerability to Harm or Illness	Worries continually that catastrophe will befall him or her; repeatedly asks others for reassurance.	Engages in phobic avoidance of "dangerous" situations.	Employs magical thinking and compulsive rituals; engages in reckless, dangerous behavior.
Enmeshment/ Undeveloped Self	Imitates behavior of significant other, keeps in close contact with "enmeshed other"; does not develop a separate identity with unique preferences.	Avoids relationships with people who stress individuality over enmeshment.	Engages in excessive autonomy.

(cont.)

TABLE 5.1. *(cont.)*

Schema	Surrender	Avoidance	Overcompensation
Failure	Sabotages work efforts by working below level of ability; unfavorably compares his or her achievement with that of others in a biased manner.	Procrastinates on work tasks; avoids new or difficult tasks completely; avoids setting career goals that are appropriate to ability level.	Diminishes achievements of others; tries to meet perfectionistic standards to compensate for sense of failure.
Entitlement/ Grandiosity	Has unequal or uncaring relationships with partners and significant others; behaves selfishly; disregards needs and feelings of others; acts superior.	Avoids situations in which he or she cannot excel and stand out.	Gives extravagant gifts or charitable contributions to make up for selfish behavior.
Insufficient Self-Control/Self-Discipline	Performs tasks that are boring or uncomfortable in a careless way; loses control of emotions; excessively eats, drinks, gambles, or uses drugs for pleasure.	Does not work or drops out of school; does not set long-term career goals.	Makes short-lived, intense efforts to complete a project or to exercise self-control.
Subjugation	Chooses dominant, controlling partners and significant others; complies with their wishes.	Avoids relationships altogether; avoids situations in which his or her wishes are different from those of others.	Acts in a passive–aggressive or rebellious manner.
Self-Sacrifice	Engages in self-denial; does too much for others and not enough for him- or herself.	Avoids close relationships.	Becomes angry at significant others for not reciprocating or for not showing appreciation; decides to do nothing for others anymore.
Negativity/ Pessimism	Minimizes positive events, exaggerates negative ones; expects and prepares for the worst.	Does not hope for too much; keeps expectations low.	Acts in an unrealistically positive, optimistic, "Pollyanna-ish" way (rare).

(cont.)

TABLE 5.1. (cont.)

Schema	Surrender	Avoidance	Overcompensation
Emotional Inhibition	Emphasizes reason and order over emotion; acts in a very controlled, flat manner; does not show spontaneous emotions or behavior.	Avoids activities involving emotional self-expression (such as expressing love or showing fear) or requiring uninhibited behavior (such as dancing).	Acts impulsively and without inhibition (sometimes under the influence of disinhibiting substances such as alcohol).
Approval-Seeking/ Recognition-Seeking	Draws the attention of others to his or her accomplishments related to status.	Avoids relationships with admired individuals out of fear of not gaining their approval.	Acts flagrantly to gain the disapproval of admired individuals.
Punitiveness	Acts in an overly punishing or harsh way with significant others.	Avoids situations involving evaluation to escape the fear of punishment.	Acts in an overly forgiving manner while being inwardly angry and punitive.
Unrelenting Standards/ Hypercriticalness	Attempts to perform perfectly; sets high standards for self and others.	Avoids taking on work tasks; procrastinates.	Throws out high standards altogether and settles for below-average performance.

READINESS FOR BEHAVIORAL PATTERN-BREAKING

How does the therapist know when it is time to shift the focus of treatment to behavioral pattern-breaking? The answer is when patients have successfully mastered the cognitive and experiential parts of treatment. If patients are able to label their Early Maladaptive Schemas when they are triggered, to understand the origins of their schemas in childhood, and to participate in schema dialogues in which they consistently defeat their schemas utilizing their healthy sides—both cognitively and emotionally—then they are probably ready to begin behavioral pattern-breaking.

DEFINING SPECIFIC BEHAVIORS AS POSSIBLE TARGETS OF CHANGE

The first step is for the therapist and patient to develop an extensive list of specific behaviors to serve as potential targets of change. The therapist and patient can refer to many sources of information to develop this list: the case conceptualization developed in the Assessment Phase, detailed descriptions of problematic behaviors, imagery of problematic situations, the therapy relationship, relationships with significant others, and schema questionnaires.

Refining the Case Conceptualization

The therapist and patient can start by refining the case conceptualization they developed in the Assessment Phase, elaborating on the processes of schema surrender, avoidance, and overcompensation. Working with these coping styles, they can begin to develop a list of specific behaviors or life circumstances that require change. It is important for the therapist to cover each major life area separately, such as intimate relationships, work, and social activities, because the patient may have different schemas and coping styles linked to different life areas. For example, a patient with an Emotional Deprivation schema may be warm and nurturing with close friends but cold and distant with romantic partners; a patient with a Subjugation schema may be passive with authority figures but domineering and controlling with younger siblings or children; or a patient may have a Defectiveness schema that is activated when meeting strangers in a social situation but not when meeting significant others one-to-one.

Detailed Descriptions of Problematic Behaviors

Perhaps the most important step in identifying self-defeating behavioral patterns is for the therapist and patient to develop detailed descriptions of problematic situations in the patient's life. When the patient reports a situation that is a consistent schema trigger, the therapist helps the patient clarify specific behaviors by asking questions. The goal is to get a blow-by-blow account of what happened. Sometimes the therapist encounters difficulty during this effort. As part of the schema perpetuation process, the patient distorts what happened to fit the schema and ignores contradictory data. The therapist must push through the patient's reluctance to recall what happened in an objective, rather than emotional, schema-driven fashion.

Case Illustration

A young female patient named Daphne comes to a session and reports that she had a fight with her husband the previous evening. Daphne has an Abandonment/Instability schema as a result of growing up in a household filled with strife. Her parents fought nearly every night, often to the point of threatening divorce. Daphne remembers watching them shouting at each other and feeling helpless to stop them, then hiding in her closet with her hands over her ears. Now she is married to Mark, a medical resident. He works long hours and comes home haggard and depleted. His homecoming sparks a fight nearly every night.

Daphne tells the story of their latest fight:

DAPHNE: Mark and I had another fight last night.

THERAPIST: What started the fight?

DAPHNE: Oh, the same old thing. He was late. I don't know. (*Tosses her head.*)

THERAPIST: How did the fight begin?

DAPHNE: The same way it always does. It doesn't matter. All we do is argue. We should probably get divorced.

THERAPIST: Daphne, I see how hopeless you feel, but it's still important for us to understand what happened. Think back to the beginning of the fight. How did it start?

DAPHNE: I had a really hard day. I couldn't seem to get any of my freelance work done. The baby was crying all day. Mark came home late again, and I let him have it.

THERAPIST: How did you let him have it?

DAPHNE: I told him I can't possibly earn money for us when I have to take care of a screaming baby all day. How am I supposed to work? When the baby's up I have to take care of him, and when's he's sleeping I'm so tired that I have to sleep, too. I mean, Mark gets to leave for the whole day, and I'm stuck here.

THERAPIST: What did Mark say?

DAPHNE: He said it wasn't his fault that the baby was crying and that he works hard, too.

THERAPIST: What happened next?

DAPHNE: I told him, "You leave us alone all day and night. You're a rotten husband and father."

THERAPIST: How were you feeling at that point?

DAPHNE: Angry. Really angry and scared. I was scared that he didn't care about me and the baby and might leave us forever.

THERAPIST: What about Mark? What do you think he was feeling?

DAPHNE: At the time I thought he couldn't care less, because he left the room. Later he told me he was devastated that I said he was a rotten husband and father.

By recounting her interaction with her husband in such detail, Daphne and her therapist are able to identify her problematic behaviors. Mark's lateness triggers her Abandonment/Instability schema, and she becomes panicked and angry. When he finally gets home, instead of expressing her vulnerability and fear, she lashes out at him, trying to hurt him as much as she can. In coping with her schema by overcompensating,

Daphne perpetuates her schema. She ends up feeling even more afraid that Mark will leave her, recreating just the kind of unstable atmosphere that frightened her so much when she was a child.

Imagery of Trigger Events

If patients have difficulty remembering details of a problematic situation, the therapist can help them use imagery to replay the situation. The therapist asks them to close their eyes and picture an image of the situation. The therapist asks questions about what is happening in the image, coaxing patients to remember the details of their behavior. The therapist says, "What are you thinking? What are you feeling? What do you wish you could do? What do you do next?" Through imagery, patients can often access thoughts, feelings, and behaviors that were previously inaccessible.

Case Illustration

Henry is a college student at a competitive school. His presenting problem is that he procrastinates doing his schoolwork and thus is performing below his ability level.

Henry is the only child of professional parents who value achievement above all else. He was the valedictorian of his small high school class—a feat he achieved without exerting much effort. He was also a star athlete in high school, but he realized in his freshman year of college that he was not talented enough to pursue a career in professional sports. "I felt like a failure," he said, "but I figured that my academic success was guaranteed." Henry expected his schoolwork to replace sports as the main source of his self-esteem. Now, however, he was not doing his schoolwork, and his grades were mediocre.

In the Assessment Phase of treatment, Henry identified Unrelenting Standards and Insufficient Self-Control/Self-Discipline as the principal schemas that interfered with his studying. After battling these schemas with cognitive and experiential strategies, the therapist and Henry turned to behavioral pattern-breaking. In the following excerpt, the therapist uses imagery to help Henry identify his behaviors while he was putting off doing his schoolwork.

THERAPIST: Do you want to do an imagery exercise to help you pinpoint the problem?

HENRY: OK.

THERAPIST: Good, then close your eyes and get an image of yourself sitting down to work last night.

HENRY: OK. (*Closes eyes.*)

THERAPIST: What do you see?

HENRY: I'm in my room. It's pretty messy, with papers all over the place. I have my books in front of me and my computer to the side. (*Pause.*)

THERAPIST: What happens when you start to think about doing your work?

HENRY: Well, it's kind of late. I told myself all day I could work later. Now I have a paper due and I haven't even started.

THERAPIST: What are you thinking?

HENRY: I don't want to do my paper. I'm too wound up to focus. I don't know where to start. Just thinking about it gives me a stomachache. I'd rather play computer games, so I do.

THERAPIST: What happens next?

HENRY: I play computer games for a while, and then I listen to music. By then it's really late and I know I have to work.

THERAPIST: What are you feeling?

HENRY: Anxious and depressed. The more anxious I get, the harder it is to concentrate.

THERAPIST: What goes through your mind?

HENRY: It's too late.

THERAPIST: It's too late to write the paper?

HENRY: No, it's too late to get an A. I could have gotten an A if I had done the work. What's the use? I've failed already.

THERAPIST: What do you do?

HENRY: I set my alarm for four in the morning, thinking I'll get up then and write the paper. I sleep through the alarm and through all my classes the next day.

Henry uses avoidant behavioral strategies such as distraction to cope with his mounting anxiety. Note that, while investigating Henry's behaviors, the therapist also elicits information about his cognitions and emotions. The more vividly the patient recalls the image, the more clearly he is able to recall specific behaviors.

The Therapy Relationship

The patient's behavior in the therapy relationship is a further source of information about behaviors that require change, especially concerning relationships with significant others. This source of information is particularly advantageous because the therapist can observe the behaviors directly, perceiving subtleties that might be lost if the patient were merely reporting about relationships outside of therapy.

The therapist can observe the patient's schemas, as well as the patient's coping styles. Each set of schemas and coping styles has its own presentation. For example, a young female patient demonstrates her Emotional Deprivation schema and avoidant coping style by leaving sessions early. Unwilling to face the fact that she shares the therapist with other patients, she leaves the session before the next patient arrives in the waiting room.

A young male patient demonstrates his Defectiveness schema and his coping style of overcompensation by repeatedly correcting the therapist's manner of speech. A young female patient shows her Enmeshment schema and her coping style of surrender by imitating the therapist's style of dress. (In the Chapter 6, we elaborate further on the presentation of schemas and coping styles within the therapy relationship.)

Case Illustration

The case of Alicia illustrates how schemas and coping styles manifest themselves in the therapy relationship and how they can subvert therapy. Alicia grew up in a strict, moralistic family. Her mother taught her that people were inherently evil and weak and that, to be good, one must watch oneself vigilantly. Forsaking family members in their time of need was the worst transgression. Alicia was dutiful and responsible and tried to fill her mother's wishes. "I wanted to please her but I never could," she says. Her father was an alcoholic, and her mother taught her that it was her duty to help him maintain self-control. Alicia tried to be very good so that she would not upset her father and "make him drink." She emptied his whiskey bottles, begged and cajoled him not to go out at night, and got him into bed when he was drunk.

Alicia's primary schemas were Defectiveness and Punitiveness. She could not forgive herself for having "bad" impulses and wishes. She also had schemas of Emotional Deprivation (from the cold emotional atmosphere of the family), Self-Sacrifice (from her mother's demands that she serve the needs of family members, especially her father), and Unrelenting Standards (from the impossibility of being "good enough" to please her mother). As she grew up, Alicia lived in ways that perpetuated her schemas. She chose troubled partners and friends. She chose one boyfriend after another who was a substance abuser. She stayed in these relationships because she felt it was her moral obligation to do so. As her mother taught her, one does not desert loved ones in their time of need. In addition, as with her father, Alicia felt it was her fault when her boyfriends abused drugs. Somehow she had failed to prevent them.

Among other therapy goals, Alicia wanted to lose weight. She began reporting to the therapist during sessions how much she had eaten the previous week. At first it seemed as though Alicia wanted attention for her weight-loss efforts, and the therapist tried to give it (hoping to counter the patient's Emotional Deprivation schema). However, it soon became clear that Alicia assumed that the therapist condemned her for the extra weight. Her Defectiveness and Punitiveness schemas were being triggered. Alicia was confessing to the therapist as she had confessed her "bad" behavior to her mother as a child. When she realized this, Alicia burst into tears, saying that she had been considering dropping out of therapy. Weight loss was not *her* goal, it was her mother's goal. Alicia believed that, if she did not do what her mother said she should do, she was a bad person. Weight loss was a promise to her mother that she had to keep. Another side of her, however—her Vulnerable Child—felt that eating was her only pleasure, and she could not bear to limit herself. (Eating was a form of overcompensation for her Emotional Deprivation and Self-Sacrifice schemas.) Reporting her eating to the therapist, Alicia turned the therapist into another punitive figure in her mind, one she had to labor endlessly to please.

The therapist helped Alicia uncover other areas of her life in which she "confessed" her "bad" behavior under the assumption that the other person was judging her negatively. Changing this pattern became one of her goals in behavioral pattern-breaking.

Reports of Significant Others

Sometimes the therapist does not rely solely on patients' self-reports to identify their problematic behaviors. There are bound to be flaws and gaps in patients' self-observations. This is especially true when patients are overcompensating for their schemas. For example, narcissists are notoriously poor observers of their own behavior and its impact on others. Consultations with partners, family members, and friends can supply additional perspectives. When it is workable for the therapist to meet with them, significant others can often provide information that the patient cannot provide. The therapist explores the points of view of these significant others and asks them for specific examples that shed light on the patient's maladaptive behavior patterns. If the therapist is unable to meet with significant others, the patient can ask them for feedback and then discuss their responses in therapy.

Taking careful histories of relationships with significant others can also furnish information. The therapist focuses on problematic behaviors. What schemas were triggered in these relationships? How did the patient cope? What exactly did the patient do? What were the self-defeating behaviors that perpetuated the schemas?

Case Illustration

Monique presents for therapy, complaining that her husband, Lawrence, will not have sex with her.

THERAPIST: Why do you think he won't have sex with you?

MONIQUE: I don't know.

THERAPIST: If you had to guess?

MONIQUE: I don't know. He's just not a sexual person.

Monique says that she pleads with her husband: "I tell him I'm lonely. I tell him I miss him." Further inquiry determines that the two of them had a good sex life before they were married. She is certain that there is no one else: Neither she nor her husband is having an affair. As far as she knows, her husband is not angry with her. In fact, she is the one who is angry with him for abandoning their sexual life. Monique is wrestling with the temptation to cheat on Lawrence. The therapist is unable to learn from her why Lawrence appears so uninterested in sex with her.

The therapist asks if Lawrence can come in for a session alone. Monique agrees, and her husband comes in. Lawrence reports that Monique criticizes his sexual performance and compares his skill as a lover unfavorably to other lovers she had before they were married. Over the years, this has made him feel increasingly anxious and inadequate as a lover. He has thus taken the route of avoiding sex with her. Thus the therapist learns what problematic behaviors on Monique's part are contributing to the break in their sexual relationship.

Schema Inventories

The Young Schema Questionnaire is an excellent source of problematic "surrender" behaviors tied to schemas. In addition, the Young–Rygh Avoidance Inventory and the Young Compensation Inventory list other forms of schema coping behaviors.

PRIORITIZING BEHAVIORS FOR PATTERN-BREAKING

Once the therapist and patient have made a list of problematic behaviors and life patterns, they deliberate about which are the most important and which should be targets of change. Looking at the most significant problematic behaviors, they explore what the healthy behavior would be for the patient in each case. Often patients are not aware that their behaviors are problematic, and they do not know what healthy behaviors are. The therapist and patient generate alternative behaviors, discussing the advantages and disadvantages of each one. They come up with healthy responses to replace maladaptive ones, and these become the behavioral goals for treatment.

The therapist helps the patient select one specific behavior to change first. The patient works on one behavior at a time, not the whole pattern at once. How do the therapist and patient select this first behavior to change? We present some rules of thumb.

Changing Behaviors versus Making Life Changes

Our general approach in schema therapy is to attempt to change behaviors *within* a current life situation before recommending major life changes, such as leaving a marriage or job. (This, of course, does not apply to dangerous or intolerable situations, such as an abusive spouse.) Changing behaviors entails staying in a situation and learning to respond more appropriately. We believe patients have a lot to gain by first learning how to handle a difficult situation before deciding whether to leave it. Rather than jumping to conclusions about the impossibility of change, patients first make sure they cannot get what they want from the current state of affairs by improving their own behavior. In addition, they build skills for future difficult situations. If, after improving their behavior, patients eventually decide to leave the current situation, they can do so knowing they have done their part in trying to make it work.

Start with the Most Problematic Behavior

We believe that the therapist should start with the most problematic behavior. This is the behavior that causes the patient the most distress and that most interferes with the patient's interpersonal or occupational functioning. The exception is cases in which the patient feels too overwhelmed to proceed. In that case, the therapist picks the most problematic behavior that the patient feels capable of changing.

Our approach contrasts with cognitive-behavioral therapy, which typically begins with the easiest behavior. In cognitive-behavioral therapy, patients only gradually approach their most difficult behaviors. The therapist and patient construct hierarchies of behaviors ranked in order of increasing difficulty, and the patient starts from the bottom and works up. For example, if a patient comes to treatment because she cannot say "no" to her boss at work, a cognitive-behavioral therapist might have her start by practicing assertiveness with strangers and service people and gradually work her way up through friends and family members, finally addressing the problem with her boss.

In schema therapy, however, the therapist begins with core schemas and coping styles. Our goal is to help patients feel substantially better as quickly as possible. Only if patients are unable to make changes in their primary presenting problem do we shift to a secondary problem.

BUILDING MOTIVATION FOR BEHAVIORAL CHANGE

Once the therapist and patient have settled on a specific target behavior, the therapist works on helping the patient build motivation for behavioral change.

Link the Target Behavior to Its Origins in Childhood

In order to help patients feel more empathic and supportive toward themselves and thus more able to make positive changes, the therapist helps them link the target behavior to its origins in childhood. Patients understand why the behavior developed in the first place and learn to forgive themselves instead of blaming themselves for the behavior. For example, a patient who is about to give up alcohol might connect the urge to drink to his Defectiveness schema, which began in childhood with his critical and rejecting father. It is to escape feelings of worthlessness and unlovability that the patient drinks. Instead of viewing himself as weak for becoming an alcoholic, the patient can understand why it happened. Drinking was his way of avoiding the painful emotions connected to his Early Maladaptive Schema.

In addition, linking the behavior to childhood helps the patient connect the behavioral component to the prior cognitive and experiential work.

Review the Advantages and Disadvantages of Continuing the Behavior

To strengthen motivation, the therapist and patient review the advantages and disadvantages of continuing the maladaptive behavior. Unless patients believe it is worth the effort, they are not going to undertake behavioral change.

Case Illustration

Alan comes to therapy at the urging of his fiancée, Nora, who is expressing uncertainty about going ahead with their wedding. Alan does not understand what is wrong with their relationship. From his point of view, everything is fine. "The only problem is that Nora isn't happy," he says. At the therapist's request, Nora comes in for a session. She tells the therapist that she feels as though her relationship with Alan is "missing something." "We don't have real intimacy," she says.

In the Assessment Phase, the therapist and Alan agree that he has an Emotional Inhibition schema that is preventing him from connecting deeply with Nora. Alan goes through the cognitive and experiential components of treatment and then begins behavioral pattern-breaking. His goal is to express more emotions—both positive and negative—in his relationship with Nora.

Alan is intensely ambivalent about this goal. In his view, his emotional inhibition is an intrinsic part of who he is. To help him build motivation to change, the therapist asks Alan to list the advantages and disadvantages of remaining unemotional toward Nora. The list of advantages include such items as (1) avoiding discomfort; (2) being true to myself; (3) I like to stay in control; and (4) I don't like confrontations. The list of disadvantages includes one item only: (1) Nora will be unhappy and may even leave me. However, contemplating this one disadvantage helped Alan build the motivation to change his behavior. Knowing that, unless he changes, he will lose Nora is enough to motivate Alan to change.

DEVELOP A FLASH CARD

The therapist and patient often compose a flash card for the patient regarding the problematic behavior. They can use the Schema Therapy Flash Card as a guide, adapting it to focus more specifically on behavior. The flash card describes the situation, identifies the schemas that have been triggered, states the reality of the situation, and describes the healthy behavior.

Case Illustration

Justine has a Subjugation schema that developed from her childhood interactions with her tyrannical father. She is engaged to marry Richard, who is loving but domineering, like her father. Justine is working on replacing her overly aggressive response to Richard's "bossiness" with more effective, less confrontational behavior. Following is the flash card Justine and her therapist developed to help her change her overcompensatory style to one of appropriate assertiveness.

> Right now I'm feeling like Richard is controlling me, telling me what to do, and not listening to me. I want to scream at him to leave me alone; I want to throw things; I want to run into the bedroom and slam the door; I want to hit him. However, I know that I'm overreacting because of my Subjugation schema, which I learned as a little girl with my domineering father. Even though I believe Richard is *intentionally* disregarding my feelings, in reality he's just being himself and doesn't mean to hurt me. Even though I feel like yelling at him and hurting him, instead I'm going to calmly tell him

how I feel and what I want to do. I'm going to say what I want in a mature way that I won't regret later.

Patients can read the flash card when they are preparing for a situation and want to remind themselves why changing their behavior is important or when they are in the situation and have the urge to revert to the old maladaptive behavior.

REHEARSE THE HEALTHY BEHAVIOR IN IMAGERY AND ROLE-PLAYS

The patient practices healthy behaviors in therapy sessions, using both imagery and role-playing. The patient runs through imagery rehearsals of the problematic situation and role-plays the situation with the therapist. The patient visualizes managing the situation in imagery, successfully navigating potential stumbling blocks. Following is an imagery scene with Justine.

THERAPIST: Close your eyes and get an image of Richard coming home. He's late and the baby's crying and you're at the end of your rope. Can you see it?

JUSTINE: (*with eyes closed*) Yes.

THERAPIST: What's happening?

JUSTINE: I'm waiting for him, walking around, watching the clock.

THERAPIST: What are you feeling?

JUSTINE: One minute I'm feeling scared to death that he's never coming home, the next minute I want to kill him for doing this to me.

THERAPIST: What happens when he walks in the door?

JUSTINE: He gives me this look, questioning, to see what kind of mood I'm in.

THERAPIST: What do you want to do?

JUSTINE: I don't know if I want to scream at him and beat his chest with my fists, or run up to him and hug him.

THERAPIST: How do you handle the two parts?

JUSTINE: Well, I talk to the angry part. I tell her, "Listen, you love Richard, and you don't want to hurt him. You're just upset because you thought he wasn't coming home anymore, but here he is! You can be happy."

THERAPIST: And what does the angry part say back?

JUSTINE: She says, "OK." She feels OK.

In talking to her angry side, Justine is doing mode work. She is conducting a dialogue between the Angry Child and the Healthy Adult modes.

In role-plays, the therapist typically models the healthy behavior first, with the patient playing the other person in the problematic situation. Then the therapist and patient switch roles, with the patient practicing the healthy behavior, while the therapist plays the other role. The therapist and patient work through the most likely stumbling blocks so that the patient feels well prepared.

AGREE ON A HOMEWORK ASSIGNMENT

The next step is for the therapist and patient to agree on a homework assignment relevant to the new behavioral pattern. The patient agrees to carry out the healthy behavior in a life situation, recording what happens.

The patient writes down the homework assignment, keeping the original and giving a copy to the therapist. The assignment is concrete and specific. For example, a homework assignment might be: "This week I'm going to ask my boss if I can take my vacation at the end of May. Just before asking him, I'm going to read my flash card, and then visualize asking him, just the way I planned it. Afterward, I'll write down what happened, how I felt, what I was thinking, what I did, and what my boss did."

REVIEW THE HOMEWORK ASSIGNMENT

Referring to the written copy of the assignment, the therapist and patient review the previous homework assignment at the start of the next session. It is vital that the therapist follow up on homework assignments. If the therapist forgets about the homework, then the patient gets the message that the homework is not important and that the therapist does not value the patient's efforts. This makes it less likely that the patient will follow through on future assignments. Attention and praise from the therapist are probably the most important reinforcers for completing homework assignments, especially in the early stages of behavioral pattern-breaking.

A CASE ILLUSTRATION OF BEHAVIORAL PATTERN-BREAKING

Alec is a 35-year-old attorney. He was recently divorced from Kay after 7 years of marriage. Although he was unhappy in his marriage and had been struggling with a sexual attraction to a coworker, Alec was completely surprised when Kay told him she wanted a divorce. She would not tell him why she wanted the divorce other than to say she was unhappy. She refused his request to try marital therapy and moved out of the house that same day. The couple had no children. After a year's separation, their divorce was finalized, and Kay dropped out of his life entirely. A few months later, Alec came to therapy.

Alec's presenting problem was his difficulty initiating a relationship with a woman, particularly one that would lead to marriage and a family. He was finding it difficult to enter the dating scene. In addition, he did not understand why Kay had ended their marriage, nor why the woman he was attracted to at work refused to date him. He was obsessed with this woman and devoted a large part of each workday to thinking about her and trying to see her, so that his performance at work was steadily declining.

Alec is the youngest of three brothers. His mother died when he was 8 years old, and his grief-stricken father raised him. His brothers grew up and left home to go to college, leaving Alec to take care of his father. (He has felt estranged from his brothers ever since.) Outside of the home, Alec felt like a "social misfit." He excelled at his schoolwork but had trouble making friends. His grim life seemed so different from the seemingly care-free lives of the other children. Whereas they seemed to have happy homes, his home life was empty and bleak. His father was chronically depressed. Alec says, "My father slept most of the time, or watched television. He pretty much was in bed or on the couch. He never went out, wouldn't see anyone. And except to say, you know, 'Pass the salt,' he hardly ever spoke to me."

In the Assessment Phase of treatment, Alec and his therapist identify his schemas as Abandonment/Instability (from the death of his mother and the fact that his brothers left home); Emotional Deprivation (from his distant, apathetic father and unconcerned brothers); Social Isolation/Alienation (from his unusual home life that led him to feel different from peers); and Self-Sacrifice (from taking care of his father).

His primary coping style is schema avoidance: Early in life, he became a workaholic. He threw himself into his schoolwork and, later, into his law career; he is highly successful. He met Kay at law school and married her a few years later. Although he was not in love with her, she was steady and sensible, and he was afraid to face the world alone. Like his father, Kay was chronically depressed. Although Alec wanted children, she refused. Their life together was stable but monotonous and without passion. (Alec's marriage to Kay represented his surrender to his Emotional Deprivation schema. In his marriage to her, he replicated the emotionally vacant family life of his childhood.)

In recent years, Alec had become sexually attracted to Joan, his coworker. She flirted with him while he was still married, but she would not date him after his divorce. Although Alec asked her to go out with him a number of times, she always said no. Although Joan accepted gifts and favors from Alec, she clearly was not interested in him romantically, and he was having a great deal of trouble accepting this fact. When asked what was so alluring about Joan, Alec said: "When we're alone, she makes me feel like I'm the only one in the world. She's very intense and attentive. But when other people are around, she's distant." Alec finds Joan's inconsistency toward him exciting. The therapist speculates that Alec's attraction to Joan is schema-driven—that is, generated largely by his Abandonment/ Instability schema. In addition, it seems likely that Self-Sacrifice is a linked schema driving the attraction, as Alec has given a lot to Joan and gotten little in return.

Alec and his therapist agree that the first target of behavioral pattern-breaking should be his "Joan-centered" activities at work, such as daydreaming about her, calling her on the phone, thinking up e-mails to send her, grilling other people about her, looking for newspaper articles of interest to her and bringing them to her, and arranging to "accidentally" run into her. Alec was spending virtually his entire workday obsessed with these activities, even though the activities were torturous for him and he regretted them afterward. Moreover, as we have noted, his performance at work was seriously impaired.

The therapist begins by helping Alec link the target behavioral pattern to its origins in childhood. The therapist asks him to close his eyes and picture an image of being at work and missing Joan.

THERAPIST: What do you see?

ALEC: I see myself at work. I'm sitting at my desk. I'm trying to work, but I can't stop thinking about her. I know I should really concentrate on my work, but I want to see her. I want to give her this article I found, I know she'll be interested in it, it's about. . . .

THERAPIST: (*interrupting*) The part of you that wants to see her, what's that part saying?

ALEC: It's saying that I can't stand feeling this way.

THERAPIST: Can you get an image of when you felt this way as a child?

ALEC: Yes.

THERAPIST: What do you see?

ALEC: I see myself alone in bed as a child, crying for my mother. It was after she died. No matter how much I wanted her, she never came.

Missing Joan at work triggers Alec's Abandonment schema, evoking feelings connected to his mother's death. To escape these feelings, Alec goes in search of Joan. The therapist and Alec compose a flash card for Alec to read when his schema is triggered at work. Rather than seeking out Joan, the flash card advises him to give the child part of him a voice by writing out a dialogue between his Abandoned Child and Healthy Adult modes (Alec calls his Healthy Adult mode his "Good Mother.") If the Healthy Adult in Alec can partially meet the unmet emotional needs of the Abandoned Child, then his Vulnerable Child will not have to go in search of Joan to meet these needs.

To further prepare Alec for behavioral change, the therapist asks him to conduct a dialogue between the schema side, which wants him to stay focused on Joan, and his healthy side, which wants him to forget Joan, focus on his work, and attempt to meet new available women. Alec plays both sides, switching chairs to signify the change. As the excerpt starts, the therapist has asked Alec to imagine being at work, fighting the desire to look for Joan.

ALEC: (*as schema side*) "Go find her. When you're with her, it can feel so good. It feels so much better than anything has for such a long time. It's worth losing some work time—it may even be worth losing everything—to be with her one more time."

THERAPIST: OK, good, now play the healthy side.

ALEC: (*switching chairs*) OK. (*as healthy side*) "You're wrong. It won't feel good. It'll feel bad. Worse than anything you've felt for a long time. There's nothing there for you, except more loneliness."

THERAPIST: And now the schema side.

ALEC: (*switching chairs, as schema side*) "Do you know what your life's like without her? Well, I'll tell you. It's boring, that's what it is. There's nothing to look forward to. You're more dead than alive."

THERAPIST: And now the healthy side.

ALEC: (*switching chairs, as healthy side*) "No, you're wrong. It doesn't have to be that way. You could meet someone else, someone who returns your feelings."

The dialogue continues until Alec feels that the healthy side has defeated the schema side.

Alec's first homework assignment for behavioral pattern-breaking is to stop his "Joan-centered" activities, replacing them with reading his flash card and writing out dialogues. He has moderate success with this homework assignment. At his next session, he reports that he was able to stop many of the activities he was doing from his desk, such as calling and e-mailing Joan. However, although every morning Alec promised himself that he would not seek her out, by the end of almost every day, he had gone back on this promise and arranged some pretext for seeing her. The therapist helps Alec work through his block to changing this behavior. Alec lists the advantages and disadvantages of continuing to seek her out.

The main advantage is that, as long as he continues to see her, there is a chance he might win her over and get what he wants. The main disadvantage is that the behavior keeps him stuck in a place of hurt and loss.

Another behavior Alec and his therapist select for pattern-breaking is overworking. They agree that Alec should spend weekends engaged in activities through which he might meet available women, rather than working all weekend in his office, as was his usual custom. In the following excerpt, Alec and his therapist design a behavioral homework assignment with this purpose in mind.

THERAPIST: So what do you want the activity to be? Where might you meet a woman you'll like?

ALEC: I don't know. It's been so long since I've gone anywhere other than my office.

THERAPIST: Well, what would you want to spend the weekend doing?

ALEC: Besides working? (*Laughs.*)

THERAPIST: Yeah. (*Laughs also.*)

ALEC: Let's see, watching a game. Going to a bar and watching a game, maybe. But I'm not likely to meet anyone there.

THERAPIST: Anything else you'd like to do?

ALEC: Maybe bike riding. If it's nice out. . . .

THERAPIST: Where would you do that?

ALEC: I could go in the park.

THERAPIST: Would you like that?

ALEC: Yeah. I'd like it. Some people at work meet Saturday mornings to go riding together. I've never gone with them.

THERAPIST: Why not?

ALEC: I don't know, I feel funny.

THERAPIST: What does it remind you of? Can you connect that feeling back to childhood?

ALEC: Yeah. I used to stay in the classroom during recess and work instead of playing outside. It feels like that.

THERAPIST: Well, tell me, if you were to walk into that classroom as you are now, as an adult, and see your "child self" sitting there during recess while all the other children played outside, what would you say to the child?

ALEC: I would say, "Don't you want to go outside and play? Don't you want to be outside with the other children?"

THERAPIST: And what does the child answer?

ALEC: (*as child*) "Oh, I want to, but I feel like I don't belong."

THERAPIST: And what do you say back?

ALEC: (*as adult*) I say, "How about if I come with you? If the other kids got to know you, I'm sure they'd like you. I'll come with you and help you figure it out."

THERAPIST: And what does the child say?

ALEC: The child says, "OK."

THERAPIST: OK, now get an image of being at work, asking someone about the bike riding. What do you see?

ALEC: I go up to Larry at lunch, and I say, "Larry, I'm thinking about joining the bike ride this Saturday. Could you tell me the details?" That's all I'd have to do.

THERAPIST: How about doing that for homework?

ALEC: OK.

The patient writes out the homework assignment, with instructions to self-monitor thoughts, feelings, and behaviors. At the next session, Alec reports the results. The therapist praises Alec for doing the homework and displays interest in the outcome. In addition, the therapist reiterates the benefits of completing the assignment.

OVERCOMING BLOCKS TO BEHAVIORAL CHANGE

Changing schema-driven behaviors is difficult, and, despite a patient's desire to change, the process has many pitfalls. Early Maladaptive Schemas are deeply rooted and drive entire life patterns. They fight for survival in both obvious and subtle ways. We have developed several approaches to overcoming blocks to behavioral change.

Understand the Block

Once patients have made a commitment to behavioral pattern-breaking, they may still have difficulty initiating new behaviors. When patients do not follow through on behavioral homework assignments, the first step is to understand why. Is the patient aware of the nature of the block? Sometimes patients know what is blocking them from complying with the homework, and they can say it directly. If not, the therapist can ask questions. Is the patient afraid of the consequences of changing? Is the patient angry that change is necessary or so hard? Is the patient having trouble tolerating the discomfort or struggle involved in changing? Did the patient uncover beliefs or feelings that are difficult to overcome? Does the patient believe that a positive outcome is impossible? Although the patient and therapist have gone over the advantages and disadvantages of changing the behavior, the patient may have minimized the power of a deterrent, or a new deterrent may have arisen once the patient attempted to change.

If the patient cannot state what the block is, or the patient's answer appears implausible, then the therapist uses other methods to explore the nature of the block.

Imagery

In the previous chapter, we discussed the use of imagery for behavior change in considerable detail. Here we review some of those strategies to highlight their importance in behavioral pattern-breaking.

The therapist can use imagery to investigate the block. The therapist asks the patient to visualize the problematic situation and to describe what happens when he or she attempts the new behavior. The therapist and patient explore the point at which the patient becomes stuck. What is the patient thinking and feeling at that moment? What are the other "characters" thinking and feeling? What does the patient want to do? In this way, the therapist and patient can often discern the nature of the block.

The therapist can use imagery in other ways. For example, the therapist might ask the patient to imagine carrying out the new behavior and investigate what happens afterward. Does the patient feel guilty or incur the wrath of a family member? Does the patient foresee some dreadful outcome? Alternatively, the therapist can ask the patient to picture an image of the block and imagine pushing through it. For example, the block might look like a dark weight pressing down on the patient. On questioning, the patient reveals that the block conveys the same message as a pessimistic parent. The patient pushes this message away by pushing away the block. Or the therapist might tie the moment of the block back to childhood by asking the patient to picture an image of feeling the same way as a child. The therapist can then use the opportunity to reparent the patient's Vulnerable Child. Thus imagery can be used both to discover the nature of blocks and to overcome them.

Dialogues between the Block and the Healthy Side

The therapist can help the patient conduct dialogues between the side of the patient that wants to avoid the new behavior and the side that is willing to try the new behavior. The patient can conduct the dialogue in imagery or role-play the two sides by switching chairs. The therapist coaches the healthy side when necessary.

The therapist works to identify the mode that is blocking change. It could be a child mode, too timid or furious to attempt change. Or it could be a Maladaptive Coping mode, tempting the patient to resort to the old maladaptive coping behavior. Or it could be a Dysfunctional Parent mode, breaking the patient's spirit by punishing the patient or demanding too much. Once the therapist knows which mode is interfering with the new behavior, he or she can start a dialogue with this mode and try to resolve its specific concerns. We discuss this kind of mode work in later chapters.

Flash Cards

The therapist and patient can write a flash card addressing the block. In the flash card, they fight the relevant schemas and maladaptive coping styles. For example, if the patient's block consists of anger, the flash card might read: "Right now I feel too angry to practice being less aggressive in my close relationships, as I agreed to do in my therapy sessions." The flash card summarizes the advantages and disadvantages of continuing the maladaptive coping style, spells out the healthy behavior, and provides solutions to practical problems. For anger, the flash card could suggest self-control techniques: "I'll take slow, deep breaths until I feel calm, and then I'll envision doing the healthy behavior." Reading the flash card gives the patient the opportunity to work through the anger before responding in the situation.

Reassign the Homework

Once the therapist and patient have identified the block and attempted to work through it, then the patient tries the new behavior again as a homework assignment. The therapist may consider reducing the difficulty of the assignment or breaking the assignment into smaller, graduated steps. If, after reassigning the homework, the patient is still unable to comply, the therapist may shift the focus to another behavioral pattern and come back to this one later. However, it is important for the therapist not to become sidetracked in the pursuit of behavioral change. Whatever happens, the therapist continues to use empathic confrontation to push for behavioral change. Sometimes it can be quite challenging for the therapist to keep empathically confronting the patient's difficulty in making behavioral changes.

Contingencies

If the preceding strategies do not work, the therapist can consider setting contingencies that reward the new behavior. For example, patients could reward themselves for carrying out the new behavior as part of the homework assignment. What serves as a reward varies from patient to patient, depending on what the patient views as pleasurable. Some possibilities include buying oneself a small gift, engaging in a fun activity or doing something self-nurturing. One especially powerful reinforcer for many patients is calling the therapist and leaving a message on the answering machine reporting that the homework is complete.

If the patient seems unalterably resistant to behavioral change over a long period of time, the ultimate contingency is for the therapist to suggest a break from therapy. For example, the therapist might introduce the idea of a time-limited effort: The therapist and patient decide how much longer to work on behavioral change, and, if no change is forthcoming during that period, they agree to cease therapy temporarily. The therapist lets the patient know that therapy can resume as soon as the patient is ready to attempt behavioral change. The therapist presents this as an issue of "readiness"—the therapist will wait for the patient to signal readiness for change. This is an extreme measure for the therapist to take and is meant for extremely resistant cases. Sometimes patients are simply not ready to change. They need time to pass or life circumstances to change before risking new behaviors. Sometimes they need to experience a greater level of distress. Staying stuck must feel worse than changing before some patients can summon enough motivation to change.

It is important to point out that we carefully weigh whether there are other benefits of remaining in therapy—such as reparenting a patient with BPD—that might outweigh the absence of behavioral change. Thus we sometimes continue treatment for a considerable period of time without behavioral change if there is a compelling rationale for doing so with a particular patient.

The therapist could introduce the idea of a time-limited effort followed by a break as follows:

> "I think you're trying very hard, but your schemas are very powerful. Perhaps at this point we've gone about as far as we can go in terms of change. Sometimes life events occur that enable people to change their behavior. How would you feel about this idea: We could continue to meet for one more month to see if you're able to make any changes. If not, we could discontinue meeting for a while, and you could call me when you feel ready to resume treatment and work on these behavioral changes. What do you think about this as a possible plan?"

Case Illustrations

Spencer: A Conflict of Modes

Spencer is 31 years old. He has come to therapy because he is dissatisfied with his job. Although he has a master's degree in fine arts, since leaving school he has held a job as a graphic designer that is far below his level of competence. Although he feels bored and unappreciated at his job, he finds himself unable to look for other work. No job seems quite right: Either the job does not seem good enough or he does not feel qualified enough. In the Assessment Phase, Spencer identifies his Defectiveness and Failure schemas. He goes through the cognitive and experiential stages of treatment and undertakes behavioral change. Week after week, he is unable to carry through with behavioral homework assignments. Time passes, and he stays frozen where he is. However, something unexpected happens: Spencer loses his job. Even though he finds his financial reserves dwindling, he is still unable to look actively for work. His survival is threatened.

The therapist theorizes that Spencer's paralysis points to a conflict in modes. When patients must take steps to ensure their very survival, yet still find themselves unable to act, then conflicting modes is a likely hypothesis. The therapist helps Spencer identify the two modes locked in conflict: the Defective Child, who feels too helpless and hopeless to proceed, and the Healthy Adult, who wants to find more fulfilling work. Conducting dialogues between these two modes helps Spencer resolve the conflict. The Healthy Adult assuages the fears of the Vulnerable Child and promises to handle whatever difficulties arise.

Rina: When the Patient Lacks Motivation to Change

Patients feel at one with their Early Maladaptive Schemas: Their schemas are part of who they are. They believe in the truth of their schemas to such an extent that many times they cannot grasp the possibility of change. In some cases, the patient has not yet gotten sufficiently angry at the schema. In other cases, such as often happens with patients with narcissistic personality disorder, the disadvantages of the dysfunctional behaviors are not sufficiently motivating. Many narcissistic behaviors upset significant others far more than they upset the patients themselves, and patients are not motivated to change until a significant other does something drastic, such as threatening to end the relationship. The therapist addresses this problem by emphasizing the long-term negative consequences of maintaining the narcissistic behavior.

Rina has an Entitlement schema. Having been spoiled as a child, she believes she deserves special treatment. Among the privileges she accords to herself but not to others is to explode in anger whenever she does not get her way. She comes to therapy because her fiancé, Mitch, is threatening to call off their engagement unless she learns to control her temper. Rina experiences difficulty carrying through on behavioral homework assignments. For example, she and the therapist agree that she will take a "time out" when she is about to lose her temper with Mitch, but each time she decides that what she wants in that instance is more important. "I want what I want," she says, and "giving in just isn't me." Hence, she continues to lose her temper. Rina does not have an Insufficient Self-Control/Self-Discipline schema, because the problem of self-control only arises when she cannot get her own way.

The therapist helps her overcome her block. Rina lists the advantages and disadvantages of continuing to lose her temper. She conducts dialogues between her healthy side and her entitled side. She and the therapist compose a flash card reminding her why it is important to learn to control her temper: She is endangering her relationship with Mitch every time she loses control of her anger, and keeping Mitch is more important to her than momentarily getting her way. Rina practices controlling her anger in imagery and role-plays. She gradually learns to control her anger and express herself more appropriately in her relationship with Mitch.

MAKING MAJOR LIFE CHANGES

Even when patients successfully change their behaviors, a problematic situation may remain painful and destructive. In such cases, patients may decide that major life changes are necessary, such as changing schools or jobs, finding new careers, moving to new places, disengaging from family members or friends, or ending romantic relationships. The therapist provides support as patients choose the path that is right for them.

When patients contemplate leaving a problematic situation, it is important for the therapist to determine whether their reasons for leaving are healthy or schema-driven. Schema-driven reasons are usually forms of avoidance or overcompensation. For example, a young male patient named Jim decides to leave his job in the financial district and move to the beach. Although this move is financially possible for him, on reflection he realizes that it is driven by his Subjugation schema. The move represents both schema avoidance and overcompensation: By moving, Jim could avoid facing conflicts with his clients and coworkers, and he could overcompensate for his schema by doing what *he* wants to do. Jim concedes that, if he did not have the conflicts with clients and coworkers, he would want to remain at his job.

Whenever patients introduce life changes that appear drastic or sudden, the therapist should assess the situation carefully. The "flight to health" noted in the psychotherapy literature is probably schema overcompensation. Even if their behaviors look healthy, patients may be behaving in an uncharacteristic manner without sufficient preparation. In such cases, the therapist empathically confronts the schema avoidance and overcompensation.

If the change the patient proposes does not seem to be a manifestation of avoidance or overcompensation, the next step is to explore alternative courses of action. The therapist and patient list the advantages and disadvantages of each alternative and then evaluate which is best. The therapist asks, "If you didn't have your schemas, what would you do?" This question helps patients identify the right course. In addition, the therapist and patient weigh the advantages and disadvantages of changing versus not changing. Sometimes the decision rests on pragmatic considerations. Can the patient afford the change financially? Is the patient likely to find another, better job? Will the patient find a more satisfying relationship? Can the person obtain the necessary resources to carry out the change?

The therapist helps patients prepare for the challenges of major life changes. These include such potential hardships as tolerating frustration and disappointment, dealing with the disapproval of significant others, and grappling with unanticipated problems.

SUMMARY

In the behavioral pattern-breaking stage of treatment, patients attempt to replace schema-driven patterns of behavior with more adaptive patterns. The behavior patterns that are the focus of change are the maladaptive coping styles patients use when their schemas are triggered. These maladaptive coping styles are generally surrender, avoidance, or overcompensation, although each Early Maladaptive Schema has its own characteristic coping responses.

Behavioral pattern-breaking begins with defining specific behaviors as possible targets of change. The therapist and patient accomplish this in a number of ways: (1) refining the case conceptualization they developed in the Assessment Phase; (2) developing detailed descriptions of problematic behaviors; (3) conducting imagery about trigger events; (4) exploring the therapy relationship; (5) obtaining reports from significant others; and (6) reviewing the schema inventories.

Next, the therapist and patient prioritize behaviors for pattern-breaking. We believe that it is important for patients to attempt to change behaviors within a current life situation before making major life changes. Unlike traditional cognitive-behavioral therapy, patients begin with the most problematic behavior they are able to tackle.

In order to build motivation for behavioral change, the therapist helps the patient link the target behavior to its origins in childhood. The therapist and patient review the advantages and disadvantages of continuing the behavior. They develop a flash card that summarizes the main points. In sessions, the therapist and patient rehearse the healthy behavior in imagery and role-plays. They agree on a behavioral homework assignment. The patient carries out the homework, and the therapist and patient discuss the results thoroughly in the next session.

We make several suggestions for overcoming blocks to behavioral change. First, the therapist and patient develop a concept of the block. The block is usually a mode, and the therapist and patient can ally in facing this mode. The patient conducts dialogues between the block and the healthy side. The therapist and patient compose a flash card for the patient to read. If, after reassigning the homework, the patient is still unable to comply, then the therapist can set contingencies for not completing behavioral homework assignments.

Chapter 6

THE THERAPY RELATIONSHIP

The schema therapist views the therapy relationship as a vital component of schema assessment and change. Two features of the therapy relationship are characteristic of schema therapy: the therapeutic stance of *empathic confrontation* and the use of *limited reparenting*. Empathic confrontation—or empathic reality-testing—involves expressing understanding of the reasons that patients perpetuate their schemas while simultaneously confronting the necessity for change. Limited reparenting involves providing, within the appropriate boundaries of the therapy relationship, what patients needed but did not get from their parents as children.

This chapter describes the therapy relationship in schema therapy. We focus on how the therapy relationship is helpful first in the assessment of schemas and coping styles and second as an agent of change.

THE THERAPY RELATIONSHIP IN THE ASSESSMENT AND EDUCATION PHASE

In the Assessment and Education Phase, the therapy relationship is a powerful means to assess schemas and to educate the patient. The therapist establishes rapport, formulates the case conceptualization, decides what style of limited reparenting is appropriate for the patient, and determines whether the therapist's own schemas are likely to interfere with therapy.

The Therapist Establishes Rapport

As in other forms of psychotherapy, the therapy relationship begins with establishing rapport with the patient. The therapist strives to embody the empathy, warmth, and genuineness identified by Rogers (1951) as the nonspecific factors of effective therapy. The goal is to create an environment that is accepting and safe, in which the patient can form an emotional bond with the therapist.

Schema therapists are personal rather than detached and aloof, in their manner of relating to patients. They try not to appear as though they are perfect, nor as though they have knowledge they are withholding from the patient. They let their natural personalities come through. They share their emotional responses when they believe it will have a positive effect on the patient. They self-disclose when it will help the patient. They aim for a stance of objectivity and compassion.

Schema therapists ask patients for feedback about themselves and the treatment. They encourage patients to express negative feelings about therapy so that these feelings do not build up and create distance and resistance. The goal in responding to negative comments is to listen without becoming defensive and to try to understand the situation from the patient's point of view. (Of course, the therapist does not let the patient behave abusively—by yelling or making personal attacks—without setting limits.) To the extent that the patient's negative feedback is a schema-driven distortion, the therapist attempts to acknowledge the kernel of truth while helping the patient identify and fight the schema through empathic confrontation. To the extent that the patient's negative feedback is accurate, the therapist acknowledges mistakes and apologizes.

Schema therapy is an approach that finds what is healthy and supports it. The basic model is one of empowering the patient. The therapist forms an alliance with the patient's healthy side against the patient's schemas. The ultimate goal of treatment is to strengthen the patient's Healthy Adult mode.

The Therapist Formulates the Case Conceptualization

The therapy relationship illuminates the patient's (and the therapist's) schemas and coping styles. When one of the patient's schemas is triggered in the therapy relationship, the therapist helps the patient identify the schema. The therapist and patient explore what happened—what actions of the therapist triggered the schema and what the patient thought, felt, and did. What was the patient's coping response? Was the style one of surrender, avoidance, or overcompensation? The therapist uses imagery to help the patient link the incident to childhood—so that the patient realizes who it was in childhood that promulgated the schema—and to current life problems.

When the therapy relationship triggers one of the patient's Early Maladaptive Schemas, then the situation is similar to Freud's concept of transference: The patient is responding to the therapist as though the therapist were a significant figure from the patient's past, usually a parent. In schema therapy, however, the therapist discusses the patient's schemas and coping styles openly and directly, rather than tacitly working through the patient's "transference neurosis" (Freud, 1917/1963).

Case Illustration

We present an excerpt from an interview Dr. Young conducted with Daniel, a patient discussed in previous chapters. At the time of the interview, Daniel had been in schema therapy with another therapist, named Leon, for approximately 9 months. Daniel's Mistrust/Abuse, Defectiveness, and Subjugation schemas had already been identified. He typically utilized schema avoidance as his coping style.

During the session, the therapist leads Daniel through a number of imagery exercises. In the final 20 minutes of the interview, Dr. Young asks Daniel about his therapeutic relationship with Leon. Next, Dr. Young explores whether Daniel's schemas were triggered during the current interview. The therapist begins by asking Daniel about his Mistrust/Abuse schema.

DR. YOUNG: When you first started working with your therapist, Leon, did you feel mistrust toward him?

DANIEL: I've always felt trusting and accepted by Leon. I get irritated at times when he tries to force me to get away from my avoidance, because in therapy I avoid even talking about some of these things. So he tries to get me back on the track, and sometimes that bothers me, but I know that I'm wasting my time when I just ramble on about other things. He tries to get me to do the work at hand.

Next, the therapist asks about Daniel's Subjugation schema.

DR. YOUNG: Do you ever feel controlled by Leon, like he's pushing you and trying to control you. . . .

DANIEL: Yes.

DR. YOUNG: Because one of the schemas here (*points to the Young Schema Questionnaire*) is Subjugation. . . .

DANIEL: Yes.

Dr. Young moves on to his own relationship with Daniel. He inquires whether Daniel's schemas were triggered during the interview. He begins by asking about Subjugation.

DR. YOUNG: Did you feel that at all in here—the issue of my trying to control you?

DANIEL: No.

DR. YOUNG: There was nothing that irritated you at all or set you off . . .

DANIEL: Well, when you were *forcing* the imagery, even though it seemed to go smoother than it normally does, I resisted, because I felt a little controlled, like you were telling me what to do.

DR. YOUNG: I see. And did you feel angry or irritated with me?

DANIEL: Irritated.

DR. YOUNG: How did you override that? How did you keep going? Did you just ignore it, or. . . .

DANIEL: Um, it seemed to have a natural flow to it, so, even though there was a momentary feeling of irritation, it seemed to flow.

DR. YOUNG: So, once you could see that you could do it, the resistance was gone.

DANIEL: Yeah.

DR. YOUNG: But there was an initial resistance. . . .

DANIEL: And even a lack of faith in my ability to bring up the images.

DR. YOUNG: So it's two things. One is feeling insecure that you can do it, the other is feeling that I'm controlling you.

DANIEL: Yes.

The therapist asks Daniel about other times his Subjugation and Defectiveness schemas were triggered during the session.

DR. YOUNG: Were there any other times during the session that you felt I controlled you, or that you wondered whether you could do it well enough?

DANIEL: During the time that you were trying to get me to think of images at the social setting and get to feel some of the feelings involved. It seemed hard for me to drum that up, to put into words.

DR. YOUNG: And you felt insecure, or you felt controlled, or both?

DANIEL: Um, a little of both.

DR. YOUNG: If you could have expressed the irritated side of you at the time, what would it have said? Could you be the irritated side, just so I can hear what it would say?

DANIEL: (*as the "irritated side," speaking disdainfully*) "I don't like to be forced into this silly little game we're playing here."

DR. YOUNG: And what would the other side say? The healthy side . . . ?

DANIEL: Um, it would say that (*as the "healthy side"*) "This is important stuff, it's important for your growth as a person to face your fears and face the things that are unpleasant, so that you might overcome them."

DR. YOUNG: And what does the schema side say back to that?

DANIEL: (*as the "schema side," speaking coldly*) "That's a bunch of baloney, because it's not going to work anyway. Obviously, you haven't been too successful up to now, and who's to say it's going to be any more successful after this? And besides, who's he to tell you what you need or what you need to do?"

The therapist makes explicit that Daniel's Mistrust/Abuse schema has also been operating in their relationship during the session, along with his Defectiveness and Subjugation schemas.

DR. YOUNG: Also, in the way you said, "silly little game," there was a sense that I might be manipulating you, if I heard it right. Was there an element of feeling manipulated in that?

DANIEL: Yeah.

DR. YOUNG: Like it was a *game*. What would the game have been? Be the suspicious part of you for a second. . . .

DANIEL: The game would be artificially creating a social scene, which is not real.

DR. YOUNG: Was it as if it was for my benefit rather than for yours, or somehow it was to hurt you?

DANIEL: To uncover me.

DR. YOUNG: To expose you?

DANIEL: Yes.

DR. YOUNG: In a way that wasn't going to help?

DANIEL: Yes. In a way that would hurt me by exposing me.

DR. YOUNG: Almost like humiliating you.

DANIEL: Yes.

The therapist links what Daniel felt during the session to other encounters in his life.

DR. YOUNG: So there was almost a momentary sense, when I started to ask you to do some imagery work, that I might be trying to expose you and humiliate you, even though it was just a fleeting feeling.

DANIEL: Yes.

DR. YOUNG: And then you were able to override that and say, "No, it's for my own good," but there's still that part of you. . . .

DANIEL: Yes.

DR. YOUNG: And that's what you're having to deal with every day when you meet women or meet people, that schema side of you, that even in a few seconds mistrusts or feels controlled or feels insecure, and you're not always sure how to respond to it.

DANIEL: Yes.

This excerpt provides a good example of how the therapist can utilize the therapy relationship to educate patients about their schemas. In addition, it is noteworthy that Dr. Young specifically asked the patient about whether his schemas were triggered in the therapy relationship. The patient would not have raised the subject without direct questioning on the therapist's part.

There are typical session behaviors for each schema. For example, patients who have Entitlement schemas might ask for extra time or special consideration in scheduling appointments; patients who have Self-Sacrifice schemas might try to take care of the therapist; patients who have Unrelenting Standards schemas might criticize the therapist for minor errors. The patient's behavior with the therapist suggests hypotheses about the patient's behavior with significant others. The same schemas and coping styles that the patient exhibits with the therapist probably appear in other relationships outside the therapy.

The Therapist Assesses the Patient's Reparenting Needs

Another task the therapist faces in the Assessment and Education Phase is assessing the patient's reparenting needs. Throughout treatment, the therapist will use the therapy relationship as a partial antidote to the patient's schemas. This "limited reparenting" provides a "corrective emotional experience" (Alexander & French, 1946) specifically designed to counteract the patient's Early Maladaptive Schemas.

The therapist uses a variety of sources to ascertain the patient's reparenting needs: childhood history, reports of interpersonal difficulties, questionnaires, and imagery exercises. Sometimes the richest source of information is the patient's behavior in the therapy relationship. Whatever sheds light on the patient's schemas and coping styles supplies clues about the patient's reparenting needs.

Case Illustration

Jasmine is a young woman who begins therapy wary of becoming "dependent" on the therapist. She tells her therapist that she has just started college and is accustomed to making her own decisions without relying on her parents or anyone else for guidance. She does not want that to change. In the first few weeks of therapy, it becomes apparent that Jasmine's core schema is Emotional Deprivation as a result of her childhood with emotionally cold parents who shamed her when she asked for help. "They expected me to deal with my problems by myself," she says. Guidance is exactly what Jasmine needs from her therapist—it is one of her unmet emotional needs. For Jasmine, limited reparenting involves giving her some of the guidance she never got from her parents as a child. Recognizing her Emotional Deprivation schema helps the therapist know what form of reparenting she needs. (One of the barriers to reparenting Jasmine will be to help her accept help and caring, as she has learned that it is shameful to do so.)

Had Jasmine's therapist taken her at her word and viewed her problem as one of preserving her independence, the therapist might have refrained from giving her the guidance she needed. Jasmine was not too dependent. Rather, she had never been permitted to be dependent enough. Emotionally, she had always been alone. By reparenting her in accord with her core Early Maladaptive Schema, the therapist could help her recognize that her dependency needs were normal and that establishing autonomy was a gradual process.

Ideal Therapist Qualities in Schema Therapy

Flexibility is a key feature of the ideal schema therapist. Because the type of limited reparenting required depends on each patient's unique childhood history, therapists must adjust their styles to fit the emotional needs of the individual patient. For example, depending on the patient's schemas, the therapist has to focus on generating trust, providing stability, giving emotional nurturance, encouraging independence, or demonstrating forgiveness. The therapist must be able to provide in the therapy relationship whatever is a partial antidote to the patient's core Early Maladaptive Schemas.

Like a good parent, the schema therapist is capable of partially meeting—within the limits of the therapy relationship—the patient's basic emotional needs we described in Chapter 1: (1) secure attachment; (2) autonomy and competence; (3) genuine self-expression of needs and emotions; (4) spontaneity and play; and (5) realistic limits. The goal is for the patient to internalize a Healthy Adult mode, modeled after the therapist, that can fight schemas and inspire healthy behavior.

Case Illustration

Lily is 52 years old, and her children are grown and out of the house. She has an Emotional Deprivation schema. As a child, no one connected with her emotionally. She became increasingly withdrawn, preferring to study or play her violin rather than interact with others. She had few friends, and they were not really close. Lily has been married to her husband, Joseph, for 30 years. She has lost interest in her marriage and spends most of her time at home isolated with her books and her music. In the Assessment Phase, Lily and the therapist agree that her core schema is Emotional Deprivation and that her main coping style is avoidance.

As the weeks pass, Lily begins to have sexual feelings for her male therapist. She becomes aware of how emotionally empty her life is. No longer satisfied to read and play music alone, she begins to want more. Alarmed and ashamed of her needs, she copes by withdrawing psychologically from the therapist. The therapist observes her withdrawal. He theorizes that her Emotional Deprivation schema has been triggered in the therapy relationship and that she is responding with schema avoidance. Knowing her core schema and main coping style points the way to understanding for the therapist.

The therapist points out Lily's withdrawal and helps her explore it. Although not able to talk about her sexual feelings, she is able to say that she is experiencing feelings of caring for the therapist and that this is making her extremely uncomfortable. She has not really cared about anybody for a long time. The therapist asks Lily to close her eyes and link the feeling of discomfort with him to times in the past that she had similar feelings. She connects the feeling first to her husband in the early days of their marriage and then to her father when she was a child. She remembers walking home from school and seeing a little boy run into his father's arms and feeling a wave of longing to do the same with her own remote father. In her memory, Lily went up to her room when she got home and spent the rest of the day practicing her violin.

The therapist helps Lily see the schema-driven distortion in her view of the therapy relationship. Unlike her father, the therapist welcomes her feelings of caring (when they are expressed within the appropriate limits of the therapy relationship). In the therapy relationship, she is allowed to care and to want caring; the therapist will not reject her for it. She is allowed to talk about her feelings directly and does not have to withdraw. Although this kind of communication was not possible with her father, it is possible with the therapist and, by implication, with other people in the world. (We encourage patients to verbalize sexual feelings to the therapist as well, although we gently, in a nonrejecting way, indicate that acting on these feelings with the therapist is not possible. We emphasize that patients can eventually share these same feelings with someone in their lives who will be in a position to respond in kind)

When a patient engages in behaviors during the session that reflect overcompensation, the schema therapist responds objectively and appropriately, utilizing empathic confrontation. The therapist expresses understanding of the reasons for the patient behaving in such a way but points out the consequences of the behavior in the therapy relationship and in the patient's outside life. The following example illustrates this process.

Case Illustration

Jeffrey is 41 years old. He comes to therapy because Josie, his girlfriend of 10 years, has broken up with him. He is realizing that, this time, he is not going to get her back. Throughout their relationship, Jeffrey repeatedly cheated on Josie. She would break up with him, he would beg for her forgiveness and promise to reform, and she would take him back. But no more. Consequently, Jeffrey has fallen into a major depression.

Jeffrey has narcissistic personality disorder, a personality type that is discussed much more fully in Chapter 10. His core schema is Defectiveness, and his primary coping style is schema overcompensation. In his relationships with women, Jeffrey overcompensates for his feelings of defectiveness by winning them over sexually. Even though he loved Josie as much as he was capable of, he was not able to give up cheating on her (a major source of narcissistic gratification).

Jeffrey overcompensates in the therapy relationship by getting angry whenever the therapist evokes feelings of vulnerability. He is uncomfortable being vulnerable with the therapist because of his Defectiveness schema: Being vulnerable causes him to feel ashamed and exposed. In one session, Jeffrey relates a childhood incident concerning himself and his emotionally rejecting mother (from whom Jeffrey is currently estranged). The therapist comments that, based on this incident, it seems that Jeffrey loved his mother, even though he was angry with her as a child. Jeffrey lashes out at the therapist, calling him a "momma's boy." In a serious tone, the therapist leans forward and asks Jeffrey why he just lashed out like that. What was he feeling underneath? When Jeffrey denies feeling anything underneath, the therapist suggests that Jeffrey may have felt vulnerable. "I understand," says the therapist. "As a child you loved your mother. I loved my mother as a child, too. It's natural for children to love their mothers. It's not a sign of weakness or inadequacy." The therapist communicates that Jeffrey does not have to feel inferior to anyone, including the therapist, for loving his mother. Next, the therapist conveys that Jeffrey's overcompensation—lashing out at the therapist—has the effect of making the therapist want to pull away from Jeffrey, instead of giving him the understanding that he needs.

Schema therapists can also tolerate and contain a patient's strong affect—including panic, rage, and grief—and provide appropriate validation. They have realistic expectations of the patient. They can set limits on their own behavior and on the patient's behavior. They can handle therapeutic crises appropriately. They can maintain appropriate boundaries between themselves and the patient, neither too distant nor too close.

Another task of the therapist in the Assessment Phase is to determine whether his or her own schemas and coping styles have the potential to be destructive to the therapeutic relationship.

The Therapist's Own Schemas and Coping Styles

Ted comes to his first therapy session saying he wants help in his career as a broker in the financial district. He wants to develop the focus and discipline he believes are necessary for him to succeed. Ted is friendly and talkative. He tells amusing stories about his life. He compliments the therapist and does not complain, even when the therapist mispronounces his last name twice. The therapist feels it is all "too much": Ted is too friendly, too talkative, too complimentary. (This sense of "too muchness" is often a sign of schema overcompensation.) Instead of feeling warm and close to Ted as one might expect with a friendly person, the therapist feels taken aback. The therapist hypothesizes that underneath Ted's amiable style is an Early Maladaptive Schema. As the weeks progress, it becomes clear that the therapist's hypothesis is correct. Underneath Ted's friendliness, he feels insecure and alone. He has a Social Isolation schema, for which he overcompensates with "hyperfriendliness."

The therapist's reactions to the patient can be a valuable resource in assessing the patient's schemas. However, therapists must be able to distinguish their valid intuition about a patient from the triggering of their own schemas. Early in therapy, it is important for therapists to become aware of their schemas in regard to the individual patient. Knowledge of one's own schemas and coping styles can help therapists avoid mistakes. Therapists can ask themselves basic questions about the patient. Does the therapist genuinely care about the patient? If not, why not? Is working with the patient triggering any of the therapist's schemas? Which ones? How is the therapist coping? Is the therapist doing anything that is potentially damaging to the patient? How would the therapist feel about doing imagery work with the patient? How would the therapist feel about dealing with the patient's raw emotions, such as panic, rage, and grief? Can the therapist empathically confront the patient's schemas as they appear? Can the therapist provide the kind of limited reparenting the patient needs?

In the following pages, we provide several examples of scenarios in which the therapist's schemas have a negative impact on the therapy relationship. Each example is followed by one or more case illustrations.

1. *The patient's schemas clash with the therapist's schemas.* One risk is that the patient's schemas might clash with the therapist's schemas in such a way that they trigger each other in a self-perpetuating loop. Here are some examples of schema clashes between therapist and patient.

Case Illustration

Maddie has a core Emotional Deprivation schema. She copes with her schema by becoming overly demanding; that is, she overcompensates through her Entitlement schema.

Maddie begins therapy with a male therapist with a Subjugation schema. Maddie is a demanding patient in many ways. She calls frequently between sessions, keeps changing her appointment time, and makes other requests for special treatment. The therapist accedes to her demands, his Subjugation schema preventing him from setting limits. Inwardly he feels a burgeoning sense of resentment. In sessions with Maddie, he becomes distant and withdrawn (employing a coping style of schema avoidance). This further triggers Maddie's Emotional Deprivation schema, and she becomes even more demanding; the therapist's Subjugation schema becomes reactivated, and so on, in a reciprocal triggering of schemas with the potential to demolish the therapeutic alliance.

If the therapist recognizes that his Subjugation schema is being triggered in his sessions with Maddie and preventing him from responding to her therapeutically, then he can work to correct the problem. He can set appropriate limits and transform his maladaptive coping response of avoidance into one of empathic confrontation. He can tell Maddie he understands that, underneath, she feels emotionally deprived in her relationship with him, just as she did in childhood; nevertheless, the way she is expressing her feelings is having the opposite effect from the one she wants. It is making it more difficult for the therapist to give her the nurturance she needs.

Case Illustration

An older male patient, Kenneth, has an Unrelenting Standards schema, and his younger female therapist has a Defectiveness schema (resulting from her childhood with her critical father). When the therapist makes even a minor mistake, Kenneth devalues her. "I'm really disappointed in you," he tells her sternly, triggering her Defectiveness schema and making her blush.

Depending on the therapist's coping style, at that moment her performance as a therapist becomes impaired by schema surrender, avoidance, or overcompensation. She either denigrates herself (schema surrender), retreats from the issue by changing the subject (schema avoidance),
or becomes defensive and blaming (schema overcompensation). Noticing
any of these "imperfect" behaviors further triggers Kenneth's Unrelenting
Standards schema, provoking him to disparage her more, and so on.
Eventually, convinced of the therapist's ineptitude, Kenneth leaves therapy.

Case Illustration

Alana, a younger female patient, begins therapy with an older female therapist. Alana has a Mistrust/Abuse schema, which began in childhood as a
result of contacts with her sexually abusive uncle. Her main coping style is
schema surrender: She repeatedly assumes a victim role with others. Her
therapist has a Subjugation schema. As a therapist, her main coping style is
overcompensation. She dominates patients in order to cope with underlying feelings of being overly controlled in other areas of her life, such as her
marriage and family of origin.

As therapy progresses, Alana assumes an increasingly passive role,
and the therapist increasingly comes to dominate her. The therapist gets
pleasure from controlling Alana, and Alana, who never learned how to resist, submits to whatever the therapist demands. The therapist unknowingly uses Alana to reduce her own feelings of subjugation, ultimately reinforcing Alana's Mistrust/Abuse schema.

Numerous variations of schema clashes arise in the therapy relationship. The patient might have a Dependence schema and the therapist a
Self-Sacrifice schema. The therapist does too much for the patient, maintaining the patient's dependence. Alternatively, the patient might have a
Failure schema and the therapist an Unrelenting Standards schema. The
therapist has unrealistic expectations of what the patient should accomplish, subtly communicates impatience, and confirms the patient's sense of
failure. Or the patient might adopt an obsessive and controlling coping
style in order to overcompensate for an underlying Negativity/Pessimism
schema, whereas the therapist has an Insufficient Self-Control/Self-
Discipline schema. The therapist appears disorganized and impulsive,
causing the patient to worry. The patient eventually leaves therapy even
more demoralized and downcast.

2. *A mismatch exists between the patient's needs and the therapist's
schemas or coping styles.* The patient might have needs that the therapist is
not able to meet. Because of the therapist's own schemas or coping styles,
the therapist cannot give the patient the right kind of reparenting. (Often

the therapist resembles the parent who originally engendered the schema in the patient.) Here are several examples.

Case Illustration

Neil enters therapy for depression and marital problems. Although it is not immediately apparent, Neil's core schema is Emotional Deprivation, based on his childhood with neglectful, self-involved parents and his marriage to a self-involved woman. It is Neil's emotional deprivation that is keeping him depressed. In terms of limited reparenting, Neil needs caring and empathy from his therapist.

Unfortunately, his therapist has an Emotional Inhibition schema and is unable to provide emotional warmth. As therapy progresses, Neil, now emotionally deprived by his therapist as well, becomes even more depressed.

Case Illustration

Edward has a Dependence/Incompetence schema. Rather than going to college after graduating from high school 6 years ago, Edward went to work for his domineering father, who owns a successful textile business. His father makes all the business decisions, and, as he had done before Edward came to work for him, he exerts a large influence on Edward's personal life.

Edward enters therapy for help with his chronically high anxiety. Even the small decisions he makes on his own torment him. Faced with a decision, he becomes frozen with anxiety and usually opts to reduce the anxiety by consulting his father.

In terms of reparenting, Edward needs a therapist who will promote gradually increasing levels of autonomy. However, Edward's therapist has an Enmeshment schema and becomes overly involved. Edward ends up weaning himself from his father's input, only to become dependent on the therapist.

Case Illustration

Max has an Insufficient Self-Control/Self-Discipline schema. He comes to therapy because his schema is holding him back in his career as a journalist. Because he is generally not accountable for his time, Max is having trouble getting his stories done. He needs a therapist who will confront him empathically and provide structure.

Max begins therapy with a female therapist who has a Subjugation schema in regard to men based on her childhood with her strict father. When she did something "bad" as a child, her father often flew into an uncontrolled rage. As with her father, the therapist assumes an avoidant coping style with Max. When Max fails to follow through on homework assignments or drifts away from difficult session material, she keeps quiet. In order to avoid conflict, she fails to confront him and set limits. She cannot give him the structure he needs and thus perpetuates, rather than heals, his schema.

3. *Overidentification takes place when the patient's and therapist's schemas overlap.* If the patient and therapist have the same schema, the therapist might overidentify with the patient and lose objectivity. The therapist colludes with the patient in reinforcing the schema.

Case Illustration

Richie, the patient, and his female therapist both have Abandonment schemas. Richie's parents divorced when he was 5 years old. He stayed with his father, and his mother became a distant figure in his life. He comes for therapy after his girlfriend leaves him. He is in a major depression and experiencing panic attacks.

The therapist lost her own mother in an automobile accident when she was 12 years old. When Richie talks about the loss of his mother, the therapist is filled with grief. When Richie mourns the end of his relationship with his girlfriend, the therapist feels overcome by his pain. She becomes too involved in his life and cannot set proper boundaries. She tells him to call her anytime, day or night, that he feels overwhelmed, and she spends hours on the phone talking to him each week. She is slow to recognize his cognitive distortions, agreeing with him rather than encouraging reality-testing when he interprets minor separations from his friends as instances of major abandonment. She supports his maladaptive coping responses rather than helping him change.

Self-Sacrifice is perhaps the most common schema among therapists. When working with patients who share this schema, therapists must be careful not to collude with the patients' schemas. These therapists must make a conscious effort to model appropriate levels of "give and take," neither giving too much to nor taking too much from their self-sacrificing patients. Unrelenting Standards is another schema common among therapists. When treating patients who share the schema, therapists must deliberately set reasonable expectations, both for themselves and for their perfectionistic patients.

4. *The patient's emotions trigger the therapist's avoidance behavior.* Sometimes the intensity of the patient's emotions overwhelms the therapist and prompts him or her to become avoidant. The therapist withdraws psy-

chologically, or changes the subject, or otherwise communicates to the patient that it is not acceptable to have intense emotions.

Case Illustration

Leigh comes to therapy following the death of her father. She tells the therapist that she was her father's "pride and joy" and that he was the only one who ever loved her. Leigh feels crushed by the loss and has stopped functioning. She has taken a leave of absence from work and spends her nights drinking at bars and her days sleeping or watching television. Since the death of her father, she has had sex with several men, all while she was drunk. She blacked out during some of these encounters and thus does not remember them.

Leigh's male therapist has a Self-Sacrifice schema. The therapist has added Leigh to an already overcrowded schedule of patients. In addition, he is doing almost all of the housework, shopping, and cooking for his pregnant wife. Confronted with the fierceness of Leigh's grief and the enormity of her emotional needs, he feels overwhelmed. He is too depleted to be there for her. He shuts down emotionally. He cannot bear to experience Leigh's neediness, so he ignores it. He denies her the forum she needs to express her pain. Feeling he does not care about her, Leigh leaves therapy after a few months.

Case Illustration

Hans is 55 years old. He has just lost his job as an executive in a small corporation. Although he made hundreds of thousands of dollars each year for the 3 years he held the position, he did not save any money. In fact, he is in debt. Hans has a history of getting fired from jobs. His main problem is managing his anger. Hans has a Defectiveness schema, and whenever he feels criticized, he overcompensates by making loud, cutting remarks. Because he often perceives slights where none are intended, almost everyone he encounters eventually falls prey to his sarcastic and insulting comments.

Hans comes to therapy for help in working through his anger over getting fired and in settling down to find a new job. In his sessions, he goes on long tirades about the series of events that led up to his getting fired and about the people at work who betrayed and plotted against him. His anger seems boundless.

When time passes and he is not able to settle down and look for work, he becomes angry with the therapist as well. He begins to spend sessions raging at the therapist for not helping him. The therapist, who has a Subjugation schema, cannot withstand the force of Hans's anger and becomes defensive. The more defensive the therapist becomes, the more angry Hans becomes.

When a patient is very vulnerable or angry a lot of the time, the therapist is at risk for engaging in some form of avoidance behavior. This is especially prone to happen with patients with BPD when the therapist cannot tolerate the patient's intense affect and suicidality. The therapist withdraws, triggering the patient's Abandonment schema, and thus further increases the intensity of the patient's affect and suicidality in a vicious cycle that can quickly spiral into crisis. This issue is discussed further in Chapter 9.

5. *The patient triggers the therapist's schemas, and the therapist overcompensates.* When the patient's emotions alarm the therapist, some therapists overcompensate. For example, when patients with BPD are very emotional or suicidal, some therapists become avoidant and withdraw, as we just described. Other therapists, however, who tend to overcompensate, may retaliate. They become angry with the patient; they attack and blame the patient. What these patients need is a sign that the therapist truly cares about them, and such a sign will almost always calm them down. Neither the therapist who avoids nor the therapist who overcompensates gives patients with BPD what they need in times of crisis, and both thus tend to respond in ways that make matters worse.

Case Illustration

Victor, the patient, and his male therapist have Defectiveness schemas, and both tend to overcompensate under perceived attack. Victor begins treatment by saying that his childhood was "blissful" and that both his parents were "totally supportive." In imagery of childhood, however, Victor recalls feeling that his father's support was fake and that he never really pleased his father at all. "My father wanted me to be like him, athletic. But sports was my weakest area. I did well at school, I got straight A's, I was Phi Beta Kappa in college, but that really didn't matter to my father."

Victor asks his therapist whether he was a good athlete in high school. The therapist, feeling envious that Victor was apparently a better student than he was, cannot resist bragging inappropriately about his own athletic record. He tells Victor that he was a state champion in wrestling. Feeling put down, Victor makes a disparaging remark about "jocks," and the therapist retorts with a hostile comment about Victor's "jealousy." Thus, rather than healing the patient's feeling of defectiveness, the therapist perpetuates it.

If the patient has an Entitlement schema and the therapist has a Self-Sacrifice schema, the therapist might give too much extra support for too long, and then, when the patient makes some entitled request, suddenly overcompensate by lashing out in anger against the patient.

6. *The patient triggers the therapist's Dysfunctional Parent mode.* The patient behaves like a "bad child," triggering a Disapproving Parent mode in the therapist. The therapist reprimands the patient like a scolding parent.

Case Illustration

Dan comes to therapy because he is failing in college. After going through the assessment, Dan and his female therapist agree that he has an Insufficient Self-Control/Self-Discipline schema. The therapist gives Dan homework assignments to self-monitor, but he does not comply. She sets up one assignment after another to foster discipline, but all of them fail. The therapist, who has a Defectiveness schema, begins to feel inadequate. She overcompensates by assuming the role of a "punitive parent." She loses empathy and chastises Dan, just as his parents did when he was a child (and, we might add, just as her parents did when she was a child). Dan feels bad about himself but still finds himself unable to complete homework assignments or adhere to agreements. Feeling punished but not getting any better, Dan leaves therapy.

Case Illustration

Lana has a Defectiveness schema. She comes to therapy because, even though she is a highly successful actress, inside she feels worthless and unlovable. Unfortunately, her male therapist has an Unrelenting Standards schema. Like her father when Lana was a child, he assumes the attitude of a "demanding parent." He sets ever higher standards for her to reach. Lana stays in therapy for years, striving to become "good enough" to win his approval.

7. *The patient satisfies the therapist's schema-driven needs.* Therapists who do not monitor their own schemas are at risk to inadvertently exploit patients. Rather than focusing on the patient's welfare, these therapists unintentionally use patients to fill their own unmet emotional needs.

Case Illustration

The female therapist has an Emotional Deprivation schema (another schema common among therapists). Throughout her life, she has received little nurturing. One of the ways she copes with her schema is by nurturing others in her work life. In this way, she symbolically nurtures her own inner child.

The patient, Marcie, has a Self-Sacrifice schema. She comes to therapy because she is depressed and does not know why. It becomes apparent that Marcie is so swept up in taking care of the members of her family, especially her mother, that she has little time for herself.

Like most people with Self-Sacrifice schemas, Marcie is empathic, self-denying, and solicitous. She notices when the therapist is looking fatigued or dejected. Even though she is bursting with things to say, she suppresses her own needs and asks the therapist what is wrong. Rather than pointing out what Marcie is doing, as she should, the therapist answers her, telling Marcie her troubles. Marcie is sympathetic. Over time the therapist increasingly allows Marcie to become her caretaker. With another person to care for, Marcie becomes even more depressed.

There are endless possibilities. Consider a patient who has an Enmeshment schema and fuses with a therapist who has a Social Isolation schema and who likes the closeness so much that she cannot help the patient individuate. Or consider an approval-seeking patient who, eager to please, compliments the therapist frequently and a therapist with a Defectiveness or Dependence schema who responds to the praise with obvious enjoyment. Unfortunately, the therapist's positive response to the patient's behavior reinforces it.

8. *The therapist's schemas are triggered when the patient fails to make "sufficient progress."* Often therapists with Defectiveness, Failure, or Dependence/Incompetence schemas respond improperly to patients who do not improve in therapy. Such therapists express anger or impatience toward the patient, often perpetuating the patient's schemas.

Case Illustration

A male therapist is treating Beth, a young patient with BPD who is depressed about her relationship with her boyfriend, Carlos. Beth is obsessed with Carlos. When the relationship first started, Beth and Carlos were inseparable. Gradually Carlos began to want more "space," and Beth became frantic. She became clingy and controlling, getting upset whenever Carlos wanted to separate and demanding an accounting of all his time away from her. By the time she started therapy, it was clear that Carlos wanted out of the relationship, but Beth was not letting him go. Rather, she was calling him repeatedly—crying, promising to change, begging him to reconsider. Carlos spoke to her, but he steadfastly refused to go back with her and started dating other women

The therapist has a Dependence/Incompetence schema. Nervously, he tries to help Beth let go of her boyfriend. He points out how self-destructive it is to try to hold onto Carlos, and Beth agrees. He teaches her thought-stopping and distraction techniques to use when she is obsessing about Carlos. He helps her identify alternative activities when she has urges to call Carlos. However, no matter what he does, nothing changes. Beth is still just as obsessed with Carlos and is still calling him and begging him to take her back. The therapist begins to feel inept and resentful. When Beth expresses feelings of hopelessness, he blames her. He insinuates that she does not want to get better. When she talks about calling Carlos, he berates her. Beth ends up feeling that she is not good enough for Carlos and not good enough for her therapist, either.

Therapists with Defectiveness, Failure, or Dependence/Incompetence schemas might respond to a patient's lack of progress in other destructive ways. Therapists who surrender as a coping style might appear agitated and lacking in confidence, thus undermining the patient's faith in therapy. Therapists who avoid might impulsively propose that the patient seek another, better therapist.

9. *The therapist's schemas are triggered when the patient has crises, such as high suicidality.* Crises have a high likelihood of triggering the therapist's schemas. They test the therapist's ability to cope in positive ways.

Case Illustration

The female therapist has a Subjugation schema based on her childhood with a controlling mother. Starting when she was a young child, her mother threatened to abandon her if she was "bad"—"bad" meaning not doing what her mother wanted.

Jessica, the patient, begins therapy. Jessica gives a confusing account of her childhood: At one point she says her aunt and uncle sexually abused her and her little brother; at another point she says it never happened. Jessica's boyfriend is a substance abuser. His drugs of choice are cocaine and alcohol. When he is on a binge, he disappears, often for days. The last time it happened, Jessica cut her ankles with a razor.

A few weeks into therapy, the boyfriend has a date to meet Jessica for dinner, but he never shows up. Jessica goes home, cuts her ankles, and calls the therapist, waking her up. "How could he do this to me?" Jessica wails over the phone. Jessica tells the therapist that she cut her ankles. Rather than feeling empathic, the therapist is furious. She thinks Jessica is trying to manipulate and control her, just as her own mother did in her childhood. "That was a very hostile thing to do!" she exclaims, throwing Jessica into a panic.

In order to handle crises effectively, the therapist must remain empathic and objective and not become critical or punitive. (We discuss the management of acute suicidality and other crises in Chapter 9.

10. *The therapist envies the patient on an ongoing basis.* If the therapist is narcissistic, the therapist might envy the patient. In such cases, the pa-

tient has access to a source of gratification that the therapist has longed for but never had, such as beauty, wealth, or success. Or, as in the following example, the patient fulfills in her own life one of the therapist's unmet needs.

Case Illustration

Jade, the patient, is 19 years old. She comes to therapy because her mother is dying of cancer. Her father brings her to her first session. It is obvious that her father loves her. Jade is soft and sweet. She talks to the therapist about her dying mother and cries.

The female therapist tells Jade she will help her cope with her mother's illness. But, despite these kind words, inside she feels jealous of Jade. The therapist grew up in a state of almost total emotional deprivation. Even though Jade's mother is dying, she still has so much more than the therapist ever had. The therapist is especially jealous of Jade's relationship with her father. Jade's father is the kind of father the therapist always dreamed of having—loving and kind, not at all like her own unapproachable father. Thus envious of Jade, the therapist is unable to be genuinely caring, open, and empathic. Sensing that something is wrong, Jade leaves therapy after a short time.

Envy might prompt the therapist to focus on the relevant material and behave in a jealous manner (schema surrender), to avoid talking about important material (schema avoidance), or to try to live vicariously through the patient (schema overcompensation).

Therapists must struggle to know their own limits. When patients trigger their Early Maladaptive Schemas, they must decide whether they can cope well with anticipated challenges and continue to behave in a therapeutic and professional manner. Therapists can use the techniques of schema therapy to address the problem, either on their own or in supervision. They can conduct dialogues between the schema and the healthy side. What is the schema saying in the therapy with the patient? What is the schema directing the therapist to do? How does the healthy side—the "good therapist"—respond? In addition, the therapist can use experiential techniques to explore and remediate the problem. For example, the therapist can recall an image of a moment during the session in which the therapist's own schemas were triggered. When in childhood did the therapist feel the same way? What does the therapist's Vulnerable Child say in the image? How does the Healthy Adult answer? The therapist can carry out dialogues between modes. Finally, the therapist can practice behavioral pattern-breaking. Rather than acting out maladaptive coping responses with the patient, the therapist can delineate homework assignments that entail the use of empathic confrontation and limited reparenting.

If there are problems that cannot be resolved through consultation or supervision, then the therapist should consider referring the patient to another therapist.

The Role of the Therapy Relationship in Educating the Patient

The therapist tailors the educational material to the patient's personality. Some patients want to learn as much as possible, whereas others tend to feel overwhelmed. Some want to read books, and others prefer to watch films or plays. Some want to show the therapist photographs from their childhoods, whereas others find this prospect unappealing. However, the therapy relationship plays an important role in educating almost all patients about their schemas and coping styles. Patients often derive great benefit from recognizing instances of schema activation right there in the session with the therapist. Such immediate examples are especially instructive. Current thoughts, feelings, and behaviors are vivid and clear and are more readily processed by patients due to the presence of affect.

In accord with the collaborative nature of schema therapy, the therapist tells the patient that, when the patient's schemas are triggered in the therapy relationship, the therapist will confront the patient empathically. In addition, the therapist will try not to reinforce the patient's maladaptive coping styles. The therapist says this in a way that communicates to the patient that it is a sign of caring.

Case Illustration

Bruce begins therapy with a therapist named Carrie. Bruce has a Mistrust/ Abuse schema, based on his childhood with a sadistic older brother. When Bruce was vulnerable as a child, his brother took the opportunity to torture and humiliate him. Now, whenever Bruce feels vulnerable in the session with Carrie, he starts to joke. He is funny, and he makes Carrie laugh. However, as time goes on, Bruce continues to avoid becoming vulnerable in therapy. At last Carrie tells him that she is going to try not to laugh at his jokes anymore in session when he is using them to avoid important material. Although she appreciates his jokes, and although she understands why it is hard for him to be vulnerable, she also knows that the vulnerable child in him deserves a chance to speak.

Case Illustration

A 52-year-old patient named Clifford comes to his first session. He says that he wants the therapist to restore his self-confidence so that he can achieve even greater success in his career. In the course of the interview it becomes clear that Clifford has lost his most important relationships—

with his wife, his children, his siblings, his best friend—but his aggressively upbeat manner does not permit appreciation of these losses. Ed, the therapist, attempts to reframe the presenting problem to include interpersonal relationships, but Clifford balks. "I'm paying the bills here," he says, "I'll pick what we talk about." In the second session, Ed again raises the issue of interpersonal relationships, including examples of how Clifford treated him in the first session. Ed says directly to the patient, "Although you think what you have is a self-confidence problem, what you have is a deeper problem. It is called narcissism, and it keeps you from getting close to others and from knowing your true emotions." For this patient, use of the diagnostic term "narcissism" was helpful. In fact, Clifford said that other therapists had stopped working with him without ever telling him why. (For other patients who are less well defended, a diagnosis might feel pejorative and be harmful rather than helpful.)

Later in treatment, Ed found it necessary to tell Clifford that he was not going to allow him to spend session time recounting his career accomplishments. He understood that Clifford's accomplishments were important to him, but because the focus of therapy was intimate relationships, this kind of self-aggrandizing was not a productive use of session time.

THE THERAPY RELATIONSHIP IN THE CHANGE PHASE

During the Change Phase, the therapist continues to confront the patient's Early Maladaptive Schemas and coping styles within the context of the therapy relationship. Empathic confrontation and limited reparenting are the two primary ways in which the therapy relationship fosters change.

Empathic Confrontation (or Empathic Reality-Testing)

Empathic confrontation is the therapeutic stance of schema therapy. The therapist takes this stance throughout the Change Phase to promote the patient's psychological growth. However, empathic confrontation is not a technique; rather, it is an approach to the patient that involves a true emotional bond. The therapist must genuinely care about the patient for the approach to work.

In empathic confrontation, the therapist empathizes with the patient and confronts the schema. The therapist expresses understanding of the reasons the patient has the schema and how hard it is to change, while simultaneously acknowledging the importance of that change, striving for the optimum balance between empathy and confrontation that will enable the patient to change. The therapist uses empathic confrontation whenever the patient's schemas are triggered in the context of the therapy relationship. The triggering of a schema is apparent in the patient's over-reactions, misinterpretations, and nonverbal behaviors.

The first step is allowing patients to freely express their "truth." The therapist encourages patients to state their points of view, fully sharing their thoughts and feelings. To help the patient, the therapist asks questions: What is the patient thinking and feeling? What does the patient have the urge to do? What actions on the therapist's part triggered the schema? Which schema is it? Who else makes the patient feel this way? Who in the patient's past made the patient feel this way? What happened? With whom did the patient feel this way in childhood? The therapist can use imagery to help the patient link the incident to past events.

Next, the therapist empathizes with the patient's feelings, given the patient's perspective on the situation, and acknowledges the realistic component of the patient's point of view. If it is appropriate, the therapist apologizes for anything he or she has said or done that was hurtful or insensitive. Once the patient feels understood and validated, the therapist moves on to reality-testing. The therapist confronts flaws in the patient's viewpoint, using logic and empirical evidence. The therapist offers an alternative interpretation, often using self-disclosure about the interaction. The therapist and patient evaluate the patient's reactions to the therapy situation. This process usually yields a kernel of truth combined with a schema-driven distortion.

Case Illustration

Lysette is a 26-year-old woman who comes to therapy following the breakup of a love relationship. Her core schema is Emotional Deprivation, which originated in her childhood with wealthy but emotionally unavailable parents. Her father and mother traveled throughout her childhood, leaving her with nannies or at boarding schools. Lysette remembers once throwing herself down the stairs to prevent her parents from leaving on a trip. In the course of a therapy session, Lysette feels that the therapist is not getting the point she is making. This triggers her Emotional Deprivation schema, and she rails at the therapist. "You never understand me," she says with rage.

The therapist utilizes empathic confrontation. First, the therapist helps Lysette express her view of what just happened. Lysette tells the therapist how angry she is and says that, underneath the anger, she is afraid the therapist will never understand her. At bottom she is afraid that she will always be alone. The therapist expresses understanding of Lysette's reason for feeling as she does and apologizes for misunderstanding her. Once Lysette feels heard, they move on to reality-testing. It is true that the therapist did not understand Lysette perfectly; however, the therapist does understand her most of the time and does genuinely care about her. When Lysette covers up her fear with anger, however, it has the effect of pushing the therapist away and making it harder for the therapist to give her what she needs.

When employing empathic confrontation in the context of the therapy relationship, therapists use appropriate self-disclosure. They share their own thoughts and feelings about the interaction when it is likely to benefit the patient. If the patient has attributed judgments, motives, or emotions to the therapist that are false, then the therapist can choose to tell the patient so outright.

For example, a young woman comes to therapy. She has an Abandonment schema and asks her therapist: "Am I too needy for you? Are you going to stop seeing me because I'm too needy?" The therapist answers directly: "No, you're not too needy for me. I don't feel that way." The therapist uses the therapy relationship to contradict the schema. (Of course, the therapist only says this if it is true.) The therapist thus assures the patient that normal expressions of neediness are fine.

As another example, a young man with a Defectiveness schema says to his therapist, "The people in my family see me as selfish. Do you see me as selfish?" The therapist answers truthfully, "No. I don't see you as selfish. I see you as very giving." Thus the therapist's self-disclosure provides a partial antidote to the patient's schemas.

Case Illustration

Bill, the patient, has a Failure schema. He comes to therapy to work on his career as a corporate manager, which is not advancing as he had hoped. At the end of the first session, Eliot, the therapist, gives Bill the homework assignment of filling out the Young Schema Questionnaire. Bill comes to the next session with the assignment undone. He enters the session with a belligerent attitude, angrily pacing about and making excuses.

Eliot waits a while until Bill calms down enough to take part in a discussion. They analyze what just happened. "I thought you were going to yell at me," Bill explains. Eliot then explores the origins of this expectation in Bill's childhood and its effects on his work life. Bill grew up on a farm, and, as a child, his father punished him harshly for not completing his chores quickly enough. (Bill also has a Punitiveness schema.) The therapist sympathizes with Bill's childhood experience. Underneath his angry exterior, there is a vulnerable child who is afraid of failing and getting punished. Eliot then helps Bill trace the effects of his schemas on his work life. It emerges that Bill has a history of antagonizing coworkers and bosses, thus hindering the growth of his career. Once Bill understands his underlying schemas (Failure and Punitiveness) and his maladaptive coping style (he overcompensates by behaving angrily), Eliot moves onto reality-testing. He self-discloses about the effects of Bill's angry behavior: When Bill behaved that way, Eliot wanted to distance himself from Bill.

By analyzing their schemas as they are triggered naturally in the therapy relationship, patients gain insight into how they perpetuate their schemas and set the stage for their difficulties in their lives outside therapy.

Therapists can anticipate schema activation, and they can teach patients to do the same. One might easily predict that a patient's Abandonment schema will be triggered when the therapist goes on vacation. Such knowledge enables the therapist to address the patient's fears ahead of time and to help the patient develop a healthy coping response. For example, the therapist and patient could construct a flash card for the patient to read in the therapist's absence.

Similarly, one might predict that a patient with a Subjugation schema will be reluctant to follow directions from the therapist. The therapist can prepare for this eventuality and give the patient suggestions rather than directions on such matters as session exercises and homework assignments. Instead of instructing the patient, the therapist asks the patient to choose the exercise or design the homework.

Limited Reparenting in the Change Phase

Limited reparenting is especially valuable for patients who have schemas in the Disconnection and Rejection domain; that is, patients who were abused, abandoned, emotionally deprived, or rejected in childhood. The more severe the trauma, the more important the reparenting aspect of therapy becomes. Nevertheless, patients with schemas in other domains also benefit from limited reparenting. With these patients, limited reparenting focuses on such issues as autonomy, realistic limits, self-expression, reciprocity, and spontaneity.

The reparenting is "limited" in that the therapist offers an approximation of missed emotional experiences within ethical and professional boundaries. The therapist does not actually try to become the parent, nor does he or she regress the patient to childlike dependency. Rather, limited reparenting is a consistent way of interacting with a patient that is designed to heal that patient's specific Early Maladaptive Schemas.

In order to fit the reparenting style to the individual patient, the therapist needs to take into account the patient's developmental stage. Patients with BPD have more childlike needs. Losing object constancy, they frequently require extra contact in the form of additional appointments or phone calls between sessions. Therapists must balance the patient's needs with their own limits and model healthy limit-setting. We discuss limit-setting further in Chapter 9.

Like empathic confrontation, limited reparenting includes genuine self-disclosure on the part of the therapist. In order to be helpful, the self-disclosure must be sincere and truthful. For example, praise for a patient with a Defectiveness schema is appropriate reparenting only if it is based on realistic positive qualities of the patient that the therapist authentically appreciates. Sometimes, with hostile or negative patients, it is difficult for the therapist to find positive qualities. In such instances, a statement that conveys understanding can counteract a schema. Such a statement to a mistrustful patient, for example, might be, "When you feel safe, you let me get closer to you." Thus the therapist acknowledges how hard it is for the patient to get close to others but explains the patient's guardedness as a form of avoidance and not as the patient's "true self."

Another type of therapist self-disclosure is answering the patient's questions directly if they are not too personal. For example, a patient with a Mistrust/Abuse schema wants to know about the therapist's record-keeping. The therapist answers her questions directly, rather than interpreting them or questioning them. Limited reparenting in this case involves being forthright with the patient about the contents of her file.

In another case, a patient with a Defectiveness schema notices that the therapist has a scale in her office and asks why. The therapist replies that she treats patients with eating disorders. Rather than weighing themselves daily (or several times a day), these patients have agreed to weigh themselves only at weekly therapy sessions with her. The patient replies, "Oh, I thought you were trying to tell me I was fat." A direct answer on the part of the therapist increases the patient's sense of trust. The therapist is not sending her indirect negative messages.

In contrast, however, patients with Dependence schemas tend to ask the therapist's opinions when they could be making decisions for themselves. In such cases, the therapist combines limited reparenting with empathic confrontation and gently declines to answer. The therapist says, for example, "I know you feel anxious deciding on your own. Your Dependence schema is preventing you from trying to figure things out for yourself, but you can do it. Instead of telling you what to do, I'll support you while you find your own answer."

It is important for therapists to remember that it is not their job to avoid activating the patient's schemas in the therapy relationship. First of all, it is probably impossible to avoid doing so, especially when working with fragile patients. The therapist's task is to work on the patient's schemas when they are triggered. Rather than minimizing the importance of what is happening, the therapist uses the activation of schemas as an opportunity to maximize the patient's potential for psychological growth.

Limited reparenting is interwoven throughout the experiential work, especially imagery. When the therapist enters patients' images to serve as the "Healthy Adult" and allows patients to say aloud what they needed but did not get from their parents as children, then the therapist is reparenting. The therapist is teaching patients that there are other ways a parent might have treated them. As children, they had needs that were not met, and other parents might have met them. By first modeling the Healthy Adult in imagery, then bringing patients into the imagery to serve as the Healthy Adult, the therapist teaches patients to reparent their own inner child.

We have elaborated specific limited reparenting strategies for each Early Maladaptive Schema. The strategies take into account the coping styles that typically characterize the schema. The limited reparenting strategies are designed to provide a partial antidote to the schema within the therapy relationship.

1. *Abandonment/Instability.* The therapist becomes a transitional source of stability, eventually helping the patient to find other stable relationships outside of therapy. The therapist corrects distortions about how likely the therapist is to abandon the patient. The therapist helps the patient accept the therapist's departures, vacations, and unavailability without shutting down or behaving self-destructively.

2. *Mistrust/Abuse.* The therapist is completely trustworthy, honest, and genuine with the patient. The therapist asks about trust and intimacy regularly and discusses any negative feelings the patient has toward him or her. The therapist asks about vigilance in sessions. In order to build up the patient's trust, when necessary the therapist postpones the experiential work and proceeds through traumatic memories slowly.

3. *Emotional Deprivation.* The therapist provides a nurturing atmosphere, with warmth, empathy, and guidance. The therapist encourages patients to ask for what they need emotionally and to feel entitled to have emotional needs. The therapist helps the patient express feelings of deprivation without lashing out or remaining silent. The therapist helps the patient accept the therapist's limitations and tolerate some deprivation while appreciating the nurturing that is available.

4. *Defectiveness.* The therapist is accepting and nonjudgmental. The therapist cares about the patient despite the patient's flaws. The therapist is willing to be imperfect, sharing minor weaknesses with the patient. The therapist compliments the patient as often as possible without seeming phony.

5. *Social Isolation.* The therapist highlights ways in which the patient and therapist are similar and ways in which the patient and therapist are different yet compatible.

6. *Dependence/Incompetence.* The therapist resists attempts by patients to take on a dependent role with the therapist. He or she encourages patients to make their own decisions. The therapist praises the patient's good judgments and progress.

7. *Vulnerability to Harm or Illness.* The therapist increasingly discourages the patient's dependence on the therapist for reassurance about the dangerousness of moving about in the world. The therapist expresses calm confidence in the patient's ability to handle phobic situations and feared illnesses.

8. *Enmeshment/Undeveloped Self.* The therapist helps the patient by setting appropriate boundaries that are neither too close nor too distant. The therapist encourages the patient to develop a separate sense of self.

9. *Failure.* The therapist supports the patient's work or school successes. The therapist provides structure and sets limits.

10. *Entitlement.* The therapist supports the patient's vulnerable side and does not reinforce the patient's entitled side. The therapist empathically confronts entitlement and sets limits. The therapist supports emotional connectedness more than status or power.

11. *Insufficient Self-Control/Self-Discipline.* The therapist is firm in setting limits. The therapist models appropriate self-control and self-discipline and rewards patients for gradually developing these abilities.

12. *Subjugation.* The therapist is relatively nondirective rather than controlling. He or she encourages patients to make choices about therapy goals, treatment techniques, and homework assignments. The therapist points out deferential or rebellious behavior and helps patients recognize anger, vent it, then learn to express it appropriately.

13. *Self-Sacrifice.* Therapists help patients to set appropriate boundaries and to assert their own rights and needs. The therapist encourages the patient to rely on the therapist, thereby validating the patient's dependency needs. The therapist discourages the patient from taking care of the therapist, pointing out the pattern with an empathic confrontation.

14. *Negativity/Pessimism.* The therapist avoids playing the positive side to the patient's negative side. Rather, the therapist asks the patient to play both the positive and negative roles. The therapist models healthy optimism.

15. *Emotional Inhibition.* The therapist encourages the patient to express affect spontaneously in the sessions. The therapist models the appropriate expression of affect.

16. *Unrelenting Standards.* Therapists model balanced standards in their approach to therapy and their own lives. Rather than maintaining an atmosphere of unbroken seriousness, therapists reward patients for playfulness. Therapists value the therapy relationship more than "getting things done" and encourage imperfect behavior.

17. *Punitiveness.* Therapists assume a forgiving attitude toward the patient and toward themselves and acknowledge the patient for forgiving others.

18. *Approval-Seeking.* The therapist emphasizes the patient's core self over such superficial attainments as status, appearance, or wealth.

The same patient behavior requires different therapist responses, depending on the underlying schema. The following scenario is an example:

A young female patient repeatedly comes inordinately late to therapy sessions (i.e., she arrives when there are only 10 minutes left to the session).

If the patient has a *Mistrust/Abuse* schema and is coming late because she is afraid the therapist is going to abuse her, then reparenting entails empathizing with the "Abused Child" and helping the child mode to feel safe. The therapist might say, "I know that it's hard for you to come to sessions, that underneath you're scared of me. I also know there's a reason you feel this way, because of the way people you trusted treated you when you were a child. I'm glad you're able to come at all, and I hope that, gradually, you'll trust me enough to come for the whole session."

If the patient has an *Abandonment/Instability* schema and is coming late because she is afraid to attach to the therapist, only to inevitably lose him or her, then reparenting involves reassuring the Abandoned Child about the stability of the therapeutic relationship. The therapist might say: "I know you think I'm mad at you for coming late. I want you to know that I'm not mad and that I know there's a reason you're coming late that has to do with your childhood. Even when you come late, I still feel a bond with you."

If the patient has an *Emotional Deprivation* schema and is late as a result of an overcompensatory feeling of entitlement, then reparenting consists of empathizing with the Deprived Child, who now will miss the support of a full session, but insisting, nevertheless, on ending the session on time. The therapist might say: "I regret that you're late and we'll only get to spend a few minutes together. I want to give you the opportunity to express your feelings about that. Let's spend the rest of the session talking about it."

If the patient has a *Defectiveness* schema and is late because she is afraid that the therapist will see her "true" self and despise her, then reparenting concerns empathizing with the Rejected Child, emphasizing that the therapist accepts her whether she is late or not. The therapist might say, "I want to acknowledge you for coming, even though it's so difficult for you. It's important to me that you know I accept you and value our relationship, even when you come late."

If the patient has a *Failure* schema and is late because she is sure she will fail in therapy, then reparenting encompasses empathizing with the underlying expectation of failure but confronting the consequences of the behavior. The therapist might say: "I know it's hard for you to believe therapy's going to work because a lot of things haven't worked for you in the past. But let's look at what's going to happen if you don't come on time, compared to what could happen if you do."

If the patient has a *Dependence/Incompetence* schema and is late because she cannot plan and navigate on her own, then reparenting involves building strengths and teaching skills. The therapist might say, "Let's look at what you did right to get here and where you went wrong. That way we can plan together how you might get here on time next week."

If the patient has a *Self-Sacrifice* schema and is late because she was waylaid by an acquaintance on the way to therapy and could not break away, then reparenting consists of pointing out the negative consequence to the patient of her self-sacrifice and building assertiveness skills. The therapist might say: "It cost you most of your therapy session to stay in that conversation, and you gained nothing. Let's talk about how you might have broken out of the conversation. Would you like to do some imagery about it? Close your eyes and picture an image of meeting your friend and getting stuck in the conversation."

Knowledge of the patient's underlying schemas helps the therapist reparent the patient in the most effective way.

SUMMARY

In schema therapy, the therapist–patient relationship is an essential element of schema assessment and change. Two features of the therapeutic relationship are emblematic of schema therapy: empathic confrontation and limited reparenting. Empathic confrontation is expressing understanding about the patient's schemas while simultaneously confronting the need for change. Limited reparenting is fulfilling, in a limited way, the unmet emotional needs of the patient's childhood.

In the Assessment and Education Phase, the therapy relationship is an efficacious way to assess schemas and educate the patient. The therapist establishes rapport, formulates the case conceptualization, decides what style of limited reparenting is appropriate for the patient, and determines whether the therapist's own schemas and coping styles are likely to interfere with the course of therapy.

Empathic confrontation and limited reparenting blend and alternate throughout the cognitive, experiential, and behavioral pattern-breaking stages of the Change Phase. Therapists adapt their reparenting styles to match the patient's schemas and coping styles. Self-knowledge of one's own schemas and coping styles helps therapists stay focused on reparenting the patient in the most helpful manner.

Chapter 7

DETAILED SCHEMA
TREATMENT STRATEGIES

In this chapter, we discuss each of the 18 schemas individually, including the clinical presentation of the schema, the goals of treatment, the strategies we emphasize, and special problems. We also present specific treatment strategies, including cognitive, experiential, and behavioral strategies, and aspects of the therapy relationship.

We do not include descriptions of how to implement the strategies—for example, how actually to conduct imagery dialogues or design exposure exercises. We assume that readers have already learned these strategies in previous chapters. Rather, we describe how to *tailor* the treatment strategies to each particular schema.

DISCONNECTION AND REJECTION DOMAIN

Abandonment

Typical Presentation of the Schema

These patients constantly expect to lose the people closest to them. They believe these people will abandon them, get sick and die, leave them for somebody else, behave unpredictably, or somehow suddenly disappear. Therefore, they live in constant fear and are always vigilant for any sign that someone is about to leave their lives.

The common emotions are chronic anxiety about losing people, sadness, and depression when there is an actual or perceived loss, and anger at the people who have left them. (In more intense forms, these emotions become terror, grief, and rage.) Some patients even become upset when people leave them for short periods of time. Typical behaviors include clinging to significant others, being possessive and controlling, accusing others of abandoning them, jealousy, competitiveness with rivals—all to prevent the other person from leaving. Some patients with an Abandonment schema avoid intimate relationships altogether, in order to avoid experiencing what they anticipate to be the inevitable pain of loss. (One patient with this schema, when asked why he could not make a commitment to the woman he loved, answered: "What if she dies?") Consistent with the schema perpetuation process, these patients typically choose unstable significant others, such as uncommitted or unavailable partners, who are a highly likely to abandon them. They usually have intense chemistry with these partners, and often fall obsessively in love.

The Abandonment schema is frequently linked with other schemas. It can be linked with the Subjugation schema. Patients believe that if they do not do what the other person wants, then he or she will leave them. It can also be linked with the Dependence/Incompetence schema. Patients believe that if the other person leaves, they will be unable to function in the world on their own. Finally, the Abandonment schema can be linked with the Defectiveness schema. Patients believe the other person will find out how defective they are and will leave.

Goals of Treatment

One goal of treatment is to help patients become more realistic about the stability of relationships. Patients who have been successfully treated for an Abandonment schema no longer worry all the time that reliable significant others are about to disappear. In object relation terms, they have learned to internalize significant others as stable objects. They are far less likely to magnify and misinterpret behaviors as signs that other people are going to abandon them.

Their linked schemas are usually diminished as well. Because they feel less subjugated, or dependent, or defective, abandonment is not as frightening to them as it used to be. They feel more secure in their relationships, so they do not have to cling, control, or manipulate. They are less angry. They select significant others who are consistently there for them, and no longer avoid intimate relationships. Another sign of improvement in patients with this schema is that they are able to be alone for extended periods of time without becoming anxious or depressed, and without having to reach out immediately and connect to somebody.

Strategies Emphasized in Treatment

The more severe the Abandonment schema, the more important the therapy relationship is to the treatment. Patients with BPD typically have Abandonment as one of their core schemas, and, therefore, the therapy relationship is the primary source of healing. According to our approach, the therapist becomes a transitional parent figure—a stable base from which the patient can venture into the world and form other stable bonds. First, the patient learns to overcome the schema within the therapy relationship, and then transfers this learning to significant others outside of therapy. Through "limited reparenting," the therapist provides the patient with stability, and the patient gradually learns to accept the therapist as a stable object. Mode work is especially helpful (see Chapter 9). Through empathic confrontation, the therapist corrects the patient's distorted sense that the therapist is constantly about to abandon the patient. The therapist helps the patient accept the therapist's departures, vacations, and unavailability without catastrophizing and overreacting. Finally, the therapist helps the patient find someone to replace the therapist as the primary relationship—someone stable, who is not going to leave—so the patient is not dependent forever on the therapist to be the stable object.

Cognitive strategies focus on altering the patient's exaggerated view that other people will eventually leave, die, or behave unpredictably. Patients learn to stop catastrophizing about temporary separations from significant others. Additionally, cognitive strategies focus on altering the patient's unrealistic expectation that significant others should be endlessly available and totally consistent. Patients learn to accept that other people have the right to set limits and establish separate space. Cognitive strategies also focus on reducing the patient's obsessive focus on making sure the partner is still there. Finally, cognitive strategies address the cognitions that link to other schemas—for example, changing the view that patients must do what other people want them to do or else they are going to be left; that they are incompetent, and need other people to take care of them; or that they are defective, and other people will inevitably find out and leave them.

In terms of experiential strategies, patients relive childhood experiences of abandonment or instability in imagery. Patients reexperience through imagery memories of the parent who left them, or of the unstable parent who was sometimes there and sometimes not. The therapist enters the image and becomes a stable figure for the child. The therapist expresses anger at the parent who acted irresponsibly, and comforts the Abandoned Child; then, patients enter the image as Healthy Adults and do the same. They express anger at the parent who abandoned them and comfort the Abandoned Child. Thus, patients gradually become able to serve as their own Healthy Adults in the imagery.

Behaviorally, patients focus on choosing partners who are capable of making a commitment. They also learn to stop pushing partners away with behaviors that are too jealous, clinging, angry, or controlling. They gradually learn to tolerate being alone. Countering their schema-driven attraction to instability, they learn to walk away from unstable relationships quickly and to become more comfortable in stable relationships. They also heal their linked schemas: They stop letting other people control them; they learn to become more competent in handling everyday affairs, or they work on feeling less defective.

Special Problems with This Schema

Abandonment often comes up as an issue in therapy when the therapist initiates a separation—such as ending a session, going on vacation, or changing an appointment time. The schema is triggered, and the patient becomes frightened or angry. These situations provide excellent opportunities for the patient to make progress with the schema. The therapist helps the patient do so through empathic confrontation: Although the therapist understands why the patient is so scared, the reality is that the therapist is still bonded to the patient while they are apart, and the therapist is going to return and see the patient again.

Alternatively, patients may be overly compliant in therapy to make sure the therapist does not ever leave them. They are "good patients," but they are not authentic. Patients may also overwhelm the therapist by constantly seeking reassurance or calling between sessions in order to reconnect. Avoidant patients may miss sessions, be reluctant to come on a regular basis, or drop out of therapy prematurely because they do not want to become too attached to the therapist. Patients with the Abandonment schema may also repeatedly test the therapist—for example, by threatening to stop therapy or accusing the therapist of wanting to stop. We address these issues in detail in our chapter on treating patients with borderline disorder (see Chapter 9). Briefly, the therapist approaches the problem through a combination of setting limits and empathic confrontation.

Another risk is that patients with the Abandonment schema may make the therapist the central figure in their lives permanently, instead of forming stable, primary connections with other people. The patient never terminates therapy, but just continues to let the therapist be the stable connection. Becoming dependent upon the therapist becomes the unhealthy solution to the schema. The ultimate goal of therapy is for patients to connect with others in the outside world who can meet their emotional needs.

Mistrust/Abuse

Typical Presentation of the Schema

Patients with the Mistrust/Abuse schema expect others to lie, manipulate, cheat, or in other ways to take advantage of them, and in the most extreme form of the schema, try to humiliate or abuse them. These patients do not trust other people to be honest and straightforward, and to have their best interests at heart. Rather, they are guarded and suspicious. They sometimes believe that other people want to hurt them intentionally. At best, they feel that people care only for themselves and do not mind hurting others to get what they need; at worst, they are convinced that people are malevolent, sadistic, and get pleasure from hurting others. In the extreme form, patients with this schema may believe that other people want to torture and sexually abuse them. (Isaac Bashevis Singer [1978] wrote about the holocaust—a mass expression of the Mistrust/Abuse schema—in his book *Shosha*: "The world is a slaughterhouse and a brothel" [p. 266].)

Therefore, patients with this schema tend to avoid intimacy. They do not share their innermost thoughts and feelings or get too close to others; and, in some cases, they end up cheating or abusing other people in a sort of preemptive strike ("I'll get them before they get me"). Broadly speaking, typical behaviors include victim and abuser behaviors. Some patients choose abusive partners and allow themselves to be physically, sexually, or emotionally abused, whereas other patients behave abusively toward others. Some patients become the "savior" of other abused people, or express outrage against people they perceive as abusers. Patients with this schema often come across as paranoid: They are perpetually setting up tests and gathering evidence to determine whether other people are worthy of trust.

Goals of Treatment

The main goal of treatment is to help patients with the Mistrust/Abuse schema to realize that, whereas some people are not trustworthy, many others *are* trustworthy. We teach them that the best way to live is to stay away from abusive people as much as possible, stand up for themselves when necessary, and focus on having trustworthy people in their personal life.

Patients who have healed a Mistrust/Abuse schema have learned to distinguish between people who are trustworthy and those who are not. They have learned that there is a spectrum of trustworthiness: People worthy of trust do not have to be perfect; they just have to be "trustworthy enough." With trustworthy people, patients learn to behave in a different way. They are willing to give them the benefit of the doubt, they are less guarded and suspicious, they stop setting up tests, and they no longer cheat others because they expect to be cheated. With individuals who become their partners or close friends, patients become more authentic. They share many of their secrets and are willing to be vulnerable. They eventually find that, if they behave openly, trustworthy people will generally treat them well in return.

Strategies Emphasized in Treatment

When dealing with childhood abuse, the therapy relationship is crucial to the success of the therapy. At the core of the experience of childhood abuse are feelings of terror, helplessness, and isolation. Ideally, the therapist provides the patient with the antidote to these feelings. At the core of the experience of therapy are feelings of safety, empowerment, and reconnection.

With patients who were abused as young children, the therapist must work to establish emotional safety. The goal is to provide a safe place for patients to tell their story of abuse. Most abuse survivors are intensely ambivalent about telling their story. One part of the patient wants to discuss what happened, whereas another part wants to hide it. Many of these patients alternate between the two—just as they alternate between feeling overwhelmed and feeling numb (a common characteristic of posttraumatic stress disorder). We hope that, by the end of therapy, most of the patients' traumatic secrets will have been uncovered, discussed, and understood. (The therapist is careful throughout this process to avoid suggesting or subtly pushing for memories of abuse that may never have happened.)

Cognitively, the therapist helps to reduce patients' overvigilance to abuse. Patients learn to recognize a spectrum of trustworthiness. In addition, patients work to alter the extremely common view of themselves as worthless and to blame for the abuse (a blending of the Mistrust/Abuse and Defectiveness schemas). They stop making excuses for the abuser and place blame where it belongs.

Experientially, patients relive childhood memories of abuse through imagery. Because this is usually an upsetting process, patients need a good deal of preparation and time before undertaking it. The therapist waits until the patient is ready. Venting anger is of primary importance in the experiential work. It is especially important for patients to vent anger at the people who abused them during childhood, rather than continually direct anger at the people in their current lives, or at themselves. In imagery of childhood abuse, patients express all the emotions that were strangulated at the time. The therapist enters the images of abuse to stand up to the perpetrator, and protect and comfort the Abused Child. This helps the patient internalize the therapist as a trustworthy and effective caretaker. Eventually, the patient enters the imagery as the Healthy Adult and does the same, standing up to the perpetrator, and protecting and comforting the child. Patients also work in imagery to find a safe place, away from the abuser. This could be an image from the patient's past, or an image the therapist and patient construct together, perhaps of a beautiful natural scene or of soothing lights and colors. Finally, patients visualize themselves being open and authentic with trustworthy significant others. Once again, the thrust of treatment is first to help patients make the sharp distinction between the people in the past who deserve the anger, and people in the present who do not; then, to help patients express anger in therapy sessions toward the people in the past who deserve it, while treating well those people in their current lives who treat them well.

Behaviorally, patients gradually learn to trust honest people. They increase their level of intimacy with appropriate significant others. When appropriate, they share their secrets and memories of abuse with their partner or close friends. They consider joining a support group for abuse survivors. They choose nonabusive partners. Patients stop mistreating others and set limits with abusive people. They are less punitive when other people make mistakes. Rather than avoiding relationships and remaining alone, or avoiding intimate encounters and staying emotionally distant from people, they allow people to get close and become intimate. They stop gathering evidence and keeping score about the things other people have done to hurt them. They stop constantly testing other people in relationships to see if they can be trusted. They stop taking advantage of other people, thus prompting others to respond in kind.

The patient's intimate relationships are an important focus of treatment. He or she learns to become more trusting and behave more appropriately with significant others, such as lovers, friends, and coworkers (assuming the other person is trustworthy). Patients become more selective, both in whom they choose and whom they trust in their lives outside sessions. It is often helpful to bring the partner into therapy as well, so the therapist can give the patient examples of how the patient is misconstruing the partner. Some patients with this schema have become so abusive that they are seriously mistreating others. These patients need the therapist to serve as a model of morality and to set limits. Getting patients to stop mistreating others is an important behavioral goal.

In terms of the therapy relationship, the therapist tries to be as honest and genuine as possible with the patient. He or she asks about trust issues regularly, discussing any negative feelings the patient has toward the therapist. The therapist moves slowly, postponing the experiential work, while building sufficient trust. The empowerment of the patient is a core principle of treating this schema. The therapist aims to restore to the patient the sense of a strong, active, and capable self that was broken by the abuse. The therapist encourages independence and gives the patient a large measure of control over the course of treatment.

Abuse severs the bond between the individual and other human beings. The person is torn out of the world of ordinary human relationships and thrown into a nightmare. During abuse, the victim feels utterly alone, and, after it is over, feels detached and estranged from others. The real world of current relationships seems hazy and unreal, whereas the memories of the relationship with the perpetrator are sharp and clear. (In *The Bell Jar,* Sylvia Plath [1966] wrote: "To the person in the bell jar, blank and stopped as a dead baby, the world itself is the bad dream" [p. 278].) The therapist is an intermediary between the abuse survivor and the rest of humanity: he or she serves as a vessel through which the patient reconnects to the ordinary world. By connecting to the therapist, the patient reconnects symbolically to the rest of humanity.

Adapting a term from Alice Miller, the therapist strives to become an "enlightened witness" to the patient's experience of abuse (Miller, 1975). As the patient tells the story, the therapist listens with a presence that is strong and nonjudgmental. The therapist is willing to share the emotional burden of the trauma, whatever it is. Sometimes the therapist must witness the patient's vulnerability and disintegration under extreme conditions, or the perpetrator's capacity for evil. Additionally, most survivors of abuse struggle with moral issues. They are haunted by feelings of shame and guilt about what they did and felt during the abuse. They want to understand their own responsibility for what happened to them, and to reach a fair, moral judgment of their own conduct. The therapist's role is not to provide the answers, but to provide a safe place for patients to find their own answers (correcting negative distortions along the way).

Through "limited reparenting," the therapist strives for a personal connection to the patient. Rather than relating as an impersonal expert, the therapist is a real person who cares about the patient and whom the patient can trust. The fact that the therapist strives for a close emotional bond with the patient does not mean that the therapist exceeds the limits of the therapist–patient relationship. Rather, the limits of the relationship provide a safe place for both therapist and patient to undertake the work of healing. Staying within these limits is essential for therapists when working with abuse survivors, because the work can be emotionally overwhelming. To treat survivors of abuse is to face dark truths about human fragility in the world and the human potential for evil.

Treating survivors of trauma can itself be traumatizing. Sometimes therapists even start experiencing the same feelings of fear, rage, and grief that the patient feels. Therapists may experience posttraumatic stress symptoms such as intrusive thoughts, nightmares, or flashbacks (Pearlman & MacIan, 1995). Therapists may fall into the patients' feelings of helplessness and hopelessness. Caught in all of these symptoms and feelings, a therapist might be tempted to exceed the limits of the therapist–patient relationship and become the patient's "rescuer." However, this would be a mistake: In exceeding limits, the therapist implies that the patient is helpless and runs the risk of becoming exhausted and resentful. (As we discussed in Chapter 2, schema therapy does exceed "typical" therapist–patient boundaries. However, although we extend the typical boundaries somewhat in order to provide limited reparenting, we are careful not to violate boundaries in ways that would be damaging to patients. For example, while we do provide trauma survivors with overt comforting, we do not push them to work faster on traumatic material than they want to go.)

In severe cases, it can take a long time for patients with a Mistrust/ Abuse schema to trust the therapist—to trust that he or she is not going to hurt, cheat, humiliate, abuse, or lie to them. A good deal of therapy time is devoted to helping patients observe all the ways they misconstrue the therapist's intentions, keep important facts secret, and avoid vulnerability. The goal is for patients to internalize the therapist as someone they can trust—perhaps the first close person in their lives who is both good and strong.

Special Problems with This Schema

If the Mistrust/Abuse schema developed out of early childhood trauma, it often takes a long time to treat—only the Abandonment schema usually takes as long to treat. Occasionally, the damage is so severe that the patient can never trust the therapist enough to open up and change. No matter what the therapist does, the patient keeps twisting the therapist's behavior in such a way that it seems malevolent or reflects some underlying negative motive. When the patient has strong compensatory behaviors, this can be a very difficult schema to overcome.

On a less serious level, patients may not want the therapist to take notes, may be unwilling to fill out forms, or may withhold important information because they are afraid that somehow the material will be used against them. We believe the therapist should accommodate these requests as much as possible, but also point them out to patients as examples of schema perpetuation.

Emotional Deprivation

Typical Presentation of the Schema

This is probably the most common schema we treat in our work, although patients frequently do not recognize that they have it. Patients with this schema often enter treatment feeling lonely, bitter, and depressed, but usually not knowing why; or they present with vague or unclear symptoms that later prove to be related to the Emotional Deprivation schema. These patients do not expect other people—including the therapist—to nurture, understand, or protect them. They feel emotionally deprived, and may feel that they do not get enough affection and warmth, attention, or deep emotions expressed. They may feel that no one is there who can give them strength and guidance. Such patients may feel misunderstood and alone in the world. They may feel cheated of love, invisible, or empty.

As we have noted, there are three types of deprivation: deprivation of *nurturance,* in which patients feel that no one is there to hold them, pay attention to them, and give them physical affection, such as touch and holding; deprivation of *empathy,* in which they feel that no one is there who really listens or tries to understand who they are and how they feel; and deprivation of *protection,* in which they feel that no one is there to protect and guide them (even though they are often giving others a lot of protection and guidance). The Emotional Deprivation schema is often linked to the Self-Sacrifice schema. Most patients with a Self-Sacrifice schema are also emotionally deprived.

Typical behaviors exhibited by these patients include not asking significant others for what they need emotionally; not expressing a desire for love or comfort; focusing on asking the other person questions but saying little about oneself; acting stronger than one feels underneath; and in other ways reinforcing the deprivation by acting as though they do not have emotional needs. Because these patients do not expect emotional support, they do not ask for it; consequently, usually they do not get it.

Another tendency we see in patients with an Emotional Deprivation schema is choosing significant others who cannot or do not want to give emotionally. They often choose people who are cold, aloof, self-centered, or needy, and therefore likely to deprive them emotionally. Other, more avoidant, patients become loners. They avoid intimate relationships because they do not expect to get anything from them anyway. Either they stay in very distant relationships or avoid relationships entirely.

Patients who overcompensate for emotional deprivation tend to be overly demanding and become angry when their needs are not met. These patients are sometimes narcissistic: Because they were both indulged and deprived as children, they have developed strong feelings of entitlement to get their needs met. They believe they must be adamant in their demands to get anything at all. A minority of patients with the Emotional Deprivation schema were indulged in other ways as children: They were spoiled materially, not required to follow normal rules of behavior, or adored for some talent or gift, but they were not given genuine love.

Another tendency in a small percentage of patients with this schema is to be overly needy. Some patients express so many needs so intensely that they come across as clinging or helpless, even histrionic. They may have many physical complaints—psychosomatic symptoms—with the secondary gain of getting people to pay attention to them and take care of them (although this function is almost always outside their awareness).

Goals of Treatment

One major goal of treatment is to help patients become aware of their emotional needs. It may feel so natural to them to have their emotional needs go unmet that they are not even aware that something is wrong. Another goal is to help patients accept that their emotional needs are natural and right. Every child needs nurturance, empathy, and protection, and, as adults, we still need these things. If patients can learn how to choose appropriate people and then ask for what they need in appropriate ways, then other people will give to them emotionally. It is not that other people are inherently depriving; it is that these patients have learned behaviors that either lead them to choose people who cannot give, or discourage people who can give from meeting their needs.

Strategies Emphasized in Treatment

There is a strong emphasis on exploring the childhood origins of this schema. The therapist uses experiential work to help patients recognize that their emotional needs were not met in childhood. Many patients never realized they were missing something, even though they had symptoms of missing something. Through imagery work, patients get in touch with the Lonely Child part of themselves and connect this mode to their presenting problems. In imagery, they express their anger and pain to the depriving parent. They list all their unmet emotional needs in childhood, and what they wish the parent had done to meet each one. The therapist enters images of childhood as the Healthy Adult, who comforts and helps the Lonely Child; then, the patient enters the image as the Healthy Adult, and comforts and helps the Lonely Child. Patients write a letter to the parent, for homework (which they do not send), about the deprivation uncovered through imagery work.

As with most of the schemas in the Disconnection and Rejection domain, the therapy relationship is central to the treatment of the schema. (The exception is the Social Isolation schema, which usually involves less emphasis on the patient–therapist relationship and more on the patient's outside relationships.) The therapy relationship is often the first place these patients have ever allowed anyone to take care of, understand, and guide them. Through "limited reparenting," the therapist provides a partial antidote to their emotional deprivation: a warm, empathic, and protective environment, where they can get many of their emotional needs met. If the therapist cares about and reparents the patient, then this will ease the patient's sense of deprivation. As with the Abandonment schema, the therapy relationship provides a model that patients can then transfer to others in their lives outside therapy (a "corrective emotional experience" (Alexander, 1956). Like the Abandonment schema, there is a great deal of emphasis on the patient's intimate relationships. The therapist and patient carefully study the patient's relationships with significant others. Patients work on choosing appropriate partners and close friends, identifying their own needs, and asking to have these needs met in appropriate ways.

Cognitively, the therapist helps patients change their exaggerated sense that significant others are acting selfishly or depriving them. To counter the "black or white" thinking that fuels overreactions, the patient learns to discriminate gradations of deprivation—to see a continuum rather than just two opposing poles. Even though other people set limits on what they give, they still care about the patient. Patients identify the unmet emotional needs in their current relationships.

Behaviorally, patients learn to choose nurturing partners and friends. They ask their partners to meet their emotional needs in appropriate ways and accept nurturance from significant others. Patients stop avoiding intimacy. They stop responding with excessive anger to mild levels of deprivation and withdrawing or isolating when they feel neglected by others.

In the therapy relationship, the therapist provides a nurturing atmosphere with attention, empathy, and guidance, making special attempts to demonstrate emotional involvement (e.g., remembering the patient's birthday with a card). The therapist helps the patient express feelings of deprivation without overreacting or remaining silent. The patient learns to accept the therapist's limitations and to tolerate some deprivation, while appreciating the nurturing the therapist does provide. The therapist helps the patient connect feelings in the therapy relationship with early memories of deprivation, and to work on those memories experientially.

Special Problems with This Schema

The most common problem is that patients with this schema are so frequently unaware of it. Even though Emotional Deprivation is one of the three most common schemas we work with (Subjugation and Defectiveness schemas are the others), people often do not know that they have it. Because they never got their emotional needs met, patients often do not even realize that they have unmet emotional needs. Thus, helping patients make a connection between their depression, loneliness, or physical symptoms on the one hand, and the absence of nurturing, empathy, and protection on the other is very important. We have found that asking patients to read the Emotional Deprivation chapter of *Reinventing Your Life* (Young & Klosko, 1993) can often help them recognize the schema. They can identify with some of the characters or recognize the behavior of a depriving parent.

Patients with this schema often negate the validity of their emotional needs. They deny that their needs are important or worthwhile, or they believe that strong people do not have needs. They consider it bad or weak to ask others to meet their needs and have trouble accepting that there is a Lonely Child inside them who wants love and connection, both from the therapist and from significant others in the outside world.

Similarly, patients may believe that significant others should know what they need, and that they should not have to ask. All of these beliefs work against the patient's ability to ask others to meet his or her needs. These patients need to learn that it is human to have needs, and healthy to ask others to meet them. It is human nature to be emotionally vulnerable. What we aim for in life is a balance between strength and vulnerability, so that sometimes we are strong and other times we are vulnerable. To only have one side—to only be strong—is to be not fully human and to deny a core part of ourselves.

Defectiveness/Shame

Typical Presentation of the Schema

Patients with this schema believe that they are defective, flawed, inferior, bad, worthless, or unlovable. Consequently, they often experience chronic feelings of shame about who they are.

What aspects of themselves do they view as defective? It could be almost any personal characteristic—they believe that they are too angry, too needy, too evil, too ugly, too lazy, too dumb, too boring, too strange, too overbearing, too fat, too thin, too tall, too short, or too weak. They might have unacceptable sexual or aggressive desires. Something in their very being feels defective: It is not something they *do*, but something they feel they *are*. They fear relationships with others because they dread the inevitable moment when their defectiveness will be exposed. At any moment, other people might suddenly see through them to the defectiveness at their core, and they will be filled with shame. This fear can apply to the private or public worlds: Patients with this schema feel defective in their intimate relationships or in the wider social world (or both).

Typical behaviors of patients with this schema include devaluing themselves and allowing others to devalue them. These patients may allow others to mistreat or even verbally abuse them. They are often hypersensitive to criticism or rejection, and react very strongly, either by becoming sad and downcast or angry, depending upon whether they are surrendering to the schema or overcompensating for it. They secretly feel that they are to blame for their problems with other people. Often self-conscious, they tend to make a lot of comparisons between themselves and others. They feel insecure around other people, particularly those perceived as "not defective," or those who might see through to their defectiveness. They may be jealous and competitive, especially in the area of their felt defectiveness, and sometimes view interpersonal interactions as a dance of "one up, one down." They often choose critical and rejecting partners, and may be critical of the people who love them. (Groucho Marx expressed the latter sentiment when he said, "I wouldn't want to belong to a club that would have me as a member.") Many of the characteristics of narcissistic patients—such as grandiosity and unrelenting standards—can be manifestations of a Defectiveness schema. In many cases, these characteristics serve to compensate for underlying feelings of defectiveness and shame.

Patients may avoid intimate relationships or social situations, because people might see their defects. In fact, we believe that avoidant personality disorder is a common manifestation of the Defectiveness schema, with avoidance as the primary coping style. This schema can also lead to substance abuse, eating disorders, and other serious problems.

Goals of Treatment

The basic goal of treatment is to increase the patient's sense of self-esteem. Patients who have healed this schema believe that they are worthy of love and respect. Their feelings of defectiveness were either mistaken or greatly exaggerated: Either the trait is not really a defect, or it is a limitation that is far less important than it feels to them. Furthermore, the patient is often able to correct the "defect." But, even if patients cannot correct it, it does not negate their value as human beings. It is the nature of human beings to be flawed and imperfect. We can love each other anyway.

Patients who have healed this schema are more at ease around other people. They feel much less vulnerable and exposed, and are more willing to enter relationships. They are no longer so prone to feelings of self-consciousness when other people pay attention to them. These patients regard other people as less judgmental and more accepting, and put human flaws into a realistic perspective. Becoming more open with people, they stop keeping so many secrets and trying to hide so many parts of themselves, and can maintain a sense of their own value, even when others criticize or reject them. They accept compliments more naturally and no longer allow other people to treat them badly. Less defensive, they are less perfectionistic about themselves and other people, and choose partners who love them and treat them well. In summary, they no longer exhibit behaviors that surrender to, avoid, or overcompensate for their Defectiveness/Shame schema.

Strategies Emphasized in Treatment

Once again, the therapy relationship is central to the treatment of this schema. If the therapist, knowing about the perceived defect, is able to still care about the patient, then the patient will know it and feel more worthwhile. It is important for the therapist to give a lot of direct affirmation and praise, and point out the patient's positive attributes.

Cognitive strategies aim to alter patients' view of themselves as defective. Patients examine the evidence for and against the schema, and they conduct dialogues between the critical schema and the healthy side that has good self-esteem. They learn to highlight their assets and to reduce the significance they assign to their flaws. Rather than being inherent, most of their flaws are behaviors they learned in childhood that can be changed, or they are not flaws at all, but rather manifestations of overcriticalness. We have found that most patients with this schema do not really have serious flaws, just extremely critical or rejecting parents. And even if the patient does have flaws, most of them can be addressed in therapy or through other means; if they cannot, they are not as profound as the patient considers them. Cognitive techniques help the patient reattribute feelings of defectiveness and shame to the criticalness of significant others in childhood. Flash cards listing the patient's good qualities are very helpful with this schema.

Experientially, it is important for patients to vent anger at their critical, rejecting parents in imagery and dialogues. The therapist enters childhood images of the parent criticizing and rejecting the patient, and the therapist confronts the parent and comforts, protects, and praises the Rejected Child. Eventually, patients are able to play this role themselves: They enter the image as the Healthy Adult who stands up to the critical parent and comforts the Rejected Child.

Behavioral strategies—particularly exposure—are important to treatment, especially for avoidant patients. As long as patients with Defectiveness schemas avoid intimate human contact, their feelings of defectiveness remain intact. Patients work on entering interpersonal situations that hold the potential to enhance their lives. Behavioral strategies can also help patients correct some legitimate flaws (i.e., lose weight, improve their style of dress, learn social skills). In addition, patients work on choosing significant others who are supportive rather than critical. They try to select partners who love and accept them.

Behaviorally, patients also learn to stop overreacting to criticism. They learn that, when someone gives them a valid criticism, the appropriate response is to accept the criticism and try to change themselves; when someone gives them a criticism that is not valid, the appropriate response is simply to state their point of view to the other person and affirm internally that the criticism is false. It is not appropriate to attack the other person; it is not necessary to respond in kind or to fight to prove the other person wrong. Patients learn to set limits with hypercritical people and stop tolerating maltreatment. Patients also work on self-disclosing more to significant others whom they trust. The more they can share themselves and still be accepted, the more they will be able to overcome the schema. Finally, patients work on decreasing compensatory behaviors. They stop trying to overcompensate for their inner sense of defectiveness by appearing perfect, achieving excessively, demeaning others, or competing for status.

It is especially important for the therapist to be accepting and nonjudgmental toward patients with this schema. It is also important that the therapist not come across as perfect. Like every human being, the therapist makes mistakes and acknowledges flaws.

Special Problems with This Schema

Many patients who have this schema are unaware of it. A lot of patients are avoiding or overcompensating for the pain of this schema, rather than feeling that pain. Patients with narcissistic personality disorder are an example of a group with a high probability of having the Defectiveness schema and a low probability of being aware of it. Narcissistic patients often get caught up in competing with or denigrating the therapist rather than working on change.

Patients with a Defectiveness schema might hold back information about themselves because they are embarrassed. A long time may pass before these patients are willing to share fully their memories, desires, thoughts, and feelings.

This schema is difficult to change. The earlier and more severe the criticism and rejection from parents, the more difficult it is to heal.

Social Isolation

Typical Presentation of the Schema

Patients with this schema believe that they are different from other people. They do not feel that they are part of most groups and feel isolated, left out, or "on the outside looking in." Anyone who grows up feeling different might develop the schema. Examples include gifted people, those from famous families, people with great physical beauty or ugliness, gay men and women, members of ethnic minorities, children of alcoholics, trauma survivors, people with physical disabilities, orphans or adoptees, and people who belong to a significantly higher or lower economic class than those around them.

Typical behaviors include staying on the periphery or avoiding groups altogether. These patients tend to engage in solitary activities: Most "loners" have this schema. Depending upon the severity of the schema, the patient may be part of a subculture but still feel alienated from the larger social world; he or she may feel alienated from all groups but have some intimate relationships, or be disconnected from virtually everyone.

Goals of Treatment

The basic goal of treatment is to help patients feel less different from other people. Even if they are not part of the mainstream, there are other people similar to them. Furthermore, at the core, we are all human beings, with the same basic needs and desires. Even though we have many differences, we are more alike than different. ("Nothing human is alien to me," [Terrence, trans. 1965, I, i].) There may be a segment of society in which the patient probably will never fit—such as a gay patient in a fundamentalist religious group—but there are other places where the patient will fit. The patient should walk away from unwelcoming groups and find people who are more similar or accepting. Often, the patient must make major life changes and overcome extensive avoidance in order to accomplish this.

Strategies Emphasized in Treatment

Unlike the other schemas in the Disconnection and Rejection realm, the focus is less on working experientially with childhood origins of the schema and more on improving the patient's current relationships with peers and groups. Thus, cognitive and behavioral strategies take precedence. Group therapy may be helpful for many patients with this schema, especially those who avoid even friendships. The more isolated the patient, the more important the therapy relationship is to the treatment, because it will be one of the patient's only relationships.

The aim of the cognitive strategies is to convince patients that they really are not as different from other people as they think. They share many qualities with all people, and some of the qualities that they regard as distinguishing them are in fact universal (e.g., sexual or aggressive fantasies). Even if they are not part of the mainstream, there are other people like them. Patients learn to focus on their similarities with other people, as well as their differences. They learn to identify subgroups of people who are like them—who share the ways they are different; they learn that many people can accept them even though they are different. They learn to challenge the automatic negative thoughts that block them from joining groups and connecting to the people in them.

Experiential strategies can help patients who were excluded as children and adolescents remember what it was like. (Some patients with this schema were not excluded as children. Rather, they chose solitude due to some preference or interest.) In imagery, patients relive these childhood experiences. They vent anger at the peers who excluded them; and they express their loneliness. Patients fight back against social prejudice toward people who are different. (This is one advantage of consciousness-raising groups: They teach group members to fight back against the hatred of others.) Patients can also use imagery to picture groups of people with whom they could fit in.

Behavioral strategies focus on helping patients overcome their avoidance of social situations. The goal is for patients gradually to start attending groups, connect to the people there, and cultivate friendships. In order to work toward this goal, patients undergo graduated exposure through a series of homework assignments. Anxiety management can help patients cope with their usually considerable social anxiety. Social skills training can help them work to correct any deficits in interpersonal skills. Where necessary, medication might be added to decrease the patient's anxiety.

Of course, it is positive when patients with this schema have a close relationship with the therapist. However, unless patients also focus on cognitive and behavioral strategies to overcome their avoidance of social situations, the therapy relationship is probably not going to help them sufficiently. Sometimes patients with this schema can connect to the therapist, yet still continue to feel different from everyone else. It depends on the severity of the schema: For patients on the extreme end, the therapy relationship can counter their feelings of utter aloneness and be important. But to the extent that patients can already connect to individuals but cannot connect to groups, the therapy relationship by itself will probably not be especially valuable as a corrective emotional experience. Group therapy can be extremely helpful if the group is accepting of the patient; for this reason, "special interest" groups—containing members who are similar to the patient in some significant way (i.e., children of alcoholics, incest survivors, support groups for overweight patients)—can be most valuable.

Special Problems with This Schema

The most common problem is that patients have difficulty overcoming their avoidance of social situations and groups. In order to confront the situations that they fear, patients must be willing to tolerate a high level of emotional discomfort. For this reason, their pattern of avoidance is resistant to change. When avoidance blocks progress in treatment, mode work can often help patients build up the part of themselves that wants the schema to change and talk back to the schema. For example, patients might imagine a group situation in which they recently felt alienated. The therapist enters the image as the Healthy Adult, who advises the Isolated Child (or Adolescent) about how to integrate with the group. Later, patients enter their images as their own Healthy Adult, to help the Isolated Child master and enjoy social situations.

IMPAIRED AUTONOMY AND PERFORMANCE DOMAIN

Dependence/Incompetence

Typical Presentation of the Schema

These patients present as childlike and helpless. They feel unable to take care of themselves on their own, experience life as overwhelming, and themselves as inadequate to cope. The schema has two elements. The first is incompetence: These patients lack faith in their decisions and judgments about everyday life. They hate and fear facing change alone; they feel unable to tackle new tasks on their own and believe they need someone to show them what to do. These patients feel like children too young to survive on their own in the world: Without parents they might die. In the extreme form of the schema, patients believe they will not be able to feed, clothe, and shelter themselves, navigate from one place to another, or fulfill the simple, everyday tasks of life.

The second element—dependence—follows from the first. Because these patients feel unable to function on their own, their only options are to find other people to take care of them or not to function at all. The people they find to take care of them are usually parents or substitute parents, such as partners, siblings, friends, bosses—or therapists. The parent figure either does everything for them or shows them what to do at new each step along the way. The core idea is "I am incompetent; therefore, I must depend on others."

Typical behaviors include asking others for help; constantly asking questions as they work on new tasks; repeatedly seeking advice about decisions; having difficulty traveling alone and managing finances on their own; giving up easily; refusing additional responsibilities (i.e., a promotion at work); and avoiding new tasks. Difficulty driving is often a metaphor for the schema. People with the Dependence/Incompetence schema often fear and avoid driving alone: They might get lost; their car might break down, and they would not know what to do. Something unforeseen might happen, and they would not be able to handle it. They would not be able to come up with a solution on their own. Thus, they need someone with them who can either give them the solution or handle the problem for them.

These patients usually do not come into therapy with the goal of becoming more independent or more competent. Rather, they come looking for a magic pill, or for an expert who will tell them what to do. Their presenting problems are often Axis I symptoms such as anxiety, phobic avoidance, or stress-induced physical problems. They may be depressed because they are afraid to leave an abusive, depriving, or controlling partner or parent figure, often a person resembling the parent who induced the schema, because they do not believe they can survive on their own. Their goal is typically to get rid of these symptoms rather than change their core sense of dependence and incompetence.

A small percentage of patients with the Dependence/Incompetence schema overcompensate for the schema by becoming counterdependent. Even though underneath they feel incompetent, they insist on doing everything on their own. They refuse to rely on anyone for anything. They will not be dependent, even in situations where it is normal to be dependent. Like pseudomature children who have had to grow up too soon, they manage alone, but they do it with a tremendous amount of anxiety. They take on new tasks and make their own decisions, and they may perform well and make good decisions, but inside, they always feel that, this time, they are not going to be able to pull it off.

Goals of Treatment

The goals of treatment are to increase the patient's sense of competence and decrease dependence on other people. Increasing the patient's sense of competence usually involves building both confidence and skills; decreasing his or her dependence involves overcoming avoidance of trying tasks alone. Ideally, these patients become able to stop relying on other people to an unhealthy degree.

Giving up the dependence is the key to treatment. The therapist guides patients through a kind of response prevention: Patients stop themselves from turning to others for help, handle tasks on their own, accept that making mistakes is how they will learn, persevere until they are successful, and prove to themselves that they can eventually generate their own solutions to problems. Through trial and error, they can learn to trust their own intuition and judgments rather than disregarding them.

Strategies Emphasized in Treatment

The cognitive-behavioral element of treatment is usually the most important with this schema. The focus is on helping patients change cognitions, build skills, and undergo graduated exposure to making decisions and functioning independently.

Cognitive strategies help patients alter the view that they need constant assistance in order to function. The techniques are the usual ones: flash cards, dialogues between the schema side and the healthy side, problem-solving to make decisions, and challenging negative thoughts. The therapist questions the patient's view that depending on others is a desirable way to live. Excessive dependence on others has costs, such as unfulfilled emotional needs for autonomy and self-expression, which the therapist and patient can elucidate together. Using cognitive strategies to build motivation is essential because, in order to overcome the schema, patients will have to be willing to tolerate anxiety. The therapist can graduate the tasks from low to high anxiety to decrease the patient's distress, and teach the patient relaxation, meditation, or other anxiety-reducing techniques.

As we have noted, experiential techniques are usually less important with this schema. At times, it is useful for patients to confront in imagery the parent who overprotected and undermined them in childhood, for example, if the parents are still treating them this way and they are angry about it. If patients are angry with the parent, the therapist helps them express it. However, patients with this schema often are not angry with the parent. Because the parent was often trying to help, mobilizing anger can be difficult. Nevertheless, even if the parent's intentions were good, what he or she did was damaging to the patients' independence and sense of competence. Because the parent made so many decisions for them, patients were unable to develop confidence in their own judgment; because their parent did so many tasks for them, they were unable to develop basic living skills.

The therapist conducts imagery sessions in which the patient remembers childhood situations that created the schema. The patient enters the image as the Healthy Adult, who helps the Incompetent Child cope and solve problems. When the patient is unable to come up with a healthy response, the therapist acts as coach. The therapist also conducts imagery sessions in which the patient imagines current situations that require practicing basic living skills. Again, the patient enters the image as the Healthy Adult to help the Incompetent Child. (Many patients with this schema see themselves as little children when they picture themselves—little children in a world of big adults). The Healthy Adult says to the child, "I know you are young and too scared to made decisions. But you don't have to make them. I will make them for you. I am an adult even though you are a child. I can make decisions and I can do things on my own."

The behavioral part of treatment helps patients overcome their avoidance of independent functioning. This is crucial to the success of the treatment: If patients do not change their behavior, they will not gather enough evidence to fight the schema. Because avoidance maintains a conditioned fear indefinitely, patients will not be able to heal the schema until they are willing to confront anxiety-arousing situations. Therapists help patients to set up graded assignments in which they handle everyday tasks on their own. Starting with the easiest one, they practice handling these tasks as homework assignments.

Therapists can carry out behavioral rehearsals with patients during sessions to help them prepare for homework assignments. Patients imagine or role-play themselves successfully completing the tasks, solving any problems that arise. It is helpful for patients to reward themselves whenever they complete homework assignments. Anxiety management techniques—such as flash cards, breathing exercises, relaxation techniques, and rational responding—can help patients tolerate the anxiety of functioning independently.

Sometimes the therapist involves family members in the treatment if they are still fostering dependence in the patient, especially when the patient is living with them. Family members can be an important part of the both the problem and the solution to the schema. If the patient is able to handle family members adequately alone, then the therapist does not meet with them. However, as more often happens, if the patient is unable to stop family members from reinforcing the schema, then the therapist considers intervening.

In the therapy relationship, it is important to resist attempts by patients to take on a dependent role with the therapist. Rather, the therapist should encourage patients to make their own decisions, giving them help only when necessary. The therapist should also remember to acknowledge patients whenever they make progress on their own.

Special Problems with This Schema

One of the greatest risks is that the patient might become dependent on the therapist rather than overcoming the schema. The therapist mistakenly assumes the role of parent figure and runs the patient's life. The amount of dependence the therapist allows is a delicate balancing act. If the therapist does not allow any dependence, the patient will probably not stay in treatment. Realistically, the therapist has to start by allowing some dependence and then gradually withdrawing. The therapist should strive to allow the least possible amount of dependence that will keep the patient in treatment.

One of the greatest challenges in treating patients with this schema is overcoming their avoidance of independent functioning. Patients have to become willing to trade short-term pain for long-term gain and tolerate the anxiety of functioning as adults in the world. As we have noted, building motivation is an important aspect of treatment. Mode work can help patients strengthen the healthy part of themselves that wants independence and competence. This Independence Seeker can carry out dialogues with the dysfunctional parent, and with the coping modes in the patient that are blocking motivation.

Vulnerability to Harm or Illness

Typical Presentation of the Schema

These patients live their lives believing that catastrophe is about to strike at any moment. They are convinced that something terrible is going to happen to them that is beyond their control. They will suddenly be struck with a medical illness; there will be a natural disaster; they will become victims of crime; they will get into a terrible accident; they will lose all their money; or they will have a nervous breakdown and go crazy. A bad thing is going to happen, and they are not going to be able to prevent it. The predominant emotion is anxiety, ranging from low-level dread to full-blown panic attacks. These patients are not afraid of handling everyday situations, like patients who have Dependence schemas; rather, they are afraid of catastrophic events.

Most of these patients rely on avoidance or overcompensation to cope with the schema. They become phobic, restrict their lives, take tranquilizers, engage in magical thinking, perform compulsive rituals, or rely on "safety signals," such as a person they trust, a bottle of water, or tranquilizers. All of these behaviors have the goal of stopping the bad thing from happening.

Goals of Treatment

The goals of treatment are to get patients to lower their estimations of the likelihood of catastrophic events and to raise their evaluations of their ability to cope. Ideally, patients come to recognize that their fears are greatly exaggerated and, even if a catastrophe did occur, they would be able to deal with it adequately. The ultimate goal of treatment is to convince patients to stop avoiding and overcompensating for the schema, and to face most of the situations they fear. (Of course, we do not encourage patients to confront truly dangerous situations, such as driving in heavy storms or swimming in the ocean too far from the shore.)

Strategies Emphasized in Treatment

Patients explore the childhood origins of the schema and trace its pattern through their lives. They count the costs of the schema. Patients explore the changes they would make in their current lives if they were not overly afraid. It is important to spend time building the patient's motivation to change. The therapist helps the patient stay focused on the long-term negative consequences of living a phobic lifestyle, such as lost opportunities for fun and self-exploration; and on the positive benefits of moving more freely in the world, such as a richer, fuller life. Mode work is especially helpful in battling the patient's resistance to change, helping the patient build a Healthy Adult who wants to progress, and who can guide the Frightened Child through challenging situations. Without sufficient motivation, patients will be unwilling to endure the anxiety of giving up their maladaptive coping devices. Cognitive and behavioral strategies for overcoming anxiety and avoidance are the central focus of treatment.

Cognitive strategies help patients lower their estimation of the probability of catastrophic events and raise their estimation of their capacity to cope. Patients counter their exaggerated perceptions of danger. Challenging catastrophic thoughts—or "decatastrophizing"—helps them manage panic attacks and other anxiety symptoms. Cognitive strategies also help patients build motivation by highlighting the advantages of changing.

Similarly, behavioral strategies help patients give up their magical rituals and safety signals, and face the situations they fear. Patients undergo graduated exposure to phobic situations in homework assignments between sessions. In order to prepare for these exposures, patients use imagery rehearsal in sessions: They picture themselves entering specific phobic situations and, with the assistance of the "Healthy Adult," coping well. Anxiety-management techniques such as breathing exercises, meditation, and flash cards, help patients cope with the exposures as they go through them.

Experiential strategies are important, especially imagery for rehearsal and mode work. If the schema is the internalization of a parent (having a parent who models the schema is one of the most common origins), then the patient can conduct dialogues with this parent in imagery. The patient can enter images of childhood or current situations as the Healthy Adult to reassure the Frightened Child, and to confront the parent about the negative consequences of catastrophizing. Additionally, patients can visualize the Healthy Adult leading the Frightened Child to safety in phobic situations.

The therapy relationship is not the crucial aspect of treatment with these patients. What is most important is that the therapist consistently adopt an attitude of empathic confrontation toward the patient's reliance on avoidance and overcompensation, and provide calm reassurance that the patient will be able to cope in healthier ways. In addition, the therapist models nonphobic ways of viewing and handling situations containing acceptable levels of risk.

Special Problems with This Schema

The greatest problem is that patients are too afraid to stop avoiding and overcompensating. They resist giving up these protections against the anxiety of the schema. As we mentioned earlier, mode work can help patients strengthen the healthy part of them that yearns for a fuller life.

Enmeshment/Undeveloped Self

Typical Presentation of the Schema

When patients with an Enmeshment schema enter treatment, they are often so fused with a significant other that neither they nor the therapist can say clearly where the patient's identity begins and the "enmeshed other" ends. This person is usually a parent or a parental figure, such as a partner, sibling, boss, or best friend. Patients with this schema feel an extreme emotional involvement and closeness with the parental figure, at the expense of full individuation and normal social development. (One such patient, enmeshed with his mother, told his therapist how his mother, trying to dissuade him from getting married, said: "I know what's best for you, son. After all, I've been in and out of a lot of women with you.")

Many of these patients believe that neither they nor the parental figure could survive emotionally without the constant support of the other, that they need each other desperately. They feel an intense bond with this parental figure, almost as though, together, they are one person. (Patients may feel that they can read the other person's mind, or sense what the other person wants without the other having to ask.) They believe it is wrong to set any boundaries with the parental figure, and feel guilty whenever they do. They tell the other person everything and expect the other person to tell them everything. They feel fused with this parental figure and may feel overwhelmed and smothered.

The characteristics discussed thus far represent the "Enmeshment" part of the schema. There is also the "Undeveloped Self", a lack of individual identify, which patients often experience as a feeling of emptiness. These patients often convey a sense of an absent self, because they have surrendered their identity in order to maintain their connection to the parental figure. Patients who have an undeveloped self feel as though they are drifting in the world without direction. They do not know who they are. They have not formed their own preferences or developed their unique gifts and talents, nor have they followed their own natural inclinations—what they naturally are good at and love to do. In extreme cases, they may question whether they really exist.

The "Enmeshment" and "Undeveloped Self" parts of the schema often, but not always, go together. Patients can have an undeveloped self without enmeshment. The undeveloped self can develop for reasons other than enmeshment, such as subjugation. For example, patients dominated as children may never have developed a separate sense of self, because they were forced to do whatever their parents demanded. However, patients who are enmeshed with a parent or parental figure almost always have an undeveloped self as a consequence. Their opinions, interests, choices, and goals are merely reflections of the person with whom they are merged. It is as though the parental figure's life is more real to them than their own: The parental figure is the star and they are the satellite. Similarly, patients with undeveloped selves might seek out charismatic group leaders with whom they can become enmeshed.

Typical behaviors include copying the behaviors of the parental figure, talking and thinking about him or her, staying in constant contact with the parental figure, and suppressing all thoughts, feelings, and behaviors that are discrepant from the parent figure. When patients do try to separate from the enmeshed person in any way, they feel overcome with guilt.

Goals of Treatment

The central goal of treatment is to help patients express their spontaneous, natural selves—their unique preferences, opinions, decisions, talents, and natural inclinations—rather than suppressing their true selves and merely adopting the identity of the parent figures with whom they are enmeshed. Patients who have been treated successfully for enmeshment issues are not focused to an unhealthy degree on a parental figure. They are at the center of their own lives. They are no longer fused with a parental figure and are aware of how they are similar to the parental figure and how they are different. They set boundaries with the parental figure and have a full sense of their own identity.

For patients who have avoided closeness as adults in order to avoid enmeshment, the goal of treatment is for the patient to establish connections with others that are neither too distant nor too enmeshed.

Strategies Emphasized in Treatment

Treatment focuses on patients' current lives. Cognitive and experiential techniques to help patients identify their preferences and natural inclinations, and behavioral techniques to help them enact their true self, are most important.

Cognitive strategies challenge the patient's view that it is preferable to be enmeshed with a parent figure than to have an identity of one's own. The therapist and patient explore the advantages and disadvantages of developing a separate self. Patients identify how they are both similar to and different from the parental figure. It is important to identify the similarities: The goal is not for patients to go to the opposite extreme and deny all similarities with the parental figure. Sometimes enmeshed patients say that they do not want to be like the parental figure at all now; and they cannot acknowledge even the similarities that exist. In this form of overcompensation for enmeshment, the patient does the opposite of the parental figure. In addition, patients conduct dialogues between the enmeshed side that wants to be fused with a parental figure, and the healthy side that wants to develop an individual identity.

Experientially, patients visualize separating from the parental figure in imagery. For example, patients relive moments in childhood when they disagreed with or felt different from the parent. They imagine saying what they truly felt, and doing what they truly wanted to do. They imagine telling past and current parental figures how they are different, and how they are alike. They imagine setting boundaries with past and current parental figures, such as refusing to divulge information or to spend more time together. The Healthy Adult, played first by the therapist and then by the patient, helps the Enmeshed Child accomplish the separation.

Behavioral strategies help patients identify their preferences and natural inclinations. Patients begin listing experiences they find inherently enjoyable as a behavioral experiment. They refer to their basic bodily sense of pleasure as a way of identifying what they enjoy. For homework, they may be asked to list their favorite music, movies, books, restaurants, or activities. Patients list what they like and dislike about significant others. Behavioral strategies also help patients act on their preferences even when they differ from those of a parental figure. Additionally, behavioral strategies help patients select partners and friends who do not foster enmeshment. Typically, patients with this schema select strong partners, and then submerge themselves in the partners' lives. The partner becomes the parental figure. Patients become a satellite in the orbit of their partner, another star.

The therapist sets appropriate boundaries, regulating the therapy relationship so that it is neither too merged nor too distant. If the therapist and patient are too merged, it will recreate the enmeshment of the patient's childhood; if it is too distant, the patient will feel disconnected and unmotivated to change.

Special Problems with This Schema

The most obvious potential problem is that the patient might enmesh with the therapist, so that the therapist becomes the new parental figure in the patient's life. The patient is able to give up the old parental figure, but only to replace the other person with the therapist. As with the Dependence/Incompetence schema, the therapist might have to allow some enmeshment at the beginning of treatment but should quickly begin encouraging the patient to individuate.

Failure

Typical Presentation of the Schema

Patients who have a Failure schema believe that they have failed relative to their peers in areas of achievement such as career, money, status, school, or sports. They feel that they are fundamentally inadequate compared to others at their level—that they are stupid, inept, untalented, ignorant, or unsuccessful, and that they inherently lack what it takes to succeed.

Typical behaviors or these patients include surrendering to the schema by sabotaging themselves or performing halfheartedly, avoidance behaviors such as procrastinating or not doing the task at all, and overcompensating behaviors such as working nonstop or otherwise overachieving. Overcompensators with Failure schemas believe that they are not as smart or talented as other people, but they can make up for it by working extra diligently. They are often quite successful, yet still feel fraudulent. These patients appear successful to the outside world but feel underneath that they are on the brink of failing.

It is important to distinguish between the Failure and Unrelenting Standards schemas. Patients with the Unrelenting Standards schema believe they have failed to meet their own (or their parents') high expectations, but they will acknowledge that they have done as well or better than the average person in their same occupation. Patients with the Failure schema believe they have done worse than most others in their occupation, and very often they are right. Most patients with the Failure schema have not accomplished as much as the average person in their peer group. Failure has become a self-fulfilling prophecy in their lives. It is also important to distinguish between the Failure schema and the Dependence/Incompetence schema, which has more to do with daily functioning than with achievement. The Failure schema involves money, status, career, sports, and school; the Dependence/Incompetence schema involves everyday decision-making and taking care of oneself in daily life. The Failure schema often leads to a linked Defectiveness schema. Feeling like a failure in areas of achievement, the person feels defective.

Goals of Treatment

The central goal of treatment is to help patients feel and become as successful as their peers (within the limits of their abilities and talents). This usually involves one of three scenarios. The first is increasing their level of success by building skills and confidence. Second, if they are, in fact, successful relative to their potential, it involves raising their appraisals of their level of success or changing perceptions of their peer group. The third scenario involves patients accepting unchangeable limitations in their abilities, while still feeling they have value.

Strategies Emphasized in Treatment

It is important to assess carefully the origin of the Failure schema for each patient, because the strategies the therapist emphasizes will depend on this assessment. Some patients have failed due to an innate lack of talent or intelligence. In these cases, the therapist tries to help the patient build skills and set realistic goals. Other patients have the talent and intelligence to succeed but have never applied themselves fully. Perhaps they have lacked direction or focused on the wrong areas. In these cases, the therapist aims to provide direction or to shift their focus to areas in which they have more natural talents. Perhaps patients have another disorder that has interfered with their development (such as attention deficit disorder), in which case the therapist needs to treat the other disorder. Perhaps they lack discipline:

Many patients with the Failure schema also have the Insufficient Self-Control/Self-Discipline schema. In these cases, the therapist allies with the patient to fight the Insufficient Self-Control/Self-Discipline schema. Perhaps patients are flooded with negative affect from another schema, such as Defectiveness or Emotional Deprivation, which they spend a lot of time and effort trying to avoid—by abusing drugs, drinking alcohol, playing the stock market, surfing the Internet, gambling, viewing pornography, or having sexual affairs—and the avoidance interferes with their dedication to work. In these cases, treatment involves working on the underlying schemas. It is important to assess why the patient has failed, in order to design the proper treatment for the problem. In most cases, the cognitive and behavioral aspects of the treatment take precedence.

If patients actually have failed relative to peers, then the most important cognitive strategy is to challenge the view that they are *inherently* inept and to reattribute their failure to schema perpetuation. These patients have not failed because they are inherently inept, but rather because they have inadvertently acted to defeat their attempts to succeed. It is the schema itself that has caused them to fail. Their coping styles—the ways they surrender to and avoid the schema—are the problem, not their basic ability. Patients conduct dialogues between the Failure schema and the healthy side that wants to fight the schema.

Another cognitive strategy is to highlight patients' successes and skills. Typically, patients with this schema have ignored their accomplishments and accentuated their failures. The therapist helps correct this bias by teaching patients to notice each time they are successful. The therapist also helps patients identify skills, utilizing cognitive techniques such as examining the evidence. Finally, the therapist helps patients set realistic long-term goals. Patients whose long-term goals are unrealistically high might have to lower their expectations for success, find a different comparison group, or switch to a different field.

Experiential techniques can be helpful in preparing patients to undertake behavioral change. In imagery, patients relive failure experiences from the past and express anger at the people who discouraged them, or mocked and devalued them for failing. Often, the person was a parent, older sibling, or teacher. Doing this helps patients reattribute the failure to the other person's criticalness rather than to their own lack of ability. Patients with attention-deficit/hyperactivity disorder are an example of a group often scolded as children for behaviors they usually could not control. Their parents viewed them as intentionally not learning, when, in fact, they could not learn normally. Naturally unathletic patients were often told they were not trying hard enough or practicing enough, when, in fact, they lacked the ability to perform at the expected level. Getting angry at parents and others for not recognizing and accepting their strengths and limitations is an important part of the process of letting go of the schema emotionally.

Alternatively, the patient's parents may not have wanted the patient to succeed. Although the parents may have been unaware of it, they did not want the child to become too successful. They were afraid that the child would surpass or abandon them. The parents gave the child subtle messages that they would reject him or her or withdraw emotionally if the child became too successful. The child developed a "fear of success." Experiential techniques help the patient identify this theme and relate to it emotionally. Getting angry with the Undermining Parent helps the patient understand that this was an unhealthy message, and one that the patient need no longer believe. Healthy parents do not punish their children for succeeding. Getting angry can help patients fight the view that people will reject them if they are too successful. Mode work helps patients develop a Healthy Adult mode that can encourage and guide the Failed Child. First the therapist, then the patient, plays the Healthy Adult in images of past and current achievement situations.

The behavioral part of the treatment is usually the most important. No matter how much progress patients make in the other areas, if they do not stop their maladaptive coping behaviors, they are going to keep reinforcing the schema. The therapist helps patients replace behaviors that surrender to, avoid, or overcompensate for the schema, with more adaptive behaviors. Patients set goals, set graded tasks to meet them, and then carry out the tasks as homework assignments. The therapist helps patients overcome blocks to completing the homework. If it is a skills problem, the therapist helps the patient develop skills. If it is an aptitude problem, the therapist helps the patient switch to more appropriate work. If it is an anxiety problem, the therapist teaches the patient anxiety management. If it is a problem with self-discipline, the therapist helps the patient create a structure to overcome procrastination and to build discipline. The therapist can help patients overcome blocks with behavioral rehearsal. Using imagery or role-playing techniques, they can work through whatever blocks naturally emerge.

In terms of the therapy relationship, the therapist models behaviors that are contrary to the schema: If the therapist sets realistic goals, works steadily to reach them, thinks through problems in advance, persists despite failure, and acknowledges progress, then the therapist's own professional life can serve as an antidote to the schema. (The therapist's professional success can also have the opposite effect, making the patient feel inadequate relative to the therapist. The therapist must be alert to this possibility. The key is that the therapist models a healthy approach to work, not that the actual level of the therapist's success matters.) The therapist also reparents patients by providing structure, supporting their successes, acknowledging them when they do well, setting realistic expectations, and setting limits.

Special Problems with This Schema

The most common problem is that patients persist in their maladaptive coping behaviors. They keep surrendering, avoiding, or overcompensating for the schema instead of trying to change. Patients are so convinced they are going to fail that they are reluctant to commit themselves fully to trying to succeed. Mode work can help patients strengthen the Healthy Adult, who is able and willing to fight the schema. In imagery, patients relive past and current moments of failure. The Healthy Adult helps the Failing Child cope in adaptive ways.

THE DOMAIN OF IMPAIRED LIMITS

Entitlement/Grandiosity

Typical Presentation of the Schema

These patients feel special. They believe that they are better than other people. Because they feel they are part of some "elite," they feel entitled to special rights and privileges, and do not feel bound by the principles of reciprocity that guide healthy human interactions. They try to control the behavior of others in order to meet their own needs, without empathy or concern for the others' needs. They engage in acts of selfishness and grandiosity. They insist they should be able to say, do, or have what they want, regardless of the cost to others. Typical behaviors include excessive competitiveness, snobbishness, domination of other people, asserting power in a hurtful way, and forcing one's point of view on others.

We distinguish between two types of patients with Entitlement schemas: those with "pure entitlement," and those who are typically described as "narcissistic" in the extensive literature on personality disorders. Narcissistic patients behave in an entitled way in order to overcompensate for underlying feelings of defectiveness and emotional deprivation. We refer to narcissism as "fragile entitlement." The focus of treatment is on the underlying Emotional Deprivation and Defectiveness schemas. Setting limits is important, but it is not as central. (We discuss how to treat fragile entitlement in detail later in Chapter 10.)

In contrast, patients with "pure entitlement" were simply spoiled and indulged as children and continue to act that way as adults. Their entitlement is not an overcompensation for underlying schemas—not a way of coping with a perceived threat. For patients with "pure entitlement," there are usually no underlying schemas to treat. Setting limits is the central part of the treatment. In this section, we focus on "pure entitlement," although many of the strategies can also be helpful as an adjunct in working with narcissistic personality disorder.

Another group of patients has what we call "dependent entitle-ment"—a blending of the Dependence and Entitlement schemas. These patients feel entitled to be dependent on others to take care of them. They believe other people should meet their daily needs for food, clothing, shel-ter, and transportation, and they become angry when other people fail to do so. In treating these patients, the therapist works on both the Entitle-ment and the Dependence schemas simultaneously.

Goals of Treatment

The basic goal with the Entitlement schema is to help patients accept the principle of reciprocity in human interactions. We try to teach these pa-tients the philosophy that, when it comes to basic worth, all people are created equal and deserve equal rights (unlike the entitled animals in George Orwell's (1946) *Animal Farm,* who changed the commandment to read: "All animals are created equal, but some are created more equal than others.") All people are equally valuable: One person is not inherently more valuable than another and is not entitled to special treatment. Healthy individuals do not dominate and bully others, but rather respect the other person's needs and rights; they also try their best to control their impulses so as not to hurt others, and they follow reasonable social norms most of the time.

Strategies Emphasized in Treatment

In order to help patients maintain the motivation to change, the therapist continually highlights all the disadvantages of the Entitlement schema. Of-ten, these patients have not come to therapy voluntarily. They have come because someone is forcing them, or because they are facing some negative consequence of their entitlement—loss of their job, a marriage breaking up, children who have stopped talking to them, or feelings of loneliness and emptiness. They may well be experiencing genuine pain about an im-pending loss. The therapist finds out what is causing them pain and why they have come to therapy, and uses these as leverage to keep these pa-tients in therapy. The therapist keeps saying, in essence: "If you don't give up your entitlement, if you aren't willing to change, people will continue to retaliate against you or leave, and you will continue feeling unhappy." The therapist keeps reminding patients what the consequences will be if they are not willing to change.

Working on interpersonal relationships and on the therapy relation-ship are the most important treatment strategies. The therapist encourages patients to feel empathy and concern for others—to recognize the damage they do when they misuse their power over others. Cognitive-behavioral strategies such as anger management and assertiveness training are important as well, so that the patient can learn to replace overly aggressive approaches to others with more assertive approaches. If the patient is in a love relationship with a partner, then it is often helpful to bring the partner into some therapy sessions. The therapist can then work with the couple to stop the patient's entitled behavior and to help the partner set limits, so that each member of the couple balances his or her own needs with the needs of the other person.

Patients with this schema have spent their lives selectively focusing on their assets and minimizing their flaws. They do not have a realistic view of their own strengths and weaknesses. They do not understand or accept that they have normal human frailties and limitations, as we all do. The therapist uses cognitive strategies to help patients develop a more realistic view of themselves, looking at both their strengths and their weaknesses. In addition, the therapist uses cognitive strategies to challenge their view of themselves as special, with special rights. Entitled patients have to learn to follow the same rules as everyone else. They have to treat people respectfully, as equals. The therapist and patient look at past situations in which the patient behaved in an entitled way and experienced negative consequences.

The therapist uses experiential strategies to help patients express acknowledgment of their parents' overly indulgent behavior in their childhood. The therapist enters the imagery as the Healthy Adult who confronts the Entitled Child empathically and teaches the principle of reciprocity. Eventually, patients enter the imagery as their own Healthy Adult modes.

The therapist watches for entitled behavior in the therapy relationship and confronts each instance through empathic confrontation. The therapist reparents by setting limits whenever the patient behaves in a bullying or demeaning way, or expresses anger inappropriately. The therapist uses the therapy relationship to support patients whenever they admit a flaw, view other people as equals, or experience feelings of inferiority. The therapist praises patients when they express feelings of empathy for others, and acknowledges them when they restrain their destructive impulses and hold back unreasonable anger. Finally, the therapist discourages patients' overemphasis on status and other superficial qualities in judging themselves and others.

Special Problems with This Schema

One likely difficulty is helping the patient maintain the motivation to change. A significant proportion of patients with entitlement leave therapy before they are better, because a great deal of secondary gain goes along with this schema. It feels good to get what one wants. Why should the patient change? The therapist has to find the leverage—the ways it is hurting the patient to be entitled or grandiose. Then, the therapist has to remind the patient continually about the negative consequences of the schema.

Insufficient Self-Control/Self-Discipline

Typical Presentation of the Schema

Patients who have this schema typically lack two qualities: (1) self-control—the ability to appropriately restrain one's emotions and impulses; and (2) self-discipline—the ability to tolerate boredom and frustration long enough to accomplish tasks. These patients are unable to restrain their emotions and impulses appropriately. In both their personal and work lives, they display a pervasive difficulty in delaying short-term gratification for the sake of meeting long-term goals. They seem not to learn sufficiently from experience—from the negative consequences of their behavior. They either cannot or will not exercise sufficient self-control or self-discipline. (In *Postcards from the Edge* Carrie Fisher [1989, p. 9] captured this sensibility when she wrote, "The trouble with immediate gratification is that it's not quick enough.")

At the extreme end of the spectrum of this schema are patients who seem like badly brought up young children. In milder forms of the schema, patients display an exaggerated emphasis on avoiding discomfort. They prefer to avoid most pain, conflict, confrontation, responsibility, and overexertion—even at the cost of their personal fulfillment or integrity.

Typical behaviors include impulsivity, distractibility, disorganization, unwillingness to persist at boring or routine tasks, intense expressions of emotion, such as temper tantrums or hysteria, and habitual lateness or unreliability. All of these behaviors have in common the pursuit of short-term gratification at the expense of long-term goals.

The schema does not primarily apply to substance abusers or addicts. Substance abuse is not at the crux of this schema, although it often accompanies it. Addictive behaviors in themselves—such as drug or alcohol abuse, overeating, gambling, compulsive sex—are not what this schema is meant to measure. Addictions can be ways of coping with many other schemas, not just this one: They can be a way of avoiding the pain of almost any schema. Rather, this schema applies to patients who have difficulty controlling or disciplining themselves over a broad range of situations. They fail to impose limits on their emotions and impulses in many areas of their lives and exhibit a broad range of self-control problems in several areas, not just addictive behaviors.

We believe that every child is born with an impulsive mode. A natural part of every human being, it is the failure to bring impulsivity under sufficient control and learn self-discipline that is maladaptive. Children are, by nature, uncontrolled and undisciplined. Through experiences in our families and in society as a whole, we learn how to become more controlled and disciplined. We internalize a Healthy Adult mode that can restrain the Impulsive Child in order to meet long-term goals. Sometimes another problem, such as attention-deficit/hyperactivity disorder, makes it hard for the child to accomplish this.

Often, there are no specific beliefs and feelings that go along with this schema. It is rare for patients with this schema to say, "It's right to express all my feelings" or "I should act impulsively." Rather, patients experience the schema as being outside of their control. The schema does not feel ego-syntonic in the way that other schemas do. Most patients we see with this schema want to be more self-controlled and self-disciplined: They keep trying, but they cannot seem to sustain their efforts for very long.

The impulsive mode is also the mode in which a person can be spontaneous and uninhibited. A person in this mode can play, be light, and have fun. There is a positive side to the mode, but when it is excessive—when it is not balanced by other sides of the self—the cost exceeds the benefit, and the mode becomes destructive to the person.

Goals of Treatment

The basic goal is to help patients recognize the value of giving up short-term gratification for the sake of long-term goals. The benefits of venting one's emotions or doing what is immediately pleasurable are not worth the costs in career advancement, achievement, getting along with other people, and low self-esteem.

Strategies Emphasized In Treatment

Cognitive-behavioral treatment techniques are almost always the most helpful strategies with this schema. The therapist helps patients learn to exercise self-control and self-discipline. The basic idea is that *between the impulse and the action, patients must learn to insert thought.* They must learn to think through the consequences of giving in to the impulse *before* acting it out.

In homework assignments, patients go through a series of graded tasks, such as becoming organized, performing boring or routine tasks, being on time, imposing structure, tolerating frustration, and restraining excessive emotions and impulses. Patients start with simple tasks that are only slightly difficult. They force themselves to do these tasks for a limited amount of time, then gradually increase the amount of time. Patients learn techniques that help them control their emotions, such as time-out and self-control techniques (meditation, relaxation, distraction), and flash cards listing reasons they should control themselves, and methods they can use to do it. In therapy sessions, patients can use behavioral rehearsal in imagery or role-playing to practice self-control and self-discipline. They can reward themselves when they successfully exert self-control and self-discipline in their outside lives. Rewards might include acknowledging oneself, treating oneself with a special activity or gift, or free time.

Occasionally, the Insufficient Self-Control/Self Discipline schema is linked with another schema that may be more primary. In this case, the therapist must address the more central schema, as well as the Insufficient Self-Control/Self-Discipline schema. For example, sometimes the schema erupts because patients have suppressed too much emotion for too long. This often happens with the Subjugation schema. Over long periods of time, patients with the Subjugation schema do not express anger when they feel it. Gradually, their anger accumulates, then suddenly bursts forth in an out-of-control way. When patients display a pattern of swinging between prolonged passivity and sudden fits of aggression, they often have underlying Subjugation schemas (see the later section on Subjugation). If patients can learn to express what they need and feel appropriately in the moment, then anger will not build up in the background. The less patients suppress their needs and feelings, the less likely they become to behave impulsively.

Some experiential techniques are helpful. Patients can imagine past and current scenes in which they displayed insufficient self-control or self-discipline. First the therapist, then the patient, enters scenes as the Healthy Adult, who helps the Undisciplined Child exert self-control. When Insufficient Self-Control/Self-Discipline is linked to another schema, the therapist can use experiential techniques to help patients battle the underlying schema. This is especially important in patients with BPD. Because of their Subjugation schemas, these patients feel that they are not allowed to express their needs and feelings. Whenever they do, they feel they deserve to be punished by their internalized Punitive Parent. They repeatedly suppress their needs and feelings. As time passes, their needs and feelings build up, beyond their ability to contain them, and then these patients flip into the Angry Child mode in order to express them. They suddenly become enraged and impulsive. When this happens, the therapist's general approach is to allow the patient to vent fully, empathize, and then reality-test.

In the therapy relationship, it is important for the therapist to be firm and set limits with these patients. This is especially true when the origin of the schema was not getting enough limits as a child. Some patients who have this schema were "latch-key children." Because their parents were working and they were left alone, there was no one to discipline them. When lack of parental involvement in childhood is the origin of the schema, the therapist can provide a partial antidote by reparenting the patient in an active way. The therapist sets consequences for such behaviors as being late for sessions and failing to complete homework assignments.

Special Problems with This Schema

Sometimes the schema appears to be biologically based and therefore very hard to change with therapy alone, for example, when the patient has a learning problem such as attention-deficit/hyperactivity disorder. If the schema is biologically based, then even when patients are highly motivated and expend great effort, they may be unable to develop sufficient self-control and self-discipline. In practice, it is often unclear how much the schema is linked to temperament and how much it is related to insufficient limits in childhood. Medication should be considered for patients who have persistent difficulty fighting the schema despite an apparent commitment to therapy.

THE DOMAIN OF OTHER-DIRECTEDNESS

Subjugation

Typical Presentation of the Schema

These patients allow other people to dominate them. They surrender control to others because they feel coerced by the threat of either punishment or abandonment. There are two forms: The first is subjugation of *needs*, in which patients suppress their own wishes and instead follow the demands of other people; and the second is subjugation of *emotions*, in which patients suppress their feelings (mainly anger) because they are afraid other people will retaliate against them. The schema involves the perception that one's own needs and feelings are not valid and important to other people. The schema almost always leads to an accumulation of anger, which manifests in such maladaptive symptoms as passive–aggressive behavior, uncontrolled outbursts of anger, psychosomatic symptoms, withdrawal of affection, acting out, and substance abuse.

Patients with this schema usually present with a coping style of surrendering to the schema: They are excessively compliant and hypersensitive to feeling trapped. They feel bullied, harassed, and powerless. They experience themselves as being at the mercy of authority figures: The authority figures are stronger and more powerful; therefore, the patients must defer to them. The schema involves a significant level of fear. At the core, patients are afraid that if they express their needs and feelings, something bad is going to happen to them. Someone important is going to get angry with, abandon, punish, reject, or criticize them. These patients suppress their needs and feelings, not because they feel they *should* suppress them, but because they feel they *have to* suppress them. Their subjugation is not based on an internalized value or a desire to help others; rather, it is based upon the fear of retaliation. In contrast, the Self-Sacrifice, Emotional Inhibition, and Unrelenting Standards schemas are all similar in that patients have an internalized value that it is not right to express personal needs or feelings: They believe it is in some way bad or wrong to express needs and feelings, so they feel ashamed or guilty when they do. Patients with these other three schemas do not feel controlled by other people. They have an internal locus of control. On the other hand, patients with the Subjugation schema have an external locus of control. They believe that they must submit to authority figures, whether they think it is right or not, or else they will be punished in some way.

Often, this schema leads to avoidant behavior. Patients avoid situations where other people might control them, or where they might become trapped. Some patients avoid committed romantic relationships because they experience these relationships as claustrophobic or entrapping. The schema can also lead to overcompensation such as disobedience and oppositionality. Rebelliousness is the most common form of overcompensation for subjugation.

Goals of Treatment

The basic goal of treatment is to get patients to see that they have a right to have their needs and feelings, and to express them. Generally, the best way to live is to express needs and feelings appropriately at the moment they occur, rather than waiting until later or not expressing them at all. As long as patients express themselves appropriately, it is healthy to express needs and feelings, and healthy people usually will not retaliate against them when they do. People who consistently retaliate against them when they express their needs and feelings are not beneficial people for them to choose for close involvements. We encourage patients to seek out relationships with people who allow them to express normal needs and feelings, and to avoid relationships with people who do not.

Strategies Emphasized in Treatment

All four types of treatment strategies—cognitive, experiential, behavioral, and the therapy relationship—are important in treating this schema.

In terms of cognitive strategies, subjugated patients have unrealistic negative expectations about the consequences of expressing their needs and feelings to appropriate significant others. By examining the evidence and designing behavioral experiments, patients learn that their expectations are exaggerated. Furthermore, it is important for patients to learn that they are acting in a healthy manner when they express their needs and feelings appropriately—even though their parents may have communicated that they were "bad" for doing so as children.

Experiential strategies are extremely important. In imagery, patients express anger and assert their rights with the controlling parent and other authority figures. Often, patients with this schema have trouble expressing anger, especially toward the parent who subjugated them. The therapist should persist with the experiential work until patients are able to vent anger freely in imagery or role-play exercises. Expressing anger is crucial to overcoming the schema. The more patients get in touch with their anger and vent it in imagery or role-play exercises (particularly at the controlling parent), the more they will be able to fight the schema in their everyday lives. The purpose of expressing this anger is not purely for ventilation, but rather to help patients feel empowered to stand up for themselves. Anger supplies the motivation and momentum to fight the passivity that almost always accompanies subjugation.

A vital behavioral strategy is to help patients select relatively noncontrolling partners. Usually, subjugated people are drawn to controlling partners. If they can experience attraction to a partner who wants to have an equal relationship, that is ideal. However, more typically, these patients are likely to select someone who is controlling—so they can get the "schema chemistry." We hope that the partner is not so controlling that patients cannot express their needs and feelings whatsoever. If the partner is dominating enough to create some chemistry, but willing to take the patient's needs and feelings into account, then this can provide a solution to the schema. There is enough chemistry to sustain the relationship, but also enough schema healing for the patient to live a healthy life. Patients also work on selecting noncontrolling friends. Assertiveness techniques can help patients learn to assert their needs and feelings with their partner and others.

When there is an undeveloped self as a consequence of the schema—when patients have served the needs and preferences of others so assiduously that they do not know their own needs and preferences—then patients can work to individuate. Experiential and cognitive-behavioral techniques can help patients identify their natural inclinations and practice acting on them. For example, patients can do imagery exercises to re-create situations in which they suppressed their needs and preferences. In the images, patients can say aloud what they needed and wanted to do. They can imagine the consequences. Patients can role-play expressing their needs and preferences with others in therapy sessions, and then express them *in vivo* in homework assignments.

Most subjugated patients initially perceive the therapist as an authority figure who wants to control or dominate them. They perceive the therapist as controlling even when the therapist is not. From a reparenting point of view, it is important for the therapist to be under- rather than overdirective. The therapist aims to be as nondirective as possible, allowing patients to make choices throughout the treatment process: which problems they want to address, what techniques they want to learn, and what homework assignments they want to carry out. The therapist is also careful to point out any deferential behavior on the part of patients with empathic confrontation. Finally, the therapist helps patients recognize and express anger toward the therapist, as it builds up, before it gets to the breaking point.

Special Problems with This Schema

As patients experiment with expressing their needs and feelings, often they do it imperfectly. At the beginning, they might fail to assert themselves enough to be heard, or they might swing to the opposite extreme and become too aggressive. The therapist can help patients anticipate that it is going to take some time to find the right balance between suppressing and expressing their needs and feelings, and that they should not judge themselves too harshly for this.

When subjugated patients first try to express their needs and feelings, they often say something like: "But I don't know what I want. I don't know what I feel." In cases such as these where Subjugation is linked to an Undeveloped Self schema, the therapist can help patients develop a sense of self by showing them how to monitor their wishes and emotions. Imagery exercises can help patients explore their feelings. Eventually, if they resist subjugating and continue to focus inward, most patients come to recognize what they want and feel.

Because some therapists like the deferential quality exhibited by subjugated patients, they might unwittingly reinforce the subjugation. It is easy to mistake a subjugated patient for a good patient. Both are compliant; however, it is not healthy for subjugated patients to be overly compliant. This perpetuates rather than heals their subjugation schemas.

We have found that, in most cases, this is a relatively easy schema to treat. Clinically, we have a high success rate with subjugation problems.

Self-Sacrifice

Typical Presentation of the Schema

These patients, like those with the Subjugation schema, display an excessive focus on meeting the needs of others at the expense of their own needs. However, unlike patients with the Subjugation schema, these patients experience their self-sacrifice as voluntary. They do it because they want to prevent other people from experiencing pain, to do what they believe is right, to avoid feeling guilty or selfish, or to maintain a connection with significant others whom they perceive as needy. The Self-Sacrifice schema often results from what we believe to be a highly empathic temperament—an acute sensitivity to the pain of others. Some people feel the psychic pain of others so intensely that they are highly motivated to alleviate or prevent it. They do not want to do things or allow things to happen that will cause other people pain. Self-sacrifice often involves a sense of over-responsibility for others. It thus overlaps with the concept of co-dependence.

It is common for patients with this schema to have psychosomatic symptoms such as headaches, gastrointestinal problems, chronic pain, or fatigue. Physical symptoms may provide these patients with a way to bring attention to themselves, without having to ask for it directly and without conscious awareness. They feel permission to receive care or to decrease their care for others if they are "really sick." These symptoms may also be a direct result of the stress created by giving so much and receiving so little in return.

Patients with this schema almost always have an accompanying Emotional Deprivation schema. They are meeting the needs of others, but their own needs are not getting met. On the surface, they appear content to self-sacrifice, but underneath, they feel a deep sense of emotional deprivation. Sometimes they feel angry at the objects of their sacrifice. Usually patients with this schema are giving so much that they end up hurting themselves.

Often, these patients believe that they do not expect anything back from others, but when something happens and the other person does not give as much back, they feel resentful. Anger is not inevitable with this schema, but patients who self-sacrifice to a significant degree, and have people around them who are not reciprocating, usually experience at least some resentment.

As we noted in the previous section on the Subjugation schema, it is important to distinguish self-sacrifice from subjugation. When patients have the Subjugation schema, they surrender their own needs out of fear of external consequences. They are afraid that other people are going to retaliate or reject them. With the Self-Sacrifice schema, patients surrender their own needs out of an inner sense or standard. (According to Kohlberg's [1963] stages of moral development, Self-Sacrifice represents a higher level of moral development than Subjugation.) Subjugated patients experience themselves as being under the control of other people; self-sacrificing patients experience themselves as making voluntary choices.

The origins of these two schemas are different as well. Although the two schemas overlap, they are almost opposite in their origins. The origin of the Subjugation schema is usually a domineering and controlling parent; with the Self-Sacrifice schema, the parent is typically weak, needy, childlike, helpless, ill, or depressed. Thus, the former develops from interaction with a parent who is too strong, and the latter with a parent who is too weak or ill. It is also common for a child, who as an adult develops a Self-Sacrifice schema, to assume the role of the "parentified child" (Earley & Cushway, 2002) from a young age.

Patients with the Self-Sacrifice schema typically exhibit behaviors such as listening to others rather than talking about themselves; taking care of other people, yet having difficulty doing things for themselves; focusing attention on other people, yet feeling uncomfortable when attention is focused on them; and being indirect when they want something, rather than asking directly. (One of our patients told the following story about her self-sacrificing mother: "I was making coffee one morning. My mother came down to the kitchen, and I asked her if she wanted a cup. 'No, I don't want to be a bother,' the mother said. 'It's no bother,' said the patient, 'let me make you a cup of coffee.' 'No, no,' the mother said, so the patient made only one cup. When the patient was finished, her mother said, 'So you couldn't make me a cup of coffee?' ")

There can also be secondary gain with this schema. The schema has positive aspects and is only pathological when brought to an unhealthy extreme. Patients might feel a sense of pride in seeing themselves as caretakers. They might feel that they are good for behaving altruistically, that they are behaving in a morally virtuous way. (In contrast, sometimes the schema has a "never enough" quality, so that no matter how much self-sacrificers do, they still feel guilty that it is not enough.) Another potential source of secondary gain is that the schema might draw other people to them. Many people enjoy the empathy and help of the self-sacrificer. Patients with this schema usually have many friendships, although their own needs often are not being met in these relationships.

In terms of overcompensatory behaviors, after self-sacrificing for a long time, some patients suddenly flip into excessive anger. They become enraged and cut off giving to the other person completely. When self-sacrificers feel unappreciated, they sometimes retaliate by conveying to the other person: "I'm not going to give you anything ever again." One patient with a Self-Sacrifice schema related the following incident to her therapist in describing what happened after her mother died: She was a young teenager and had begun cooking, cleaning, and doing laundry for her father. One day, while she was ironing, her father walked in and said, "From now on, button my shirts when you hang them on the hanger." The patient stopped ironing, walked out of the room, and never cleaned, cooked, or did the laundry for her father again. "I washed my own clothes and left his there in a pile on the floor," she concluded.

Goals of Treatment

One major goal is to teach patients with the Self-Sacrifice schema that all people have an equal right to get their needs met. Even though these patients experience themselves as stronger than others, in reality, most of them have been emotionally deprived. They have sacrificed themselves and have not gotten their own needs met in return. Therefore, they are needy—just as needy as most of the "weaker" people they devote them-selves to helping. The primary difference is that patients with a Self-Sacrifice schema do not experience their own needs, at least not con-sciously. They have usually blocked out the frustration of their own needs in order to continue self-sacrificing.

An important goal of treatment is to help patients with a Self-Sacrifice schema to recognize that they have needs that are not being met, even though they are not aware of them; and that they have as much right to get their needs met as anyone else. Despite any secondary gain that the schema might bring, these patients are paying a high price for their self-sacrifice. They are not getting something they need deeply, which is to be cared for by other human beings.

Another goal of treatment is to decrease the patient's sense of over-responsibility. The therapist shows patients that they often exaggerate the fragility and helplessness of other people. Most other people are not as fragile and helpless as the patient thinks they are. If the patient were to give less, the other person would usually still be fine. In most cases, the other person is not going to fall apart or experience unbearable pain if the patient gives less.

Another goal of treatment is to remedy patients' associated emotional deprivation. The therapist encourages patients to attend to their own needs, to let other people meet their needs, to ask for what they want more directly, and to be more vulnerable instead of appearing strong more of the time.

Strategies Emphasized in Treatment

All four change components are important with this schema. In terms of cognitive strategies, the therapist helps patients test their exaggerated per-ceptions of the fragility and neediness of others. In addition, the therapist helps patients increase their awareness of their own needs. Ideally patients realize that they have needs —for nurturance, understanding, protection, and guidance—that have long gone unmet. They are taking care of others but not allowing others to take care of them.

Furthermore, the therapist helps patients become aware of other schemas that underlie their self-sacrifice. As we have noted, patients with a Self-Sacrifice schema almost always have some degree of underlying emo-tional deprivation. Defectiveness is also a common linked schema: These patients "give more" because they feel "worth less." Abandonment can be a linked schema: Patients self-sacrifice in order to prevent the other person from abandoning them. Dependence can be a linked schema: Patients self-sacrifice so that the parent figure will stay connected to them and keep taking care of them. Approval-Seeking can be a linked schema: Patients take care of others to get approval or recognition.

The therapist highlights the imbalance of the "give–get ratio": the ratio of what patients are giving to what they are getting from significant others in their lives. In a healthy relationship between equals, what each person gives and gets should be approximately equal over time. This balance does not have to occur in each separate aspect of the relationship, but rather in the relationship as a whole. Each person gives and gets according to his or her abilities, but the overall balance is approximately equal. A significant imbalance in the ratio of giving and getting is usually unhealthy for the patient. (The exceptions are relationships of nonequals, such as parents and children. Patients who sacrifice for their children, for example, do not necessarily have a Self-Sacrifice schema. To have the schema, patients have to sacrifice across many relationships as part of a general pattern.)

Experientially, the therapist helps patients become aware of their emotional deprivation, both in childhood and in their current lives. Patients express sadness and anger about their unmet emotional needs. In imagery, they confront the parent who deprived them—the self-centered, needy, or depressed parent who did not nurture, listen to, protect, or guide them. They express anger about becoming a parentified child: Even if unintentional on the part of the parent, it was not fair that they were put in this role. Patients acknowledge their lost childhood. In imagery, they express anger toward significant others who deprive them in their current life, and they ask for what they need.

Behaviorally, patients learn to ask to have their needs met more directly, and to come across as vulnerable instead of strong. They learn to select partners who are strong and giving rather than weak and needy. (Patients with this schema are often drawn to weak and needy partners, such as people who are drug addicts, depressed, or dependent, instead of partners who can give to them as equals.) In addition, patients learn to set limits on how much they give to others.

One treatment strategy that would be unhealthy for patients with other schemas can be very helpful for patients with Self-Sacrifice schemas: Patients keep track of how much they are giving and getting with significant others. How much are they doing for, listening to, and taking care of each person, and how much are they getting in return? When the balance is off—as it usually is for patients with the Self-Sacrifice schema—they can aim to make the ratio more equal. They can give less and ask for more.

In a sense, this schema is the opposite of the Entitlement schema. The Entitlement schema involves self-centeredness; the Self-Sacrifice schema involves other-centeredness. These two schemas "fit" together well in relationships: Patients who have one of these schemas often end up with a partner who has the other. Another common combination is one partner with a Self-Sacrifice schema, and the other with Dependent Entitlement. The self-sacrificer does everything for the entitled partner. Therapy can help these couples pull each other toward a healthier middle ground.

When we consider the schemas of psychotherapists, Self-Sacrifice is one of the most common (the other is Emotional Deprivation). For many professionals in the mental health field, a Self-Sacrifice schema was one factor that motivated them to choose their work. If the therapist and patient both have the schema, one potential problem is that the therapist might inadvertently model behavior that is too self-sacrificing. In both the therapy relationship and when discussing other areas of their lives, therapists show that although they are giving, they are not self-denying. The therapist has needs and rights in relationships and appropriately asserts them.

It is important for therapists to be very giving to patients with this schema, because they have been given so little by their parents and others. It is important for therapists to be caring and not to allow the patient to take care of them. Whenever a self-sacrificing patient tries to take care of the therapist, the therapist points out the pattern through empathic confrontation. The therapist encourages the patient to rely on him or her as much as possible. Some of these patients have never relied on another human being. The therapist validates the patient's dependency needs and encourages the patient to stop acting so adult-like and strong, and instead to be vulnerable and, at times, even child-like with the therapist.

Special Problems with This Schema

One problem is that there is often a high cultural and religious value placed on self-sacrifice. Furthermore, self-sacrifice is not a dysfunctional schema within normal limits. Rather, it is healthy to be self-sacrificing to a certain degree. It becomes dysfunctional when it is excessive. For a patient's self-sacrifice to be a maladaptive schema, the self-sacrifice has to be causing problems for the person. It has to be creating symptoms or creating unhappiness in relationships. There has to be some way it is manifesting itself as a difficulty: Anger is building up, the patient is experiencing psychosomatic complaints, feeling emotionally deprived, or otherwise suffering emotionally.

Approval-Seeking/Recognition-Seeking

Typical Presentation of the Schema

These patients place excessive importance on gaining approval or recognition from other people at the expense of fulfilling their core emotional needs and expressing their natural inclinations. Because they habitually focus on the reactions of others rather than on their own reactions, they fail to develop a stable, inner-directed sense of self.

There are two subtypes. The first type seeks approval, wanting everyone to like them; they want to fit in and be accepted. The second type seeks recognition, wanting applause and admiration. The latter are frequently narcissistic patients: They overemphasize status, appearance, money, or achievement as a means gaining the admiration of others. Both subtypes are outwardly focused on getting approval or recognition in order to feel good about themselves. Their sense of self-esteem is dependent on the reactions of other people, rather than on their own values and natural inclinations. One young female patient with this schema said: "You know how you see women on the street who just look like they're having a great life? Their life might really be awful, but when you see them walk by, you just think everything's great. I've often thought that if I had to choose, I'd rather *look* like I'm having a great life than actually have one."

Alice Miller (1975) writes about the issue of recognition-seeking in *Prisoners of Childhood*. Many of the cases she presents are individuals at the narcissistic end of this schema. As children, they learned to strive for recognition, because that was what their parents encouraged or pushed them to do. The parents obtained vicarious gratification, but the children grew more and more estranged from their genuine selves—from their core emotional needs and natural inclinations..

The subjects in Miller's book have both the Emotional Deprivation and the Recognition-Seeking schemas. Recognition-seeking is often, but not always, linked with the Emotional Deprivation schema. However, some parents are both nurturing and recognition-seeking. In many families, the parents are very child-oriented and loving, but also very concerned with outward appearances. Children from these families feel loved, but they do not develop a stable, inner-directed sense of self: Their sense of self is predicated on the responses of other people. They have an undeveloped, or false, self, but it is not a true self. Narcissistic patients are at the extreme end of this schema, but there are many milder forms in which patients are more psychologically healthy yet still devoted to seeking approval or recognition to the detriment of self-expression.

Typical behaviors include being compliant or people-pleasing in order to get approval. Some Approval-Seekers place themselves in a subservient role to get approval. Other individuals may feel uncomfortable around them because they seem so eager to please. Typical behaviors also include placing a great deal of emphasis on appearance, money, status, achievement, and success in order to obtain recognition from others. Recognition-seekers might fish for compliments or appear conceited and brag about their accomplishments. Alternatively, they might be subtler, and surreptitiously manipulate the conversation, so that they can cite their sources of pride.

Approval-Seeking/Recognition-Seeking is different from other schemas that might result in approval-seeking behavior. When patients display approval-seeking behavior, it is their motivation that determines whether the behavior is part of this or another schema. Approval-Seeking/Recognition-

Seeking is different from the Unrelenting Standards schema (even if the childhood origins may appear similar) in that patients with the Unrelenting Standards schema are striving to meet a set of internalized values, whereas approval-seeking patients are striving to obtain external validation. Approval-Seeking/Recognition-Seeking is different from the Subjugation schema in that the latter is fear-based, whereas the former is not. With the Subjugation schema, patients act in an approval-seeking way because they are afraid of punishment or abandonment, not primarily because they crave approval. The Approval-Seeking/Recognition-Seeking schema is different from the Self-Sacrifice schema in that it is not based on a desire to help others one perceives as fragile or needy. If patients act in an approval-seeking way because they do not want to hurt other people, then they have the Self-Sacrifice schema. The Approval-Seeking/Recognition-Seeking schema is different from the Entitlement/Grandiosity schema in that it is not an attempt to aggrandize oneself in order to feel superior to others. If patients act in an approval-seeking way as a means of gaining power, special treatment, or control, then they have the Entitlement schema.

Most Approval-Seekers probably would endorse conditional beliefs such as "People will accept me, if they approve of me or admire me," "I'm worthwhile if other people give me approval," or "If I can get people to admire me, they will pay attention to me." They live under this contingency: In order to feel good about themselves, they have to gain approval or recognition from others. Thus, these patients are frequently dependent on other people's approval for their self-esteem.

The Approval-Seeking/Recognition-Seeking schema is often, but not always, a form of overcompensation for another schema, such as Defectiveness, Emotional Deprivation, or Social Isolation. Although many patients use this schema to overcompensate for other issues, many other patients with this schema seek approval or recognition simply because they were raised this way; their parents placed a strong emphasis on approval or recognition. The parents set goals and expectations that were not based on the child's inherent needs and natural inclinations, but rather on the values of the surrounding culture.

There are both healthy and maladaptive forms of approval-seeking. This schema is common in highly successful people in many fields, such as politics and entertainment. Many of these patients are skillful in intuiting what will gain them approval or recognition and can adapt their behavior in a chameleon-like way, in order to endear themselves to or impress people.

Goals of Treatment

The basic goal is for patients to recognize that they have an authentic self that is different from their approval-seeking, false self. They have spent their lives suppressing their emotions and natural inclinations for the sake of gaining approval or recognition. Because their true self has been suppressed and their approval-seeking self has been directing their lives, their core emotional needs have not been met. Compared to genuine self-expression and being true to oneself, other people's approval provides only a superficial and transient form of gratification. Here, we state a philosophical assumption of our theory: Humans are happiest and most fulfilled when they are expressing authentic emotions and acting on their natural inclinations. Most patients with this schema do not know what it means to be authentic. They do not know what their natural inclinations are, let alone how to act on them. The goal of treatment is to help patients to focus less on obtaining other people's approval or recognition, and more on who they are and what they value intrinsically.

Strategies Emphasized in Treatment

All four components of treatment play important roles in treatment: cognitive, experiential, behavioral, and the therapy relationship.

One cognitive strategy is demonstrating to patients the importance of expressing one's true self rather than continuing to seek the approval of others. It is natural to want approval and recognition, but when this desire becomes extreme, it is dysfunctional. Patients can examine the pros and cons of the schema: They weigh the advantages and disadvantages of discovering who they truly are and acting on that versus continuing to focus on gaining other people's approval. In this way, patients can make the decision to fight the schema. If they continue to put all their emphasis on money, status, or popularity, then they are not going to enjoy life fully; they will continue to feel empty and dissatisfied. It is not worth it to "sell one's soul" for approval or recognition. ("I thought I was going up, I was really going down," thinks the dying, social-climbing Ivan Ilyitch in Tolstoy's story [1986, p. 495].) Approval and recognition are only temporarily satisfying. They are addictive and not fulfilling in a deep and lasting sense.

Experiential strategies can be helpful, especially mode work. The Approval-Seeker is a mode the patient learned in childhood. The therapist helps the patient identify the Approval-Seeker and the Vulnerable Child modes (using whatever names fit for the patient). The patient relives childhood incidents of seeking approval from a parent, and alternates between the Approval-Seeking mode and the Vulnerable Child, expressing each side aloud. What did the patient truly need at significant moments in childhood? What did the child truly think? Feel? Want to do? Want the parent to do? What was demanded of the child by the parent and other authority figures? The child expresses anger at the Demanding Parent, and grieves for a childhood that was lost to approval-seeking. The Healthy

Adult, played first by the therapist, then by the patient, helps the child fight the Approval-Seeker and behave in accord with the Vulnerable Child.

Patients can conduct behavioral experiments to explore their natural inclinations. They can self-monitor their thoughts and feelings, and use behavioral techniques to practice acting on their natural inclinations more frequently in their lives. Learning to tolerate the disapproval of other people is an important behavioral goal. Patients practice accepting situations in which other people do not give them approval or recognition. To the extent that approval-seeking has become like an addiction, patients learn to give up the addiction, tolerate the withdrawal from approval or recognition, and then substitute other, healthier forms of gratification. This process can be painful for patients, especially at first, and the therapist helps by adopting a stance of empathic confrontation. The behavioral component is crucial to the success of the treatment. If patients do not actually shift their focus away from what other people think, toward becoming more true to themselves in everyday situations, especially in relationships with significant others, then the other strategies are not going to work in a lasting way.

In the therapy relationship, it is important for the therapist to watch for instances in which the patient tries to gain approval or recognition. This pattern almost always emerges in therapy with these patients. When it does, the therapist points out the behavior through empathic confrontation and encourages the patient to be open and direct rather than hiding negative reactions.

Special Problems with This Schema

One problem is that the Approval-Seeking/Recognition-Seeking schema usually provides the patient with a great deal of secondary gain. Approval and recognition can bring potent interpersonal rewards, and this schema is socially sanctioned to a high degree. Getting applause, becoming famous, achieving recognition, being successful, being liked, fitting in—there is a great deal of positive reinforcement in society for all of these. The therapist is thus asking the patient to fight or moderate something that society values heavily. Therapist and patient work together to determine that the cost of *excessive* approval- or recognition-seeking is not worth the price. Furthermore, the goal is to *moderate* the tendency, not to eradicate it altogether, because the schema has many valuable aspects when it is balanced with self-actualization.

Patients with this schema are easily mistaken for healthy individuals, and therapists often unknowingly reinforce their schema-driven behaviors. These patients work hard to get therapists to approve of them or admire them, but if what they do is based on a false rather than a true self, then it is an impediment to their progress.

OVERVIGILANCE AND INHIBITION DOMAIN

Negativity/Pessimism

Typical Presentation of the Schema

These patients are negativistic and pessimistic. They display a pervasive, lifelong focus on the negative aspects of life, such as pain, death, loss, disappointment, betrayal, failure, and conflict, while minimizing the positive aspects. In a wide range of work, financial, and interpersonal situations, they have an exaggerated expectation that things will go seriously wrong. Patients feel vulnerable to making disastrous mistakes that will cause their lives to fall apart in some way—mistakes that might lead to financial collapse, serious loss, social humiliation, being trapped in a bad situation, or loss of control. They spend a great deal of time trying to make sure they do not make such mistakes and are prone to obsessive rumination. Their "default position" is anxiety. Typical feelings include chronic tension and worry, and typical behaviors include complaining and indecision. Patients with this schema can be difficult to be around because, no matter what one says, they always see the negative side of events. The glass is always half-empty.

Treatment strategies depend on how the therapist conceptualizes the origins of the schema, which is primarily learned through modeling. In this case, the schema reflects a depressive tendency toward negativity and pessimism that the patient learned from a parent. The patient internalized the parent's attitudes as a mode. Experiential work is especially helpful with patients who acquired the schema in this manner. In imagery and role-playing exercises, first the therapist, then the patient, practices fighting this Pessimistic Parent as the Healthy Adult. The Healthy Adult confronts the Negative Parent, and reassures and comforts the child.

A second origin of the schema is a childhood history of hardship and loss. In this case, patients are negativistic and pessimistic because they experienced so much adversity early in life. This is a more difficult origin to overcome. These patients, often at a young age, lost the natural optimism of youth. One patient, a 9-year-old child whose father had died years before, said, "Don't try to tell me bad things can't happen, because I know they can." Many of these patients need to grieve for past losses. When personal misfortune is the origin of the schema, all of the treatment strategies are important. Cognitive techniques can help patients see that negative events in the past do not predict the occurrence of negative events in the future. Experiential techniques can help patients express anger and grief about traumatic childhood losses. Behavioral techniques can help patients spend less time worrying in their current lives, and more time seeking enjoyment. In the therapy relationship, the therapist expresses empathy for the patient's losses, but also models and rewards optimistic attitudes and behavior.

Alternatively, the schema might be an overcompensation for the Emotional Deprivation schema. The patient complains in order to get attention or sympathy. In this case, the therapist treats the underlying deprivation by reparenting the patient, providing nurturance, while being careful not to reinforce schema-driven complaining. For example, the therapist ignores the content of the patient's pessimistic comments, focusing instead on allaying the patient's underlying feelings of emotional deprivation. Gradually, the patient learns healthier ways to meet emotional needs, first with the therapist, and then with significant others outside of the therapy.

For some patients, the schema may have a biological component and origin, perhaps related to obsessive–compulsive disorder or dysthymic disorder. These patients might benefit from a trial of medication.

Goals of Treatment

The basic goal is to help patients predict the future more objectively, that is, more positively. Some research suggests that the healthiest way to view life is with an "illusory glow" (Alloy & Abramson, 1979; Taylor & Brown, 1994), that is, as slightly more positive than is realistic. A negative view does not appear to be as healthy or adaptive. Perhaps this is because, generally speaking, if one expects things to go wrong and is accurate, one does not feel much better. It has not helped very much to imagine the worst. It is probably healthier to go through life expecting things to go well—as long as one's expectations are not so at odds with reality that one constantly has major disappointments.

We do not realistically expect most patients with this schema to become carefree and optimistic, but at least they can move away from the extreme negative end toward a more moderate position. Some signs that patients with this schema have improved are that they worry less frequently, have a more positive outlook, and stop constantly predicting the worst outcome and obsessively ruminating about the future. They are no longer focused so obsessively on trying to avoid making mistakes. Rather, they make a reasonable effort to avoid mistakes, and focus more on fulfilling emotional needs and following their natural inclinations.

Strategies Emphasized in Treatment

The cognitive and behavioral strategies are usually the main parts of treatment, although experiential strategies and the therapy relationship can be useful as well.

Many cognitive techniques can be helpful with this schema: identifying cognitive distortions, examining the evidence, generating alternatives, using flash cards, conducting dialogues between the schema-driven and the healthy sides. The therapist helps patients make predictions about the future and observe how infrequently their negative expecta-

tions come true. Patients self-monitor their negative, pessimistic thinking, and practice looking at their lives more objectively, based on logic
and empirical evidence. They learn to stop exaggerating the negatives
and focus more on the positives in their lives. Patients note corresponding changes in mood.

When patients have a past history of negative events, cognitive techniques can help them analyze these events and learn to distinguish the
present and future from the past. If a past, negative event was controllable,
then the therapist and patient can work together to correct the problem so
that it does not happen again. If the event was not controllable, then the
event has no bearing on the future. Logically, there is no basis for pessimism about a future event, even if the patient has experienced uncontrollable negative events in the past.

When the schema is serving a protective function, cognitive techniques can help patients challenge the idea that it is better to assume a
negative, pessimistic perspective, so that they are not disappointed. This
idea is usually incorrect: If patients expect something to go wrong, and it
does go wrong, they do not feel that much better having worried about it;
if they expect something to go right and instead it goes wrong, they do not
feel that much worse. Whatever they gain by anticipating negative outcomes does not outweigh the cost of living day-to-day with chronic worry
and tension. Patients list the advantages and disadvantages of assuming
the worst. They experiment with both positions, observing the effects on
their mood.

Some patients display what Borkovec calls "the magic of worrying"
(Borkovec, Robinson, Pruzinsky, & DePree, 1983). They believe that worrying is a magical ritual that can prevent bad things from happening: As
long as they are worrying, the bad thing will not happen. (As one patient
with this schema said, "At least when I'm worrying, I'm doing *something*.")
This stance is a form of trying to gain *control* over negative outcomes.
However, in actuality, many objects of their worry are either beyond their
control or not controllable by worrying. Patients can also conduct dialogues between their negative, pessimistic side and their positive, optimistic side, which therapy is helping to develop. In this way, they come to see
the benefits of taking a more positive stance toward life.

Experiential techniques help patients connect with their Happy Child
mode. If the origin of the schema was a negativistic, pessimistic parent, patients can conduct dialogues with this parent in imagery. As the Healthy
Adult, first the therapist, then the patient, enters childhood images where
the Pessimistic Parent deflated the child's enthusiasm. The Healthy Adult
challenges the Negative Parent and reassures the Worried Child. The child
expresses anger at the Negative Parent for being such a negative and stressful presence.

Therapists can use experiential techniques to help patients resolve underlying feelings of emotional deprivation about painful events from their past. If patients express anger and grief about these events in imagery, with the therapist empathizing, then they are often able to leave these events behind them. Rather than being stuck in unresolved grief, they can begin moving forward once again in their lives. The Healthy Adult guides the patient through the process.

Patients can conduct behavioral experiments to test their distorted, negative beliefs. For example, they can predict the worst outcome and measure how much of the time they are right; they can test the hypothesis that worrying leads to a better outcome; or they can test whether predicting negative outcomes or positive outcomes feels better.

Therapists can teach patients with a Negativity/Pessimism schema "response prevention" techniques to reduce their overvigilance about making mistakes. Patients gradually learn to become less obsessive about avoiding mistakes and to engage in fewer unnecessary behaviors designed to prevent mistakes, and then observe the increase in satisfaction and pleasure they gain from implementing these changes.

Instructing patients not to complain to others can be a helpful behavioral homework assignment. When the schema is an overcompensation for the Emotional Deprivation schema, the therapist can teach patients to ask others more directly to meet their emotional needs in relationships. Many of these negativistic, pessimistic patients—especially the ones therapists call "help-rejecting complainers" (Frank et al., 1952)—are extremely difficult to treat and often have an Emotional Deprivation schema underneath. Without any conscious awareness, they complain as a means of getting people to nurture them. The reason that the chronic complaining we see in these patients is so unresponsive to logical persuasion and evidence to the contrary is because the core issue is emotional deprivation: Patients are complaining to gain nurturance and empathy, not because they want practical solutions or advice. The self-defeating aspect of their complaining is that, after a while, other people get fed up with their complaining and become impatient or avoid them. Nevertheless, in the short run, the complaining often wins patients sympathy and attention. If they learn to ask more directly for caring rather than seeking it through complaining, then they can begin to meet their emotional needs in healthier ways.

Limiting the time spent worrying by scheduling "worry time" is a behavioral strategy that helps many of these patients. They learn to notice when they are worrying, and then postpone the worrying until the prescribed time. Many of these patients also benefit from scheduling more activities for fun. Often, people with this schema have lives oriented around survival rather than pleasure. Life is not about getting "good things"—it is about preventing "bad things." Getting patients to schedule pleasurable activities can be an antidote to their tendency to spend so much time worrying. As with the treatment of depression, increasing pleasurable activities is an important component of treating the Negativity/Pessimism schema.

As we noted earlier, many patients with this schema were emotionally deprived as children and thus need a great deal of nurturing from the therapist. The therapist can focus on providing validation for past negative events, being careful not to support complaints or negative predictions about the future. If the therapist can nurture the patient regarding past losses, while not responding to excessive complaining about current events, the patient can begin to heal. This "limited reparenting" promotes grieving without reinforcing pessimism or complaining.

Special Problems with This Schema

This is usually a difficult schema to change. Often, patients cannot remember a time when they did not feel pessimistic, and cannot imagine feeling otherwise. Mode work can help them free up their Happy Child mode, long buried under mountains of worry. The Healthy Adult—first role-played by the therapist, then the patient—comes into images of upsetting past and current situations, and helps the Worried Child take a more positive view of them.

Therapists must be careful not to fall into the role of arguing with patients about their negative thinking. Rather than the therapist repeatedly playing the positive side and the patient playing the negative side, it is important for the patient to play both sides. When the therapist and patient assume opposite sides, sessions tend to become too much like debates, and the relationship is prone to becoming adversarial. If the patient plays both sides, the therapist can coach the healthy side when necessary. The therapist can help the patient identify two modes, the Pessimist and the Optimist, then carry out dialogues between them.

There can be a lot of secondary gain for the schema if the patient receives attention for complaining. The therapist should try to alter these contingencies as much as possible. The therapist can meet with family members who are reinforcing the patient's complaining and teach them a healthier response. The therapist can help them learn to ignore patients when they complain, rewarding instead expressions of confidence and hope.

When the schema is hard to change as a result of a history of extremely negative life events, it is often helpful for patients to grieve for past losses. Genuine grieving can relieve the pressure to complain. Grieving helps patients separate the present, where they (presumably) are safe and secure, from the past, where they underwent traumatic loss or damage.

As we have said, for some patients, there may be a biological component to the worrying, and medication is a potential addition to their treatment. We have sometimes found antidepressant medications, especially selective serotonin reuptake inhibitors, to be quite helpful.

Emotional Inhibition

Typical Presentation of the Schema

These patients present as emotionally constricted and are excessively inhibited about discussing and expressing their emotions. They are affectively flat rather than emotional and expressive, and self-controlled rather than spontaneous. They usually hold back expressions of warmth and caring, and often attempt to restrain their aggressive urges. Many patients with this schema value self-control above intimacy in human interactions and fear that, if they let go of their emotions at all, they might completely lose control. Ultimately, they fear being overcome with shame or bringing about some other grave consequence, such as punishment or abandonment. Often, the overcontrol is extended to significant others in the patient's environment (the patient tries to prevent significant others from expressing both positive and negative emotions), especially when these emotions are intense.

Patients inhibit emotions that it would be healthier to express. These are the natural emotions of the Spontaneous Child mode. All children have to learn to rein in their emotions and impulses in order to respect the rights of other people. However, patients with this schema have gone too far. They have inhibited and overcontrolled their Spontaneous Child so much that they have forgotten how to be natural and to play. The most common areas in which patients are overcontrolled include inhibition of anger; inhibition of positive feelings such as joy, love, affection, and sexual excitement; excessive adherence to routines or rituals; difficulty expressing vulnerability or communicating fully about one's feelings; and excessive emphasis on rationality while disregarding emotional needs.

Patients with the Emotional Inhibition schema frequently meet the diagnostic criteria for obsessive–compulsive personality disorder. In addition to being emotionally constricted, they tend to be overly devoted to decorum at the expense of intimacy and play, and are rigid and inflexible rather than spontaneous. Patients who have both the Emotional Inhibition and Unrelenting Standards schemas are especially likely to meet diagnostic criteria for obsessive–compulsive personality disorder, because the two schemas together include almost all the criteria.

The most common origin for the Emotional Inhibition schema is being shamed by parents and other authority figures when, as children, patients spontaneously displayed emotion. This is often a cultural schema, in the sense that certain cultures place a high value on self-control. (One patient told the following joke to illustrate the emotional restraint of his Scandinavian heritage: "Did you hear about the Scandinavian man who loved his wife so much he almost told her?") The schema often runs in families. The underlying belief is that it is "bad" to show feelings, to talk about them or act on them impulsively, whereas it is "good" to keep feelings inside. Patients with this schema usually appear to be self-controlled, joyless, and grim. In addition, as a result of a reservoir of unexpressed anger, they are frequently hostile or resentful.

Patients with the Emotional Inhibition schema often become romantically involved with partners who are emotional and impulsive. We believe this is because there is a healthy part of them that wants in some way to let the Spontaneous Child inside of them emerge. (One female patient, who was taught it was wrong to "show off," married a man who loved to wear fancy clothes and go to expensive places: "When I'm with him, it feels like I'm allowed to dress up," she explained.) When inhibited people marry emotional people, the couple sometimes becomes increasingly polarized over time. Unfortunately, sometimes the partners begin to dislike each other for the very qualities that first attracted them: The emotional partner scorns the reserve of the inhibited one, and the inhibited partner disdains the intensity of the emotional one.

Goals of Treatment

The basic goal of treatment is to help patients become more emotionally expressive and spontaneous. Treatment helps patients learn how to appropriately discuss and express many of the emotions they are suppressing. Patients learn to show anger in appropriate ways, engage in more activities for fun, express affection, and talk about their feelings. They learn to value emotions as much as rationality, and to stop controlling the people around them, humiliating others for expressing normal emotions, and feeling shame about their own emotions. Instead, they allow themselves and others to be more emotionally expressive.

Strategies Emphasized in Treatment

The behavioral and experiential treatment strategies are probably the most important. Behavioral strategies are directed at helping the patient discuss and express both positive and negative emotions with significant others, and engage in more activities for fun. Some education is useful; otherwise, cognitive strategies generally are not as helpful—they reinforce the patient's already excessive emphasis on rationality.

Experiential work can enable patients to access their emotions. In images of childhood, the Healthy Adult helps the Inhibited Child express the emotions that patients suppressed as children. First the therapist, then the patient, plays the Healthy Adult. The Healthy Adult confronts the Inhibiting Parent and encourages the child to express feelings such as anger and love. In images of current and future situations, the Healthy Adult helps the patient to articulate emotions, and to encourage other people to articulate their emotions as well.

The therapy relationship can also be quite helpful in healing the Emotional Inhibition schema. A therapist who is generally more expressive and emotional can "reparent" the patient and provide a model. (However, a highly rational, inhibited therapist might inadvertently strengthen the schema.) Reparenting could involve occasionally doing something spontaneously in the session just for fun (e.g., telling a joke, discussing a frivolous topic, using humor) to break up the serious tone. Most importantly, the therapist reinforces the patient for expressing rather than restraining emotions. If the patient has strong feelings about the therapist, then the therapist encourages the patient to express them aloud.

Cognitive strategies help the patient accept the advantages of being more emotional, and thereby make the decision to fight the schema. The therapist presents the process of fighting the schema as seeking a balance on a spectrum of emotionality rather than as all-or-nothing. The goal is *not* for patients to flip to the other extreme and become impulsively emotional; rather, the goal is for patients to reach a middle position.

Finally, cognitive strategies can help patients evaluate the consequences of expressing their emotions. Patients with this schema are afraid that, if they express their emotions, something bad will happen. Often, what they fear is that they will be humiliated or made to feel ashamed. Helping patients see that they can use good judgment about expressing emotions, so that this is not likely to happen, allows them to feel more comfortable and willing to experiment.

Experiential strategies help patients access and express unacknowledged childhood emotions, such as longing, anger, love, and happiness. In imagery, patients relive important childhood situations, this time expressing their emotions. They say out loud the feelings they inhibited at the time. First the therapist, then the patient, enters the image as the Healthy Adult and helps the Inhibited Child. The Healthy Adult rewards the child for expressing feelings rather than humiliating or shaming the child, as the parent figures did. The Healthy Adult confronts the parent, and consoles and accepts the child. The patient expresses anger and sadness about his or her lost Spontaneous Child.

There are a wealth of potential behavioral role plays and homework assignments. Patients can practice discussing their feelings with other people, appropriately expressing both positive and negative feelings, playing and being spontaneous, and doing activities designed for fun. They might take a dance class or experiment sexually, or do something on the spur of the moment. They might express aggression with their bodies, for example, by playing competitive sports or pounding a punching bag. If necessary, the therapist can grade behavioral tasks in terms of difficulty, so that patients gradually let go of their overcontrol. Working with the partner can be useful. The therapist encourages both the patient and the partner to express feelings in constructive ways. Finally, patients design tests of their negative predictions, writing down what they predict will happen if they express their emotions, and what actually happens. Patients role-play interchanges with significant others in imagery and with the therapist, and then carry them out for homework assignments. They compare the actual results with the predicted ones.

The therapist both models and encourages appropriate emotional expression. Group therapy can help many patients with this schema become more comfortable expressing their emotions to others.

Special Problems with This Schema

When people have been emotionally inhibited for virtually their entire lives, it is hard for them to begin acting differently. Expressing emotion feels so foreign to patients who have this schema—it is so contrary to what feels like their true nature—that they experience great difficulty doing it. Mode work can help patients access the healthy side of them that wants to battle the schema and express emotions more openly.

Unrelenting Standards/Hypercriticalness

Typical Presentation of the Schema

Patients with this schema present as perfectionistic and driven. They believe that they must continually strive to meet extremely high standards. These standards are internalized; therefore, unlike the Approval-Seeking/Recognition-Seeking schema, patients with the Unrelenting Standards schema do not as readily alter their expectations or behaviors based on the reactions of others. These patients strive to meet standards primarily because they "should," not because they want to win the approval of other people. Even if no one were ever to know, most of these patients would still strive to meet the standards. Patients often have both the Unrelenting Standards and Approval-Seeking/Recognition-Seeking schemas, in which case they seek both to meet very high standards and to win external approval. Unrelenting Standards, Approval-Seeking/Recognition-Seeking, and Entitlement are the most readily observable schemas in the narcissistic personality (although Emotional Deprivation and Defectiveness schemas often underlie these compensatory schemas). We discuss this further in Chapter 10 on treating narcissistic patients.

The most typical emotion experienced by patients with the Unrelenting Standards schema is *pressure*. This pressure is relentless. Because perfection is impossible, the person must perpetually try harder. Beneath all the exertion, patients feel intense anxiety about failing—and failing means getting a "95" rather than a "100." Another common feeling is hypercriticalness, both of themselves and of others. Most of these patients also feel a great deal of time pressure: There is so much to do and so little time. A common result is exhaustion.

It is difficult to have unrelenting standards, and it is often difficult to be with someone who has unrelenting standards. (As one of our patients said about his wife, who has unrelenting standards: "This is no good, and that's no good. Nothing's ever any good.") Another common feeling in patients with this schema is irritability, usually because not enough is getting done quickly enough or well enough. Yet another common feeling is competitiveness. Most patients who are classified as "type A"—that is, as demonstrating a chronic sense of time pressure, hostility, and competitiveness (Suinn, 1977)—have this schema.

Often, patients with the Unrelenting Standards schema are workaholics, working incessantly within the particular realms to which they apply their standards. The realms can be varied: school, work, appearance, home, athletic performance, health, ethics or adherence to rules, and artistic performance are some possibilities. In their perfectionism, these patients often display inordinate attention to detail and often underestimate how much better their performance is relative to the norm. They have rigid rules in many areas of life, such as unrealistically high ethical, cultural, or religious standards. There is almost always an all-or-nothing quality to their thinking: Patients believe that either they have met the standard exactly or they have failed. They rarely take pleasure from success, because they are already focused on the next task that must be accomplished perfectly.

Patients with this schema do not usually view their standards as perfectionistic. Their standards feel normal. They are just doing what is expected of them. In order to qualify as having a maladaptive schema, the patient must have some significant impairment related to the schema. This could be a lack of pleasure in life, health problems, low self-esteem, unsatisfying intimate or work relationships, or some other form of dysfunction.

Goals of Treatment

The basic goal of treatment is to help patients reduce their unrelenting standards and hypercriticalness. The goal is twofold: to get patients to try to accomplish less, and to accomplish it less perfectly. Successfully treated patients have more of a balance in their lives between accomplishment and pleasure. They play, as well as work, and do not worry so much about "wasting time" and feeling guilty about it. They take the time to connect emotionally to significant others and are able to allow something to be imperfect and still consider it worthwhile. Less critical of themselves and others, they are less demanding and more accepting of human imperfection, and are less rigid about rules. They come to realize that their unrelenting standards cost more than they gain: In trying to make one situation slightly better, they are making many other situations a lot worse.

Strategies Emphasized in Treatment

The cognitive and behavioral treatment strategies are usually most important. Although experiential strategies and the therapy relationship can be useful, they are usually not central to the treatment of this schema.

The therapist utilizes cognitive strategies to help patients challenge their perfectionism. They learn to view performance as lying on a *spectrum* from poor to perfect—with many gradations in between—rather than as an all-or-nothing phenomenon. They conduct cost–benefit analyses of perpetuating their unrelenting standards, asking themselves: "If I were to do things a little less well, or if I were to do fewer things, what would the costs and benefits be?" The therapist highlights the advantages of lowering their standards—all the benefits that would accrue to their health and happiness, all the ways they are suffering as a result of their unrelenting standards, and all the ways the schema is damaging their enjoyment of life and relationships with significant others. The cost of the schema is greater than the benefits: This conclusion is the leverage that can motivate patients to change. The therapist also helps patients reduce the perceived risks of imperfection. Imperfection is not a crime. Making mistakes does not have the extreme negative consequences that patients anticipate.

The Unrelenting Standards schema seems to have two different origins, with different implications for treatment. The first and more common origin is the internalization of a parent with high standards (the Demanding Parent mode). When this is the origin, experiential exercises help patients build up a part of the self that can fight the internalized Demanding Parent. This is the Healthy Adult, played first by the therapist, then by the patient. Patients express anger about the pressure and the high cost of the parent's standards; they have paid dearly for internalizing those standards.

The second origin of the Unrelenting Standards schema is as a compensation for the Defectiveness schema: Patients feel defective and then overcompensate by trying to be perfect. When this is the origin, helping patients become aware of the underlying Defectiveness schema is an important part of treatment. Experiential strategies can help patients access the underlying shame. All of the imagery exercises that apply to the Defectiveness schema become relevant. Patients can also visualize their perfectionistic side (one patient calls hers "Miss Perfect": "She has her hands on her hips and a stern, disappointed look on her face"). In imagery, the perfectionistic mode can step aside and let the Vulnerable Child speak.

Behavioral strategies can help patients gradually reduce their unrelenting standards. The therapist and patient design behavioral experiments to help rein in the perfectionism—to do less and to do it less well. Some examples of behavioral experiments include scheduling how much time they are going to spend working versus doing other things, such as playing and connecting to significant others; setting lower standards and practicing adhering to them; intentionally doing tasks imperfectly; giving praise for the imperfect yet worthwhile behaviors of significant others; or "wasting time" interacting with friends or family members purely for the sake of enjoyment or to enhance the quality of the relationships. Patients monitor their mood as a consequence of carrying out the assignments and observe the effects on the moods of significant others. They learn to fight the guilt they feel when they do not try hard enough. The Healthy Adult assures the Imperfect Child that it is acceptable to permit some imperfection.

Ideally, therapists model balanced standards in both their approach to therapy and in their portrayal of their own lives. Therapists who are themselves too perfectionistic can undermine the patient's progress in treatment. The therapist uses empathic confrontation when the patient's unrelenting standards manifest themselves in therapy, such as when the patient fills out forms too well or does the homework too perfectly. Although the therapist understands why patients feel they have to perform perfectly, because this is what was conveyed to them by their parents in childhood, in reality, they do not have to perform perfectly for the therapist. The therapist will not shame or criticize them for performing imperfectly. He or she is more interested in forming a relationship and helping the patient to heal than in evaluating the patient's performance in therapy, and wants the patient to feel the same.

Special Problems with This Schema

The biggest obstacle by far is the secondary gain that comes from the schema: There are so many benefits to doing things so well. Many patients with this schema are reluctant to give up their unrelenting standards because, to them, it seems that the benefits far outweigh the costs. In addition, many patients are afraid of embarrassment, shame, guilt, and their own self-criticalness, if they do not live up to the standards. The potential for negative affect seems so high that they are reluctant to risk lowering their standards even a little bit. Moving slowly can help these patients, as can closely evaluating the outcomes of lowering the standards. Mode work can help patients build up their healthy side that wants to trade perfectionism for greater fulfillment in life.

Punitiveness

Typical Presentation of the Schema

These patients believe that people—including themselves—should be harshly punished for their mistakes. They present as moralistic and intolerant, and find it extremely difficult to forgive mistakes in other people or in themselves. They believe that, rather than forgiveness, people who make mistakes deserve punishment. No excuses are permitted. Patients with this schema display an unwillingness to consider extenuating circumstances. They do not allow for human imperfection, and they have difficulty feeling any empathy whatsoever for a person who does something they view as bad or wrong. These patients lack the quality of mercy.

The best way to detect this schema is by the punitive, blaming *tone of voice* these patients use when someone has made a mistake, whether they are speaking about other people or about themselves. The origin of this punitive tone of voice is almost always a blaming parent who spoke in the same tone of voice. The tone conveys the implacable necessity of exacting punishment. It is the voice of the "fire and brimstone" preacher: heartless, cold, and contemptuous. It lacks softness and compassion. It is a voice that will not be satisfied until the wrongdoer has been punished. There is also the sense that the penalty the person wants to exact is too severe— that the punishment is greater than the crime. Like the Red Queen in Lewis Carroll's (1923) *Alice in Wonderland*, shouting "Off with his head!" for every minor infraction, the schema is undiscriminating and extreme.

Punitiveness is often linked to other schemas, especially Unrelenting Standards and Defectiveness. When patients have unrelenting standards and punish themselves for not meeting them, as opposed to simply feeling imperfect, they have both the Unrelenting Standards and Punitiveness schemas. When they feel defective and punish themselves for it, as opposed to simply feeling depressed or inadequate, they have both the Defectiveness and Punitiveness schemas. Most patients with borderline disorder have both Defectiveness and Punitiveness schemas: They feel bad whenever they feel defective, and they want to punish themselves for being bad. They have internalized their Punitive Parent as a mode, and they punish themselves for being defective, just as the parent used to punish them: They yell at themselves, cut themselves, starve themselves, or otherwise mete out punishment. (We discuss the "Punitive Parent" mode further in the Chapter 9 on treating patients with BPD.)

Goals of Treatment

The fundamental goal is to help patients become less punitive and more forgiving, toward both themselves and others. The therapist begins by teaching patients that, most of the time, there is little value in punishing people. Punishment is not an effective way to change behavior, particularly when compared to other methods, such as rewarding good behavior or modeling. There is a great deal of operant research on the ineffectiveness of punishment as a means of changing behavior (Baron, 1988; Beyer & Thrice, 1984; Coleman, Abraham, & Jussin, 1987; Rachlin, 1976). Other research shows that an authoritarian style of parenting is less effective than a democratic style. In an authoritarian parenting style, the parent punishes "bad" behavior; in a democratic parenting style, the parent explains why the child's behavior is wrong. Authoritarian parents tend to produce children who disobey whenever the parent is out of sight, whereas democratic parents tend to produce children who try to do what is right, whether the parent is there or not. In addition, the children of democratic parents have higher self-esteem (Aunola, Stattin, & Nurmi, 2000; Patock-Peckham, Cheong, Balhorn, & Nogoshi, 2001).

Each time the patient expresses the desire to punish someone, the therapist asks a series of questions: "Were the person's intentions good or bad? If the person's intentions were good, doesn't that count for something? Doesn't the person deserve some forgiveness? If the person's intentions were good, then how will punishment help? Isn't the person likely to repeat the behavior when you're not there to see? Even if the person behaves better next time, isn't the cost too high? The punishment will have undermined the relationship and the person's self-esteem. Is that what you want?" These questions guide the patient to discover that punishment is not the most beneficial approach.

Patients work toward building empathy and forgiveness for human beings in all their frailty and imperfection. They learn to consider extenuating circumstances and to have a balanced response when someone makes an error or fails to meet their expectations. If they are in a position of authority (e.g., if the other person is a child or employee), they do not punish the person. Rather, they focus on helping the person understand how to behave better the next time. Punishment should be reserved for those who are grossly negligent or have immoral intentions. As the saying goes, "The scales of justice must always be tempered with mercy.")

Strategies Emphasized in Treatment

Cognitive strategies are important in building patients' motivation to change. The main strategy is educational: Patients explore the advantages and disadvantages of punishment versus forgiveness. They list both the consequences of punishing a person and of being more forgiving and encouraging the person to reflect on the behavior. Exploring the advantages and disadvantages helps the patient accept intellectually that punishment is not an effective way to deal with mistakes. Patients conduct dialogues between the punitive side and the forgiving side, in which the two sides debate each other. Initially, the therapist plays the healthy side and the patient plays the unhealthy side; eventually, the patient plays both sides in the dialogue. Becoming convinced on a cognitive level that the cost of the schema is greater than the benefit can help strengthen the patient's resolve to battle the schema.

Because the schema is almost always the internalization of a parent's Punitiveness schema, much experiential work focuses on externalizing and fighting the Punitive Parent mode. In imagery, patients picture the parent talking to them in the punitive tone of voice. They talk back to the parent, saying, "I'm not going to listen to you anymore. I'm not going to believe you anymore. You're wrong, and you're not good for me." Doing imagery work with the Punitive Parent gives patients a way to distance from the schema and to make it feel less ego-syntonic. Rather than hearing the punitive voice of the schema as their own voice, they hear it as their parent's voice. Patients can say to themselves: "This is not my voice that is punishing me; this is my parent's voice. Punishment wasn't healthy for me in childhood, and it isn't healthy for me now. I'm not going to beat up on myself anymore, and I'm not going to punish other people anymore, especially the people I love."

The aim of the behavioral strategies is to practice more forgiving responses in situations where patients have urges to blame themselves or others. Patients rehearse the behaviors in imagery exercises or role plays with the therapist, then carry out the behaviors for homework. The therapist can model more forgiving responses when necessary. Patients note whether the consequences match their dire predictions. For example, as a behavioral experiment, one patient, a mother with a young daughter, changed her response to her daughter's misbehaviors for one week. Rather than yelling at her daughter when she misbehaved, the patient calmly explained why the behavior was wrong. The patient predicted that her daughter would misbehave more and found that, instead, her daughter misbehaved less.

The therapist can use the therapy relationship to model forgiveness. The "limited reparenting" the therapist provides emphasizes compassion over punishment. For example, if the patient makes a mistake, such as mixing up an appointment time or forgetting a homework assignment, the therapist does not reprimand the patient. Rather, the therapist helps the patient figure out how to avoid the mistake in the future.

Special Problems with This Schema

This can be a difficult schema to change, particularly when it is combined with the Defectiveness schema. The patient's sense of moral indignation and injustice can be very inflexible. Maintaining the patient's motivation to change is the key to the treatment. The therapist helps the patient stay focused on the costs and the benefits of the schema in terms of improved self-esteem and more harmonious interpersonal relationships.

Chapter 8

SCHEMA MODE WORK

As we stated in Chapter 1, a mode is the set of schemas or schema operations—adaptive or maladaptive—that are currently active for an individual. Our development of the concept of a mode was part of a natural progression in which we focused the model on patients with increasingly severe disorders. We started with traditional cognitive-behavioral therapy, which helped many patients with Axis I disorders. However, many other patients—especially patients with chronic symptoms and those with Axis II disorders—either went largely unhelped or were helped with their Axis I symptoms but still experienced significant emotional distress and impaired functioning—that is, significant characterological psychopathology. Similarly, schema therapy helped a majority of these patients but left a group of patients with severe disorders requiring further treatment, especially those with borderline and narcissistic disorders.

Although we originally developed mode work to treat these latter patients, we now use it with many of our higher functioning patients as well. At this point, mode work has become an integral part of schema therapy, and we blend mode work fluidly into regular schema work, rather than thinking of the two approaches as separate. The difference is whether we use mode work as the primary approach, as with patients with borderline and narcissistic disorders, or as an adjunctive method, as with healthier patients. Thus mode work is an advanced component of schema work, used whenever the therapist is blocked or feels it would be useful. All dialogues with two different modes, including the schema side and healthy side, are forms of mode work.

WHEN MIGHT WE USE A MODE APPROACH?

When might a clinician choose to use a mode approach rather than the simpler schema approach described thus far? In our practice, the higher functioning the patient, the more likely we are to emphasize "standard" schema terminology (as described in the earlier chapters of this book); the more severely disordered the patient, the more likely we are to emphasize mode terminology and strategies. For patients in the middle range of functioning, we tend to blend the two approaches together, referring to schemas, coping styles, and modes.

We might shift from a simple schema approach to a mode approach when the therapy seems stuck and we cannot break through the patient's avoidance or overcompensation to the underlying schemas. This might happen with a patient who is very rigid and avoidant or almost continuously in an overcompensating mode, such as patients with obsessive–compulsive or narcissistic disorders are likely to be.

We might also shift to a mode approach when the patient is rigidly self-punitive and self-critical. Usually this is an indication of an internalized dysfunctional parent who is punishing and criticizing the patient. The clinician and patient can then join forces, allying against this Punitive Parent mode. Labeling the mode in this way helps the patient externalize the mode and make it more ego-dystonic.

We might shift to modes with a patient who has a seemingly unresolvable internal conflict: for example, in whom two parts of the self are locked in opposition about a major life decision, such as whether to leave a long-term relationship. Each part of the self can be labeled as a mode, and the two modes can then conduct dialogues and negotiate with one another. Finally, we generally emphasize modes with patients who display frequent fluctuations in affect, such as often occurs with patients with BPD who repeatedly flip from anger to sadness to self-punishment to numbness.

COMMON SCHEMA MODES

As noted in Chapter 1, we have identified four main types of modes: Child modes, Maladaptive Coping modes, Dysfunctional Parent modes, and the Healthy Adult mode. Each type of mode is associated with certain schemas (except the Healthy Adult and Happy Child) or embodies certain coping styles.

In patients with borderline and narcissistic disorders, the modes are relatively disconnected, and the person is capable of experiencing only one mode at a time. Patients with BPD switch rapidly from mode to mode. Other patients, such as those with narcissistic personality disorder, switch less often and can be in one mode for a long time. For example, a patient with narcissistic personality disorder who is on a month-long vacation might spend the entire time in a detached self-soothing mode, pursuing novelty and excitement; in contrast, a patient with narcissistic personality disorder who is at work or at a party might spend the entire time in a self-aggrandizing mode.

Still other patients, such as those with obsessive-compulsive personality disorder, are rigidly locked in a single mode and almost never fluctuate. Regardless of where they are, who they are with, or what is happening to them, they are essentially the same: self-controlled, rigid, and perfectionistic. The frequency of shifts is important when we look at an individual patient, but it is not what defines a mode. Modes can either shift frequently for a given patient or stay relatively constant. Either extreme can lead to significant problems for the patient.

Child Modes

The Child modes are clearest in patients with BPD, who are themselves so much like children. We have identified four Child modes: the Vulnerable Child, the Angry Child, the Impulsive/Undisciplined Child, and the Happy Child (see Table 8.1). We believe that these Child modes are innate and that they represent the inborn emotional range of human beings. What

TABLE 8.1. Child Modes

Child mode	Description	Common associated schemas
Vulnerable Child	Experiences dysphoric or anxious affect, especially fear, sadness, and helplessness, when "in touch" with associated schemas.	Abandonment, Mistrust/Abuse, Emotional Deprivation, Defectiveness, Social Isolation, Dependence/Incompetence, Vulnerability to Harm or Illness, Enmeshment/Undeveloped Self, Negativity/Pessimism.
Angry Child	Vents anger directly in response to perceived unmet core needs or unfair treatment related to core schemas.	Abandonment, Mistrust/Abuse, Emotional Deprivation, Subjugation (or, at times, any of the schemas associated with the Vulnerable Child).
Impulsive/ Undisciplined Child	Impulsively acts according to immediate desires for pleasure without regard to limits or others' needs or feelings (not linked to core needs).	Entitlement, Insufficient Self-Control/Self-Discipline.
Happy Child	Feels loved, connected, content, satisfied.	None. Absence of activated schemas.

happens in the early childhood environment may suppress or enhance a Child mode, but human beings are born with the capacity to express all four of them.

A patient in the *Vulnerable Child* mode might appear frightened, sad, overwhelmed, or helpless. This mode is like a young child in the world who needs the care of adults in order to survive but is not getting that care. The child desperately needs a parent and will tolerate just about anything to get one. (Marilyn Monroe captured the defenselessness of the Vulnerable Child). The specific nature of the wound to the Vulnerable Child depends on the schema: The parent leaves the child alone for long periods of time (the Abandoned Child), hits the child excessively (the Abused Child), withholds love (the Deprived Child), or harshly criticizes the child (the Defective Child). Other schemas that can be associated with this mode include Social Isolation, Dependence/Incompetence, Vulnerability to Harm or Illness, Enmeshment/Undeveloped Self, and Failure. Most schemas are part of the Vulnerable Child mode. For this reason, we regard the Vulnerable Child as the core mode for the purposes of schema work. Ultimately it is the mode that we are most concerned with healing.

The *Angry Child* has become enraged. Virtually all young children become angry at some point when their core needs are not being met. Although the parent might punish the child or otherwise squelch the response, rage is a normal reaction for a young child in this predicament. Patients in the Angry Child mode vent anger directly in response to perceived unmet needs or unfair treatment related to associated schemas, including Abandonment, Mistrust/Abuse, Emotional Deprivation, and Subjugation, among others. When a schema is triggered and the patient feels abandoned, abused, deprived, or subjugated, the patient becomes furious and might yell, lash out verbally, or have violent fantasies and impulses.

The *Impulsive/Undisciplined Child* acts impulsively to fill needs and pursue pleasure without regard to limits or concern for others. This mode is the child in a natural state, uninhibited and "uncivilized," irresponsible and free. (Peter Pan, the eternal child, incarnates this mode.) The Impulsive/Undisciplined Child has low frustration tolerance and cannot delay short-term gratification for the sake of long-term goals. A person in this mode may appear spoiled, angry, careless, lazy, impatient, unfocused, or out of control. Associated schemas can include Entitlement and Insufficient Self-Control/Self-Discipline.

The *Happy Child* feels loved and contented. This mode is not associated with any Early Maladaptive Schemas because the child's core needs are being met adequately. The Happy Child mode represents the healthy absence of schema activation.

Maladaptive Coping Modes

The Maladaptive Coping modes represent the child's attempts to adapt to living with unmet emotional needs in a harmful environment. These coping modes were adaptive when the patient was a young child, but they are often maladaptive in the wider adult world. We have identified three broad types: the Compliant Surrenderer, the Detached Protector, and the Overcompensator (see Table 8.2). They correspond, respectively, to the coping processes of surrender, avoidance, and overcompensation.

The function of the Compliant Surrenderer is to avoid further mistreatment. The function of the other two modes, the Detached Protector and the Overcompensator, is to escape the upsetting emotions generated by schema eruption.

The *Compliant Surrenderer* submits to the schema as a coping style. Patients in this mode appear passive and dependent. They do whatever the therapist (and others) want them to do. Individuals in the Compliant Surrenderer mode experience themselves as helpless in the face of a more powerful figure. They feel they have no choice but to try to please this person to avoid conflict. They are obedient, perhaps allowing others to abuse them, neglect them, control them, or devalue them in order to preserve the connection or avoid retaliation.

The *Detached Protector* uses schema avoidance as a coping style. The coping style is one of psychological withdrawal. Individuals in the Detached Protector mode detach from other people and shut off their emotions in order to protect themselves from the pain of being vulnerable. The mode is like a protective armor or wall, with the more vulnerable modes hiding inside. In the Detached Protector mode, patients may feel numb or empty. They may adopt a cynical or aloof stance to avoid investing emotionally in people or activities. Behavioral examples include social withdrawal, excessive self-reliance, addictive self-soothing, fantasizing, compulsive distraction, and stimulation-seeking.

TABLE 8.2. Maladaptive Coping Modes

Maladaptive Coping modes	Description
Compliant Surrenderer	Adopts a coping style of compliance and dependence.
Detached Protector	Adopts a coping style of emotional withdrawal, disconnection, isolation, and behavioral avoidance.
Overcompensator	Adopts a coping style of counterattack and control. May overcompensate through semiadaptive means, such as workaholism.

The Detached Protector mode is problematic for many of our characterological patients, especially those with BPD, and is often the most difficult mode to change. When these patients were young children, development of the Detached Protector mode was an adaptive strategy. They were trapped in a traumatic environment that created too much suffering, and it made sense for them to distance themselves, to detach and not to feel. As these children matured into adults and entered a less hostile or depriving world, it would have been adaptive to let go of the Detached Protector and become open to the world and their own emotions again. But these patients have become so accustomed to being in the Detached Protector mode that it is automatic, and they no longer know how to get out of it. Their refuge has become a prison.

Overcompensators use schema overcompensation as a coping style. They act as though the opposite of the schema were true.[1] For example, if they feel defective, they try to appear perfect and superior to others. If they feel guilty, they blame others. If they feel dominated, they bully others. If they feel used, they move to exploit others. If they feel inferior, they seek to impress others with their status or accomplishments. Some overcompensators are passive–aggressive. They appear overtly compliant while secretly getting revenge, or they rebel covertly through procrastination, backstabbing, complaining, or nonperformance. Other overcompensators are obsessive. They maintain strict order, tight self-control, or high levels of predictability through planning, excessive adherence to routines, or undue caution.

Dysfunctional Parent Modes

Dysfunctional Parent modes are internalizations of parent figures in the patient's early life. When patients are in a Dysfunctional Parent mode, they *become* their own parent and treat themselves as the parent treated them when they were children. They often take on the voice of the parent in their "self-talk." In Dysfunctional Parent modes, patients think, feel, and act as their parent did toward them when they were children.

We have identified two common types of Dysfunctional Parent modes (although some patients may exhibit other parent modes as well): the Punitive (or Critical) Parent and the Demanding Parent (see Table 8.3). The *Punitive Parent* angrily punishes, criticizes, or restricts the child for expressing needs or making mistakes. The most common associated schemas are Punitiveness and Defectiveness. This mode is especially prominent in patients with BPD or severe depression. Patients with BPD have a Punitive

---

[1]Entitlement and Unrelenting Standards are schemas that often function as forms of overcompensation. However, they can also be "pure" schemas rather than forms of overcompensation.

TABLE 8.3. **Dysfunctional Parent Modes**

Dysfunctional Parent mode	Description	Common associated schemas
Punitive/Critical Parent	Restricts, criticizes, or punishes the self or others.	Subjugation, Punitiveness, Defectiveness, Mistrust/Abuse (as abuser).
Demanding Parent	Sets high expectations and high level of responsibility toward others; pressures the self or others to achieve them.	Unrelenting Standards, Self-Sacrifice.

Parent mode in which they become their own abusive parent and punish themselves: For example, they say they are evil, dirty, or bad, and often punish themselves by cutting themselves. In this mode they are not Vulnerable Children; rather, they are Punitive Parents meting out punishment to the Vulnerable Child. Actually, they shift back and forth from the Punitive Parent to the Vulnerable Child, so that at some moments they are the child who is being abused, and at other moments they are their own parent perpetrating the abuse.

The *Demanding Parent* pressures the child to achieve unrealistically high parental expectations. The person feels that the "right" way to be is to be perfect and the "wrong" way to be is fallible or spontaneous. Often the associated schemas are Unrelenting Standards and Self-Sacrifice. This mode is very common in patients with narcissistic and obsessive–compulsive disorders. Patients shift into a Demanding Parent mode in which they set high standards for themselves and drive themselves to meet them. However, the Demanding Parent is not necessarily punitive: The Demanding Parent expects a lot but may not blame or punish. Most frequently, the child recognizes the parent's disappointment and feels ashamed. Many patients have a combined Punitive and Demanding Parent mode, in which they both set high standards for themselves and punish themselves when they fail to meet them.

The Healthy Adult Mode

This mode is the healthy, adult part of the self that serves an "executive" function relative to the other modes. The Healthy Adult helps meet the child's basic emotional needs. Building and strengthening the patient's Healthy Adult to work with the other modes more effectively is the overarching goal of mode work.

Most adult patients have some version of this mode, but they vary drastically in how effective it is. Healthier, higher functioning patients have a stronger Healthy Adult mode; patients with more severe disorders usually have a weaker Healthy Adult mode. Patients with BPD often have almost no Healthy Adult mode, so the therapist must augment or help to create a mode that is extremely undeveloped.

Like a good parent, the Healthy Adult mode serves the following three basic functions:

1. Nurtures, affirms, and protects the Vulnerable Child.
2. Sets limits for the Angry Child and the Impulsive/Undisciplined Child, in accord with the principles of reciprocity and self-discipline.
3. Battles or moderates the maladaptive coping and dysfunctional parent modes.

During the course of treatment, patients internalize the therapist's behavior as part of their own Healthy Adult mode. Initially, the therapist serves as the Healthy Adult whenever the patient is incapable of doing so. For example, if a patient is able to battle the Punitive Parent on his own, the therapist does not intervene. However, if the patient is unable to battle the Punitive Parent and instead attacks himself endlessly without defending himself, then the therapist intervenes and battles the Punitive Parent for the patient. Gradually the patient takes over the Healthy Adult Role. (This is what we mean by "limited reparenting.")

THE SEVEN GENERAL STEPS IN SCHEMA MODE WORK

We have developed seven *general* steps in schema mode work. (In the following two chapters, we discuss how we adapt these broad strategies to work with the individual modes we have identified for patients with borderline and narcissistic personality disorders.)

1. Identify and label the patient's modes.
2. Explore the origin and (when relevant) adaptive value of the mode in childhood or adolescence.
3. Link maladaptive modes to current problems and symptoms.
4. Demonstrate the advantages of modifying or giving up one mode if it is interfering with access to another mode.
5. Access the Vulnerable Child through imagery.
6. Conduct dialogues among the modes. Initially, the therapist models the Healthy Adult mode; later the patient plays this mode.
7. Help the patient generalize mode work to life situations outside therapy sessions.

CASE ILLUSTRATION: ANNETTE

We illustrate the seven steps of schema mode work with the case of Annette. The following excerpts are from a consultation interview Dr. Young conducted with Annette, who was already being treated by another schema therapist named Rachel. At the time of the interview, Annette had been in therapy with Rachel for about 6 months.

Annette is a 26-year-old woman. She is single and lives alone in an apartment in Manhattan, where she works as a receptionist. At the start of therapy, her presenting problems were depression and alcohol abuse. She also reported a history of problems in relationships and at work: She had drifted from one relationship to another and from one job to another and had trouble disciplining herself to complete tasks at work.

Thus far in therapy, Rachel has approached Annette's treatment with a combination of cognitive-behavioral strategies for her depression and alcohol abuse (in combination with Alcoholics Anonymous) and schema therapy. Rachel has had only limited success. Annette has realized that she is emotionally disconnected from other people and that she uses drinking and partying to blot out her feelings and fill the emptiness. Although she has gained in self-awareness, she is still depressed, and she continues to have episodes of alcohol abuse.

We considered Annette a good candidate for mode work, mainly because the therapy seemed stuck. Annette's Detached Protector mode was so strong that she could not acknowledge any vulnerable feelings. Her inability to access her vulnerable feelings—her schemas—was blocking the therapy. This is an example of a common type of case in which the therapist can make headway through schema mode work: The patient is highly avoidant or overcompensated and cannot access schemas emotionally. In the following interview, Dr. Young uses mode work to break through the Detached Protector and reach the underlying schemas of the Vulnerable Child.

In this first segment, Annette describes her current goals in therapy.

THERAPIST: Can you tell me a little about your goals in therapy now?

ANNETTE: Well, I'd like to be happy. I'm depressed.

THERAPIST: I see. So mostly it's the depressed feeling that's bothering you?

ANNETTE: Yeah. I'm trying to change my lifestyle.

THERAPIST: Do you know what it is about your life that is making you depressed?

ANNETTE: Well, now I do.

THERAPIST: What have you learned that it is?

ANNETTE: Well, I don't know how to show my feelings or talk about them. My family, they don't discuss their feelings.

THERAPIST: So none of them can discuss, really, their feelings.

ANNETTE: Right. I'm close to my mother, but we're more like friends.

THERAPIST: But like friends who don't share feelings?

ANNETTE: Right.

THERAPIST: I see. Do you have girlfriends that you would share your feelings with?

ANNETTE: No.

THERAPIST: No. So you've always been a very private person?

ANNETTE: Uh-huh.

Without actually using mode language, Annette connects her depression to her Detached Protector mode. It is because she is emotionally disconnected from other people that she feels depressed.

THERAPIST: I see. Another thing you mentioned was not feeling good about yourself.

ANNETTE: Yeah.

THERAPIST: What are some of the ways you don't feel good about yourself?

ANNETTE: Well, when I get depressed, I drink.

THERAPIST: I see.

ANNETTE: I just don't feel good about myself.

THERAPIST: If you stop drinking, do you think you will then feel good about yourself?

ANNETTE: Well, like now I'm not drinking, but I don't feel good about myself.

THERAPIST: So what is it? What do you think is underneath that you are not happy with about yourself?

ANNETTE: It's just like, you know, my family and friends, and just, like, my lifestyle. It's just really lame.

THERAPIST: I see.

ANNETTE: I need to change it.

Annette goes on to describe her romantic life. She had been having an affair with a married man but broke it off, and she is now dating a man who is stable and loving but who bores her: "Yeah, he's like stable and normal and I lose interest."

The therapist proceeds to the first step in mode work, identifying and labeling the patient's modes.

Step 1: Identifying and Labeling the Patient's Modes

This is typically a process that arises naturally as the therapist observes the patient's thoughts, feelings, and behaviors from moment to moment. The therapist notices shifts in the patient and begins to identify modes associated with each state. As the modes appear in sessions or in the material the patient presents, the therapist starts to label the modes for the patient.

Therapists should be careful to ensure that a mode has been accurately identified before labeling it. The therapist should therefore gather a substantial amount of evidence and examples to illustrate the mode—both by repeatedly observing the mode in sessions and by listening attentively to the patient's descriptions of incidents outside the session. Once the therapist has identified a mode, he or she obtains feedback from the patient about whether it seems to fit. It is rare for patients to deny the existence of a mode that has been identified correctly by the therapist. With rare exceptions, the therapist does not try to persuade patients to accept modes that they cannot intuitively recognize. Similarly, the patient plays an integral role in naming a mode. The incorporation of a mode as a "character" in the therapy is always a collaborative process.

The therapist and patient work together to individualize the name of each mode to capture the specific strategies the individual patient utilizes. Usually we do not use the exact names for the modes that we listed previously. Rather, we work with patients to find names for modes that more precisely fit their individual thoughts, emotions, or behaviors. For example, the Compliant Surrenderer mode might be relabeled the "Good Girl." Instead of referring to the "Vulnerable Child" mode with a given patient, we might call the mode the "Abandoned Child" or the "Lonely Child." Rather than the "Detached Protector," we might call the mode the "Workaholic," the "Wall," or the "Thrill-Seeker." Rather than the "Overcompensator," we might call this mode the "Dictator," the "Bully," or the "Status-Seeker." We try to work with the patient to find a name that captures the essence of what the patient is doing or feeling in the mode.

Most patients relate well to the concept of modes. When the therapist asks the patient, "Which mode are you in right now?" the patient can say, "Right now I'm in my Compulsive mode," or "Right now I'm the Angry Child." The model tracks the patient's internal experience of shifting affective states.

In the following segment, the therapist helps Annette begin to identify and label her principal modes. As the segment begins, Annette is describing her feelings of boredom. The therapist explores what lies underneath her boredom.

THERAPIST: So you are craving some kind of stimulation all the time?

ANNETTE: Uh-huh.

THERAPIST: You always want things to be new and different. When you start to feel really bored, what does that feel like? Have you ever let it go on enough time to feel that emotion?

ANNETTE: I'm, like, really hyper. I mean I get wound up. Like if I stay home, let's say, all weekend.

THERAPIST: Yes. Let's say you stayed home all weekend.

ANNETTE: Yeah. I did that last weekend.

THERAPIST: What was that like?

ANNETTE: I was, like, a little depressed. I was losing my mind.

THERAPIST: I see. So what's interesting is that you were telling me you were bored, but now you're saying you were really depressed.

ANNETTE: Well, I was both.

THERAPIST: Yeah, I'm wondering if "bored" is the term that you use to yourself to not have to acknowledge the fact that you're really depressed underneath?

ANNETTE: Probably.

Underneath Annette's boredom lies the depression of the Vulnerable Child mode. The therapist will explain this to Annette later.

"Spoiled Annette"

The therapist helps Annette identify the mode that she and the therapist call "Spoiled Annette." (We do not usually use pejorative labels, but the patient alluded to this idea herself.) This mode is a variation of the Impulsive/Undisciplined Child. Although Annette has been somewhat successful recently in fighting this mode, it still creates problems for her by causing her to do whatever feels good in the moment—such as drinking and partying—rather than what is beneficial in the long run, such as developing more lasting intimate relationships or a career.

The therapist continues to explore the depression underneath Annette's boredom. The interchange leads to the identification of Spoiled Annette.

THERAPIST: So what's happening is that, when things are too calm, there's time to think about the depressed feelings underneath. When things are active and stimulating, it sort of pulls you away from having to think about those painful things.

ANNETTE: (*in an annoyed tone*) Well, I don't always think about them, it's just too much work.

THERAPIST: I see. (*Pause.*) When you say it's too much work, what does that mean? Is it just too much of a nuisance?

ANNETTE: (*still annoyed*) Well, because I used to, when I was bored, I would go out with my friends and get drunk and I wouldn't have to think about anything. Now it's just, I have to have all these feelings and stuff, and I'm not used to it.

THERAPIST: So, this sounds like you resent that you even have to do it.

ANNETTE: (*Laughs.*)

THERAPIST: You know what I mean, like you shouldn't have to do this. Can you tell me more about that side that shouldn't have to do this?

ANNETTE: (*half-joking*) I shouldn't have to do anything I don't want to do, right?

THERAPIST: I see. You said, "right," as if you expected me to agree.

ANNETTE: Well, aren't you going to agree?

The therapist explores the thoughts and feelings of this entitled part of Annette.

THERAPIST: You mentioned how both your parents let you do anything you wanted to do. But you said you realized it wasn't right.

ANNETTE: I wouldn't do it if I had a kid; I wouldn't do it now because I can see the damage.

THERAPIST: But, even though intellectually you see the damage, emotionally you still have the feeling that you shouldn't have to do anything you don't want to.

ANNETTE: Yeah, 'cause I have a temper. It's like, if I don't get what I want, I just have, like, a fit.

THERAPIST: I see, like a kid throws a tantrum.

ANNETTE: I don't go around throwing things.

THERAPIST: What would it be like?

ANNETTE: If I can't get my way, like with my parents, I just won't go with them. I'll go off by myself.

THERAPIST: Like you're punishing them?

ANNETTE: (*animated*) Yeah, that's it. I punish them. That's exactly it.

THERAPIST: I see. You punish them because they're not giving you what you want?

ANNETTE: Yeah. Exactly. I mean, I only spite myself. I suffer for it, nobody else does, but I do it anyway.

In the next segment, the therapist labels "Spoiled Annette" as a mode.

THERAPIST: So there is a part of you, I don't want you to hear this as a criticism, but it sounds like a spoiled part of you.

ANNETTE: (*Laughs.*)

THERAPIST: Does that seem, feel, right? There's a part of you that feels you should be able to do whatever you want to?

ANNETTE: (*Laughs.*) Are you saying that I'm a brat?

THERAPIST: No, I wasn't saying a brat. I'm saying there is a *part* of you that was spoiled by your. . . .

ANNETTE: (*Interrupts.*) Oh, yeah, I was kind of spoiled, I guess.

THERAPIST: I wasn't saying that it's the only part of you, because we're going to talk about the other parts of you. But it *is* one part of you.

ANNETTE: Yeah, definitely.

By making the "spoiled" part of Annette into a mode, the therapist is able to acknowledge this part of her while still remaining allied with her. This ability to confront patients while preserving the therapeutic alliance is an advantage of the mode approach: the therapist can confront the dysfunctional aspects of the mode without condemning the patient as a whole person.

"Tough Annette"

As the interview continues, a second mode arises that proves to be both more difficult and more important than Spoiled Annette. This is the mode the therapist calls "Tough Annette," a variant of the Detached Protector.

In the first segment following, the therapist continues speaking to Spoiled Annette. In the excerpt following that, the therapist tries to access the Vulnerable Child, but the way is blocked by Tough Annette.

THERAPIST: How did you feel about having to do this form? Did that, too, feel like a waste of time? Boring?

ANNETTE: I just felt, "Why do I have to fill out another form?" I filled out forms you already have to look at.

THERAPIST: So you felt resentful?

ANNETTE: I did it, but, you know, it was hard to get started.

THERAPIST: So you pushed yourself to do it because you knew you were supposed to?

ANNETTE: Well, because, you know, I was being nice. I was being nice because Rachel [her therapist] wants me to be nice.

In the next excerpt, the therapist tries to discuss Annette's attachment to her therapist, Rachel, as an inroad to reach the Vulnerable Child.

THERAPIST: Well, that goes back to my question, whether part of the reason you're being nice is for Rachel?

ANNETTE: Well.

THERAPIST: There's nothing wrong with that, if that's part of the reason.

ANNETTE: I don't know. I like Rachel, she helps me, so I want to change and get better.

THERAPIST: Do you want her to be proud of you?

ANNETTE: I don't know.

THERAPIST: It sounds like you're afraid to admit you have an attachment to Rachel over this time. Is it hard for you to acknowledge feeling like that?

ANNETTE: I don't know. It's just different.

The therapist identifies "Tough Annette" to the patient, the part of her that is reluctant to acknowledge that she depends on other people for help.

THERAPIST: You know, you have this kind of a tough act. I don't know what you want to call it, but you come across a little bit tough.

ANNETTE: I *am* tough. It's not an act.

THERAPIST: I see. But, on the other hand, you also look a little bit nervous.

ANNETTE: (*more vulnerable*) I am nervous.

THERAPIST: So there must be another part of you underneath that doesn't feel as tough as you look. So I'm feeling your toughness is partly an act or partly a mechanism to look strong to other people.

ANNETTE: It's just what I'm used to. I've always done this.

The therapist labels "Tough Annette" as a mode and distinguishes her from the core person. It is the Vulnerable Child—the one who is "nervous"—who is core.[2] Tough Annette is an "act" or a "mechanism to look strong to other people."

---

[2]This belief that the "Vulnerable Child" is the core mode of the person is a philosophical assumption of our model. We recognize that it is not a universal truth.

Step 2: Exploring the Origins and Adaptive Value of Modes

As part of the second step in mode work, the therapist helps patients understand and empathize with their modes. Together the therapist and patient explore the origin of each one and the function it has served. Many modes have had some adaptive value for the patient. The therapist asks questions to guide the patient: "When do you first remember feeling this way?" "Why do you think you developed this mode as a child?" "How is the mode affecting your life now?"

   We return now to Annette to illustrate this second step. Having identified Tough Annette, the therapist helps Annette explore the childhood origins of the mode.

THERAPIST: Are your mother and father tough, too?

ANNETTE: No, my father, he is, I don't know what he is, we're not really close. But my mother is nice; she doesn't have a tough act at all.

THERAPIST: When do you think you developed this sort of tough front? Do you remember at what age?

ANNETTE: I don't know. I can just always remember, I've always been just tough.

THERAPIST: Like in the crib? (*Laughs.*) A tough baby?

ANNETTE: Yeah, I was tough (*smiles*). I don't know, I mean I'm not sure, but probably 'cause I always want to protect my mother, so I have to appear that way. I don't want anybody messing with her. So that's probably why I'm like that.

THERAPIST: I see. Did your father mess with her? Did he mistreat her?

ANNETTE: No, I mean, they got married really young. So, I don't know, they're just different.

THERAPIST: What are you protecting her from then?

ANNETTE: I don't know. Everyone, I guess. She's just so nice. I don't want anyone. . . . She's kind of naive, like she'll do something out of just kindness, and people will take advantage, and I don't like it, so. . . .

THERAPIST: I see, so you're protecting her from other people who take advantage of her?

ANNETTE: Right.

THERAPIST: How do you think you got in that role of the protector?

ANNETTE: I don't know.

THERAPIST: Maybe that goes back to you and your mother being so close. You got close, and maybe it wasn't quite like a friend. Maybe she actually turned to you like you were a mother. Is that possible?

ANNETTE: Yeah. Well, you know, Rachel and I, we talked about that, if, like, I'm *her* mother.

Tough Annette originated in her childhood with her mother, who was weak and fragile, and her father, who was angry and seemed dangerous. Annette became her mother's protector. The mode began as a way of shutting down her vulnerable emotions so that she could be strong for her mother. Tough Annette does not share her vulnerable emotions with anyone—she keeps other people at a distance.

Step 3: Linking Modes to Current Problems and Symptoms

It is important to show patients how their modes are creating problems in their current lives and how their modes are linked to their presenting problems. This gives patients a rationale for treatment and helps build motivation to change.

For example, if a patient says he is coming to treatment because he is drinking too much, then the therapist links this problem to the Detached Protector mode. The therapist says that drinking is one of the ways the patient avoids experiencing his anger about the abandonment, abuse, or deprivation that he felt as a child. The patient drinks in order to avoid his negative feelings and to switch into the Detached Protector mode. If the therapist and patient can work with the patient's Vulnerable or Angry Child modes, then the patient can learn to cope with his emotions and get his needs met. He will then have much less need to drink to avoid his emotions, his schema-driven drinking will be reduced. (The therapist advocates Alcoholics Anonymous in addition, because many components of alcoholism are not schema-driven and need to be addressed independently.)

Annette connects Spoiled Annette to her difficulties sustaining a job, and the therapist uses this as an opportunity to link the mode to her current problems at work.

ANNETTE: Well, I don't have patience, you know. I don't like to have to do things I don't really want to do.

THERAPIST: Uh-huh.

ANNETTE: You know, like, say at work and stuff like that. I don't know, I just get aggravated.

THERAPIST: So, if they give you something that's boring to do, for example, and you're not interested in it, you resent having to do it?

ANNETTE: Yeah.

THERAPIST: I see. And what would you be saying to yourself to drum up your anger?

ANNETTE: I'd probably just say, "I want to get out of here. I want to leave."

The therapist helps the patient explore the mode in connection with her problems at work. The therapist sets up a dialogue in which Annette plays Spoiled Annette and the therapist plays the Healthy Adult.

THERAPIST: OK, I'm going to try to play this sort of "healthy" side. I want you to make the best case you can for this more entitled side, so I can hear what it would really say. OK, first I'm going to be like the boss telling you what you have to do. I want you to tell me what you're thinking inside as I'm saying these things, OK?

ANNETTE: OK.

THERAPIST: (as boss) "Well, Annette, you know you have to get this stuff done. It's part of your job. We're paying you money here, and you're just not working hard enough."
    (as therapist) So what's going through your mind? I want you to say out loud what you're thinking. Tell me what you're thinking to yourself.

ANNETTE: I would just think, like, you know, "Why do I have to work in general? I mean, it's all just boring anyway," you know?

THERAPIST: OK, now I'm going to be this other voice of, sort of, "health," and so I'll say, "Well, look, that's just the way the world is. The world is set up so that, if you want to get something, you have to give something. We call it reciprocity. If you expect people to give to you, you have to give them something back. So why should you get clothing, food, and a nice place to live if you're not giving anything back to the world? It's only fair that you have to work to contribute your share." Make the best case for why that's not true.

ANNETTE: I wouldn't understand. I would just say, "Why? Why does it have to be that way? Why do I have to do things? I can get things from my parents."

THERAPIST: Yeah, well, maybe your parents won't be alive forever? One of your fears is your mother dying. I think you said that.

ANNETTE: Probably.

The preceding dialogue helps Annette experience her Spoiled Annette mode. The therapist then summarizes what he believes is Annette's primary conflict related to the Spoiled Annette mode and the Healthy Adult:

THERAPIST: So there is a real struggle. Because there's a real strong part of you that really believes you should just be able to have fun and do what you want.

ANNETTE: That's why I'm so bored lately.

THERAPIST: Because?

ANNETTE: (*sulkily*) I can't do any of that stuff. I have to go to work, and I used to miss work a lot, a *lot*. Now I'm like there, and I hate it.

THERAPIST: Yes, it sounds like it's been imposed on you, the way you just said now, "I'm not supposed to."

ANNETTE: (*Laughs.*)

THERAPIST: It sounds like someone has sort of pushed you, forced you.

ANNETTE: I wonder who *that* would be? (*Laughs and looks over at Rachel.*)

THERAPIST: Is that Rachel?

ANNETTE: She has pushed me.

THERAPIST: I see. Does it feel like you're doing it to please her, or does it feel like the right thing to do and that's why you're doing it?

ANNETTE: No, I mean, I don't know what's exactly right, but I'm depressed, so I have to change, you know. I want to be different. 'Cause if I stay the same, I'm going to continue to be miserable.

THERAPIST: So the healthy part of you knows if you go in the direction you were going, you would get worse and worse and feel miserable. But this more spoiled, entitled part feels you shouldn't have to be doing that. It's a waste of time and you should be able to have fun and party.

ANNETTE: Right.

THERAPIST: And these sides are in conflict. The two sides in you are fighting each other.

ANNETTE: All the time.

THERAPIST: All the time. And what side wins most of the time lately?

ANNETTE: Lately I'm behaving. I go to work and I don't go out and have any fun. Not that I don't have fun, but I don't go out with any of my friends. You know, that side is, like, winning lately, but I'm not exactly thrilled about it. It's not that much fun.

The dialogue enables the patient to access her thoughts and feelings both when she is in the Spoiled Annette mode and when she is in the Healthy Adult mode, challenging Spoiled Annette.

Step 4: Demonstrating the Advantages of Modifying or Giving Up One Mode

In the next segment, the therapist goes from Tough Annette to Little Annette. Little Annette is the Vulnerable Child, the central figure in the mode work. The therapist has to get past Tough Annette to reach Little

Annette. As the segment begins, the therapist is discussing how Annette defended her mother against her father when she was 7 years old.

THERAPIST: You were supplying your mother with the strength she didn't have to stand up to him and to stand up to the world. So that's your role.

But now the question is, "What happened to Little Annette?" So we have this tough girl who is 7 years old protecting her mother. And then we have the spoiled part of you, too, who's able to do whatever she wants. Now what about the little girl who wants someone to hold her?

ANNETTE: She's lost.

THERAPIST: Yeah.

ANNETTE: She's nowhere.

THERAPIST: Can you feel her at all?

ANNETTE: Sometimes.

THERAPIST: When can you feel her? Can you feel her right now?

ANNETTE: A little bit. I'm a little vulnerable right now because I agreed to come here.

The therapist follows her vulnerable feelings.

THERAPIST: Actually, it *is* hard to do this in front of people. What does the vulnerable side feel about being here?

ANNETTE: I just feel like my family is all right. They're obviously messed up, but they are not that bad, you know. So I just feel like a failure, like, from my family, 'cause they would never come and do this. And they don't go to therapy, so I just feel like, I'm like the failure. I'm all messed up and they just seem to go on like everything is always OK, it doesn't seem to bother them, but it bothers me.

The patient expresses feelings of defectiveness triggered by the therapy situation. In her family she is the "identified patient." No one else is seeking therapy. The therapist allies with the Vulnerable Child against the family to offer her support.

THERAPIST: Yeah, well, let's look at that idea that everything is okay with them, though. You said your mother is being taken advantage of all the time by people. Your father is closed off, inhibited, and critical of other people. They're fighting all the time. That doesn't sound *that* great.

ANNETTE: Right, but they don't seem to get depressed by it like I do.

THERAPIST: Yes, because they let it out all the time through their anger; so, I mean, they've traded one set of symptoms for another.

ANNETTE: (*angry at herself*) They just accept it, like, for what it is, and I don't. That's the difference.

THERAPIST: (*pause*) What do *I* think is probably wrong with the way you grew up?

ANNETTE: What do you think?

THERAPIST: Yeah, what do I think is wrong?

ANNETTE: Well, my parents, they never talked about how they felt or . . . I told Rachel I can't think of one time when my mother hugged me. We don't even, I don't even go near them. I mean I don't even go this close to them 'cause I just feel strange about it.

But the way I look at it now, you see, my mother was just a kid herself when she got married and had kids. How can a kid take care of a kid?

Annette alternates between acknowledging the emotional desolation of her childhood and protecting her mother: She alternates between the Vulnerable Child in touch with her needs and the Detached Protector denying her needs are valid.

THERAPIST: Right. So that's the problem. There was no one there to take care of you. But is that your fault that there was no one to take care of you, or is that . . . ?

ANNETTE: (*Interrupts*) No, it's not my fault.

THERAPIST: So you are the victim of parents who were unable to adequately take care of your emotional needs. You grew up without affection, without empathy, without someone to listen to you and understand you. So you grew up alone, isolated in a room. That is very, very hard because really the most basic needs of children, other than food and clothing, are to be held and loved and cared for. So your most basic emotional needs never got met when you were a child. So no wonder you're unhappy underneath. And no wonder it's hard for you to reach out to other people. Does that make sense to you?

ANNETTE: Yeah, it makes sense.

Much of the progress in mode work derives from getting past the Maladaptive Coping modes, accessing the Vulnerable Child, and then reparenting the child. Because the Vulnerable Child mode contains most of the core schemas, much of the schema healing takes place during work with this mode. The therapist attempts to demonstrate the advantages to the patient of modifying or giving up modes that are interfering with access to the Vulnerable Child.

Imagery often proves the most effective way for the therapist to establish a line of communication with the Vulnerable Child. The therapist asks the patient to access an image of the Vulnerable Child; the therapist then comes into the image as the Healthy Adult and talks to the Vulnerable Child. The therapist helps patients in the Vulnerable Child mode to express their unmet needs while the therapist tries to provide for these needs—safety, nurturance, autonomy, self-expression, limits—through "limited reparenting." (We use this same exercise routinely, even when we are not doing "formal" mode work.)

The therapist asks Annette to form an image of Little Annette, the Vulnerable Child, but Annette refuses. The therapist helps her identify the sources of her resistance: Spoiled Annette and Tough Annette are refusing. Spoiled Annette does not want to work at something unpleasant; Tough Annette believes it is weak to be vulnerable and is blocking painful emotions to protect Little Annette. The therapist uses mode work to break through these two maladaptive modes to access the Vulnerable Child mode.

THERAPIST: How would you feel about trying an exercise in imagery to get to that child side of you?

ANNETTE: I can't do it.

THERAPIST: Would you be willing to try?

ANNETTE: I don't know. Rachel and I try to do it all the time. It doesn't work.

THERAPIST: Sometimes, even if it doesn't work, it might help me to figure out why, so that I can give some suggestions later on on how to get it to work for the next time. So even if it didn't work, that wouldn't be a problem.

All we need to do right now is figure out what's making you resist it. We don't necessarily have to overcome it today. Even if I could just understand why it's hard for you to do the imagery, that would be helpful. Wouldn't you like to help me to try to explore why it's hard to do imagery for you?

ANNETTE: I guess.

THERAPIST: OK, so what are you feeling right now?

ANNETTE: I just don't like to do it.

THERAPIST: Be that side of you that doesn't want to do it so I can hear it.

ANNETTE: I don't know. I just don't want to do it. I don't like to do things that I don't really want to do.

Here Spoiled Annette is resisting doing imagery, because she does not want to do anything she does not feel like doing The therapist begins a dialogue with Spoiled Annette, empathically confronting her.

THERAPIST: OK, I'm going to play the Healthy side and say, "Well, you know I know it's not easy for you, but sometimes it's only by trying hard things that you can reach something that's really important, that you can't get to otherwise." Play the other side so I can hear what it says back.

ANNETTE: I don't like to do difficult things. It's too much work.

THERAPIST: Would you try it anyway?

ANNETTE: I guess.

THERAPIST: All right. We'll do it for 5 minutes and if you really hate it. . . .

ANNETTE: (*Interrupts in a tough, defiant voice.*) If I hate it, I'll tell you, don't worry. How's that?

THERAPIST: Just keep your eyes closed for 5 minutes and then, if you hate it, you can open your eyes and stop.

ANNETTE: (*Half-laughs.*) I can't even sit still for 5 minutes, much less keep my eyes closed for 5 minutes.

THERAPIST: I think you're just saying that to resist doing it, because you've sat very still for 35 minutes already, so you'd probably be able to sit still if you wanted.

ANNETTE: I just don't want to do it.

THERAPIST: Yeah, that's what I think. And I think that the reason you don't want to do it, though, is that you don't want to get down to that other side of you, the side of you that's in pain, that's depressed and lonely. You don't want to know that side.

ANNETTE: Yeah, because it's bad.

As she refuses to try imagery, Annette alternates between being entitled and being tough—not acknowledging her Vulnerable Child, which she thinks is a bad part of her. Her feeling that her vulnerable side is bad is coming from her Defectiveness schema. The therapist persists nevertheless. In the next section, the Detached Protector proves to be the major obstacle making it difficult to connect to the Vulnerable Child. The Detached Protector does not want her to appear weak to others, because they might hurt her.

THERAPIST: Bad, like . . . ?

ANNETTE: I don't know, just bad stuff. I feel bad enough, why do I want to remember that?

THERAPIST: Because the only way you're going to get better is by getting to know those feelings and trying to heal her. My feeling is that Tough Annette is not letting Little Annette let anyone love her or be close to her. That's her role.

ANNETTE: (*Sighs deeply.*)

THERAPIST: She's keeping everyone away. So Little Annette keeps feeling lonely and lost and uncared for. Unless I can help Tough Annette let up a little bit, there's no way Little Annette is going to get the love she needs from people. She's going to keep feeling lonely. So the only way really to help is by convincing Tough Annette to step aside a little bit so we can find Little Annette and get her what she needs. But Tough Annette doesn't want to look at Little Annette.

So I want you to let go of Tough Annette enough to do the exercise. And what I think is that Tough Annette doesn't want to do the exercise because she doesn't want me to see Little Annette.

ANNETTE: What if there *is* no Little Annette?

THERAPIST: Then you wouldn't be depressed and you'd be like the rest of your family. Everything would be fine. We know there has to be a Little Annette or you wouldn't feel lonely and depressed. You wouldn't be in therapy. So Little Annette is the part of you that's sad. Tough Annette isn't sad. Spoiled Annette isn't sad. So the only one left that's feeling sad is Little Annette.

ANNETTE: (*Sighs deeply.*)

THERAPIST: But you don't want to look at her, even though she has all the pain. She carries around all the pain that you're feeling.

ANNETTE: It's not that I don't want to look at her; I don't know her. I don't know where she is.

THERAPIST: By resisting doing imagery, you're resisting looking at her. And I'm saying to you, let up a little bit on her. Let's see what she's like. Don't fight her so hard. Nothing that terrible is going to happen by looking at her and seeing what she's like. I think it's not going to be as bad as you think it's going to be to look at her and to figure out what she's feeling. We could try it.

ANNETTE: I guess.

Step 5: Accessing the Vulnerable Child through Imagery

The patient finally agrees to try to picture an image of Little Annette. Note how the therapist continues to push Annette to get her to this point—not criticizing her, but continuing to convince her—through empathic confrontation. The therapist keeps empathizing with the pain it causes Annette to access her vulnerability but nevertheless keeps pushing her to do it.

At classes and conferences, therapists often express surprise at how much we push patients to do experiential work. They believe that patients are too fragile to handle being pushed this way—that patients will decompensate or leave. However, we believe that many therapists exaggerate how fragile most patients are or how likely they are to leave if they are pushed in this way.

We would certainly not push this hard at the beginning of therapy, nor would we push this hard with more fragile patients, such as those with BPD or who have suffered serious trauma or abuse. However, we would push this hard with higher functioning patients, such as Annette, who have no history or indication that they are at risk for significant decompensation. We find that it is extremely rare for patients to decompensate or leave because we push them to do experiential work if they have been screened appropriately. On the contrary, what usually happens is that, when emotionally avoidant patients experience the more emotional parts of themselves, they experience a profound sense of relief. They feel less empty, more alive, less depressed. Finally they know why they are so numb. For the most part, we have observed that, if patients really do not want to do imagery or feel they are at high risk, they will not do it, even when they are gently but persistently pushed.

In the next segment, the therapist accesses Little Annette.

THERAPIST: All right, then, I'm going to ask you to close your eyes, and I'm going to ask you to keep them closed for five minutes.

ANNETTE: (*Closes her eyes.*)

THERAPIST: OK. After 5 minutes, if you want to open them, it's OK. But, at least for 5 minutes, try to really force yourself to get in touch with her. Close your eyes and get an image of Little Annette, the absolute youngest that you can picture her. This is yourself as a child. Just tell me what you see, OK?

ANNETTE: Like what do I see, like how?

THERAPIST: Just try to get a picture as if you're looking at her as a little child. She doesn't have to be doing anything. Just sort of picture her face or picture her body. Just picture her somehow, picture a photograph if you can't get her as a live person.

ANNETTE: OK.

THERAPIST: What do you see?

ANNETTE: I see somebody like, maybe, 5 years old.

THERAPIST: Where is she right now? Can you see where she is?

ANNETTE: She's home.

THERAPIST: I see. Can you tell me what room she's in?

ANNETTE: In her bedroom.

THERAPIST: And is she alone?

ANNETTE: Yeah.

THERAPIST: Can you look at the expression on her face and tell me how she's feeling?

ANNETTE: I don't know. She's just quiet.

THERAPIST: Can you ask her how she's feeling and tell me what she says to you? I want you, as the Adult Annette, to talk to Little Annette and ask her how she's feeling, and tell me what she says.

ANNETTE: Um, I don't know, she's nervous.

THERAPIST: She's scared about something?

ANNETTE: Yeah.

THERAPIST: I see. Can you ask her what she's scared about? Does she know?

ANNETTE: She knows.

THERAPIST: Can you tell me?

ANNETTE: Um, well, she's scared 'cause like, um, her parents, they fight a lot.

THERAPIST: Is she worried about her mother? What is she worried is going to happen?

ANNETTE: I don't know. Her father has like, sort of, a temper.

THERAPIST: How bad does the temper get?

ANNETTE: Well, I mean, he doesn't hit her or her mother, or anything like that, but he, like, yells a lot.

THERAPIST: And what is she scared will happen if her father's temper goes out of control? What is she scared will happen?

ANNETTE: She's scared of, like, I don't know, like he'll beat somebody up or kill somebody.

THERAPIST: Is she worried she'll get hurt herself?

ANNETTE: Maybe.

THERAPIST: So is she hiding in her room so she's safer?

ANNETTE: Yeah.

The therapist was able to speak indirectly to the Vulnerable Child (through Adult Annette) and find out what she was feeling. He learned that Little Annette is afraid of her father. Next, the therapist asks Annette to bring her mother into the image.

THERAPIST: Can you let her mother come into the room now and tell me what you see happening?

ANNETTE: Her mother is upset. She's always upset.

THERAPIST: Upset like sad, or upset like angry?

ANNETTE: She looks scared.

THERAPIST: And how does Little Annette feel seeing her mother so scared and upset?

ANNETTE: Scared, too.

THERAPIST: So they're, like, scared together?

ANNETTE: Uh-huh.

THERAPIST: They both would like someone to protect them?

ANNETTE: Yeah.

THERAPIST: But there is nobody strong enough, or now is Little Annette going to have to get involved?

ANNETTE: I guess she will. I don't know if she knows how. She's little.

THERAPIST: I see. What's going through her mind? Tell me out loud what's going through her mind as she sees how scared her mother is.

ANNETTE: She just thinks her mother is sad and depressed.

THERAPIST: She's worried about her?

ANNETTE: Uh-huh.

THERAPIST: Does she want to do something to help her, or does she feel she wants some help herself?

ANNETTE: No, she feels like she wants to help her mother.

THERAPIST: So to do that she has to be strong, though; she can't let herself show that she's scared. Is that right?

ANNETTE: Yeah.

THERAPIST: So she is going to have to act tough for her mother so her mother doesn't see that she is scared.

ANNETTE: Yeah. She doesn't want her, you know, to be upset. She doesn't want to upset her mother more.

Once the therapist is able to get past Tough Annette in the image, the mode that comes to the surface in the image—as commonly happens—is the Vulnerable Child. Now the therapist can work on the core schemas that are part of Little Annette: her underlying feelings, memories, needs, and beliefs. What we find underneath is the fear of her father's anger and the wish to protect her mother. There is nobody strong who can protect Annette: Her father is dangerous and her mother is weak. The core schemas are Mistrust/Abuse, Self-Sacrifice, and Emotional Deprivation.

Step 6: Conducting Dialogues among the Modes, with the Therapist as the Healthy Adult

Once the Vulnerable Child and the Healthy Adult are established as characters in the patient's imagery, the therapist brings the patient's other modes into the imagery and sets up dialogues. The therapist helps the modes to communicate and negotiate with each other. For example, the Healthy Adult might talk to the Punitive Parent, or the Vulnerable Child might talk to the Detached Protector. The therapist serves as the Healthy Adult (or Healthy Parent) whenever patients are unable to do so on their own.

To review, the Healthy Adult serves several functions in these mode dialogues: (1) to nurture, affirm, and protect the Vulnerable Child; (2) to set limits for the Angry Child and the Impulsive/Undisciplined Child; and (3) to battle, bypass, or modulate the Maladaptive Coping and Dysfunctional Parent modes. This can all be done in imagery, or the therapist can use the Gestalt technique of changing chairs. The therapist can assign each mode to a chair and have the patient switch chairs while role-playing the modes. Once again, the therapist plays the Healthy Adult whenever the patient is unable to do so. (The therapist usually plays the Healthy Adult for several months before the patient is able to take over this role.).

In the following segment, a continuation of the previous one, the therapist helps the patient conduct a dialogue between the Healthy Adult and the Vulnerable Child. As the segment begins, the patient is still in her bedroom with her mother as a little girl. The therapist asks Annette to bring Rachel into the image to talk to the Vulnerable Child rather than himself, because Rachel has a much stronger connection with Annette after many months of working together. The therapist plays the role of Rachel, even though Annette is uncomfortable showing her vulnerability.

THERAPIST: Can you bring Rachel into the image now?

ANNETTE: How?

THERAPIST: Just stick her right in the middle of that image with you.

ANNETTE: When I'm small?

THERAPIST: Yeah, and get everyone else out. Get Tough Annette out, get your mother out, so now it's just Little Annette and Rachel. Can you see that?

ANNETTE: Yeah.

THERAPIST: Can you say to Rachel what you just said to your mother?

ANNETTE: (*adamantly*) No!

THERAPIST: Why?

ANNETTE: I don't know, I just can't.

THERAPIST: What does it feel like? Like she's going to be judgmental? Or she is going to think badly of you for saying that?

ANNETTE: I don't know. She'll think I'm weird. I don't know, I don't know what she'll think.

The patient cannot imagine being so vulnerable with Rachel. Because the patient is blocked, the therapist steps in to help. The therapist shows empathy for the feelings of the Vulnerable Child by supplying the words for Rachel.

THERAPIST: Let me put Rachel in and I'll supply words for Rachel. OK?

ANNETTE: OK.

THERAPIST: (*as Rachel*) "Annette, you know it's understandable that you feel scared right now, with your family fighting and your father's temper, and you have a right to have somebody who's strong for you and cares about you and who feels you matter and listens to you and hugs you and takes care of you. You have a right to that right now, and I'd like to do that as much as I'm able to do it as your therapist, because I think you never had anyone to do that before. And if you could do that, you wouldn't have to be so tough all the time, because you could let someone else take care of you once in a while." What does Little Annette feel when I say that?

ANNETTE: I don't know. She doesn't feel comfortable.

THERAPIST: What is she feeling? Can you verbalize what she's feeling?

ANNETTE: She just feels like, "Why does she deserve all that stuff?"

The therapist affirms the rights of the Vulnerable Child, but the patient disagrees. The excerpt resumes.

THERAPIST: All right, now I'm going to be Rachel: "Because you're a good girl. You're trying so hard to help everyone. You're such a lovable girl. You're a nice girl and you're trying so hard to help the rest of your family and protect your mother. You deserve to be taken care of and to be treated nicely and you deserve affection. Every child deserves it, and you're a particularly good child."

ANNETTE: Maybe I'm not that good. Maybe I'm bad.

THERAPIST: (*as Rachel*) "If you were so bad, you wouldn't be trying so hard to protect your mother. If you were that selfish, you'd be thinking only about yourself. You'd be getting just what you needed. But that's not what's happening. You're actually sacrificing yourself for her, to keep her safe. That is what a very, very sensitive, caring child does. So I don't think you're a bad child at all. You maybe have a spoiled side of you when you're getting things, things you can buy; but when it comes to emotional things, you're not selfish at all. You're in fact very sacrificing. In fact, you're the one who has been cheated emotionally. You haven't gotten what you deserve. You haven't got very much emotionally." What are you feeling now?

ANNETTE: I just feel confused. I don't understand.

THERAPIST: Does my explanation feel right to you?

ANNETTE: No.

The therapist engages the part of Annette that rejects his explanation.

THERAPIST: Be the part of you that doesn't believe it. Is it your mother who doesn't believe that? Or is it Tough Annette that doesn't believe that?

ANNETTE: It's Annette, Tough Annette.

THERAPIST: All right. You be Tough Annette who doesn't believe this.

ANNETTE: (*as Tough Annette*) "I don't see the point to, you know, affection, and, you know, talking about your feelings. Why is it necessary, you know?"

The therapist plays the roles Annette has the most difficulty playing: the Vulnerable Child and the Healthy Adult.

THERAPIST: I'll be Little Annette, then Healthy Annette.
(*as Little Annette*) "But, look, I'm a little child, and I'm scared, too. You're an adult, and every child needs to be hugged and kissed and listened to and respected. These are basic needs of every child."
(*as Healthy Adult*) "We're born that way, and the only reason you don't feel you deserve it is because you never got it. But we all need this. And you became tough because you couldn't see any way to get it. So you said, 'I might as well be tough and pretend I don't need it.' But really, you know you need it as much as I do. You're just afraid to admit it, because you think there's no way you're ever going to get it."

ANNETTE: (*as Tough Annette*) "It's a flaw."

THERAPIST: What's a flaw?

ANNETTE: (*as Tough Annette*) "You know, being that needy."

THERAPIST: No, it's a part of human nature. Everyone's that way. Have you ever seen a little child who didn't want to be helped or didn't need to be held? Would you say that every child that wants to be held is flawed? Is every infant a flawed infant because he or she wants to be held?

ANNETTE: No, I guess not.

In the next segment, the therapist asks Annette to get angry at her mother in the image. This is done in order to help Annette battle her Emotional Deprivation schema by asserting her rights to her mother. The mother is behaving in an emotionally depriving way—she is not protecting Annette, and she is not giving her the emotional care that she needs.

THERAPIST: Can you be Little Annette now, and say to your mother what you need for yourself? Just say it out loud?

ANNETTE: What Little Annette needs?

THERAPIST: Yes. "I need. . . . "

ANNETTE: I don't know. I guess I need a hug. I'm so scared.

THERAPIST: How does it feel, saying that?

ANNETTE: I don't know. It doesn't feel good.

THERAPIST: What does it feel like?

ANNETTE: It just gives me anxiety.

THERAPIST: How does your mother react when you say you need a hug?

ANNETTE: If I was to say that?

THERAPIST: Yes, be her now.

ANNETTE: (*Speaks scornfully.*) She wouldn't say anything. She would probably just look at me.

THERAPIST: And tell me what's going through her mind as she looks at you like that.

ANNETTE: She would think, "Why does she need a hug? I'm the one who has all the aggravation. What does she need a hug for?"

In the image, the mother denies Annette's needs, focusing instead on what she regards as her own, much greater needs. The therapist remarks that the mother's response is selfish.

THERAPIST: Are you angry with your mother for saying that?

ANNETTE: (*agreeing emphatically*) Yeah.

THERAPIST: Let Little Annette get angry at your mother for saying that. (*Long pause.*) You could start with, "I'm only five years old."

ANNETTE: (*Laughs.*) Um, I don't know. You know, "I'm only five years old. I need someone to take care of *me*." (*Long pause.*)

THERAPIST: Tell her what kind of care you need. Do you need hugs?

ANNETTE: Yeah. I need hugs. I need someone to tell me how they feel about me.

THERAPIST: Do you need praise?

ANNETTE: Nah. I guess.

THERAPIST: Someone who can be strong for you, so you don't have to worry so much?

ANNETTE: She just wants someone to tell her that she matters.

The therapist helps Annette verbalize what she needed as a child from her mother. Annette was taught that she should not need or ask for anything. She should be tough. She should protect other people. She should not ask anyone for love or help. It is thus no wonder that, as an adult, she does not turn to significant others with an expectation that they will want to comfort or help her.

Step 7: Helping the Patient Generalize the Mode Work to Life Outside Therapy Sessions

The final step is to help patients generalize from working with their modes in sessions to working with their modes when they arise in their lives outside sessions. What is happening when the patient shifts into the Detached Protector or the Punitive Parent or the Angry Child? How can the patient stay centered as the Healthy Adult?

The therapist uses self-disclosure about his own childhood to help Annette accept her vulnerable side and become more willing to express it. Annette comments that her Vulnerable Child is too needy.

THERAPIST: Do you think that the little child part of you is all that different from the little child part of me, or the little child part of Rachel?

ANNETTE: Maybe. Maybe you had affection, and it's different.

THERAPIST: I didn't have much affection either as a child. That's why I know how important it is to get that affection. I know what it means to not have affection.

ANNETTE: (*Speaks accusingly.*) You're just saying that to get me to relate.

THERAPIST: You don't believe me. I don't say things just to manipulate you, believe me. I'm telling you something that's true. I didn't have that either, and I know what it feels like not to have it. And I'm telling you that everyone needs it. I grew up believing that *I* didn't need it. That all I had to do was be good in school, and be good with other people, and be socially appropriate, and do all the right things, and that's all I'd need to be happy.

Annette later told her therapist, Rachel, that this was the most important part of the session for her. The therapist's self-disclosure served as a powerful form of reparenting.

The therapist helps Annette generalize mode work to life outside therapy sessions. What are the implications of what she has learned? They discuss her love relationships and why it has been hard for her to connect to men. She has been unable to accept love. Like most people with a strong detached side, she has been drawn to men who are emotionally depriving. Even though it is uncomfortable for her, one goal of therapy is for Annette to seek and stay with men who are emotionally giving.

THERAPIST: So when someone hugs you, it feels awkward. It feels like it's not right. You have to overcome that feeling entirely.

ANNETTE: How? How do you overcome it?

THERAPIST: By letting someone do it and trying to stay there and saying to yourself, "This doesn't feel comfortable, but it's what I need. It's what's right."

ANNETTE: Even if it freaks you out?

THERAPIST: It will freak you out at first, because you've never had it. At least not since you can remember.

ANNETTE: I have nightmares of people hugging me.

THERAPIST: I don't doubt it. And I'm saying to you, if you get over that, if you would let some people do it and stay there and say to yourself, "This feels unfamiliar to me, but I need it anyway. If I could just stay with it long enough, I'll get over it. If I let the affection in, then I'll feel better." And you just fight the part of you that feels uncomfortable with it.

Ultimately, the goal is for Annette to recognize her unmet needs and ask appropriate significant others to meet them. In this way she can connect emotionally to other people at a deeper, more fulfilling level.

The therapist ends the interview by summarizing the implications of the mode work for her goals in therapy.

THERAPIST: You need to acknowledge Little Annette and believe that her needs are good and not bad and that they are normal. And you have to help her get them met, not try to pretend that she doesn't need anything. Because if you keep pretending she doesn't have any needs, you'll keep feeling depressed and lonely and isolated.

And that means that you'll have to tolerate uncomfortable feelings, like doing this imagery was uncomfortable. But if you don't tolerate the discomfort of feeling close to people, you won't get over this, and I'm saying it is a phase. The "uncomfortableness" is a phase. It's a phase you'll get over. Then eventually it will feel good to have someone hold you and touch you and listen to you.

Annette's goal is to form intimate relationships with significant others who are capable of meeting her emotional needs and then to allow them to do so. In mode terms, her goals are to build a Healthy Adult mode that can nurture, affirm, and protect Little Annette; to set limits on Spoiled Annette; and to learn to bypass Tough Annette most of the time.

SUMMARY

A mode is the set of schemas or schema operations—adaptive or maladaptive—that are currently active for an individual. We developed the concept of a mode as we focused the model on patients with increasingly severe disorders, especially those with BPD and narcissistic personality disorder. Although we originally developed mode work to treat these types of patients, we now use it with many of our higher functioning patients as well. Mode work has become an integral part of schema therapy.

In our practice, the higher functioning the patient is, the more likely we are to emphasize schemas, and the more severely disordered the patient is, the more likely we are to emphasize modes. We tend to blend the two approaches together with patients in the middle range of functioning.

A therapist can shift from a schema approach to a mode approach when the therapy seems stuck and the patient's avoidance or overcompensation cannot be broken through. A mode approach might also work when the patient is rigidly self-punitive and self-critical or has a seemingly unresolvable internal conflict: for example, when two parts of the self are locked in opposition about a major life decision. Finally, we generally emphasize modes with patients who display frequent fluctuations in affect, such as often occurs with patients with BPD.

We have identified four main types of modes: Child modes, Maladaptive Coping modes, Dysfunctional Parent modes, and the Healthy Adult mode. Each type of mode is associated with certain schemas (except the Healthy Adult and Happy Child) or embodies certain coping styles.

The Child modes are the Vulnerable Child, the Angry Child, the Impulsive/Undisciplined Child, and the Happy Child. We believe that these child modes are innate. We have identified three broad types of Maladaptive Coping modes: the Compliant Surrenderer, the Detached Protector, and the Overcompensator. They correspond, respectively, to the coping processes of surrender, avoidance, and overcompensation. We have identified two Dysfunctional Parent modes: the Punitive Parent and the Demanding Parent. The Healthy Adult mode is the part of the self that serves an "executive" function relative to the other modes. Building the patient's Healthy Adult to work with the other modes more effectively is the overarching goal of mode work. Like a good parent, the Healthy Adult mode serves the following three basic functions: (1) nurturing, affirming, and protecting the Vulnerable Child; (2) setting limits for the Angry Child and the Impulsive/Undisciplined Child, in accord with the principles of reciprocity and self-discipline; and (3) battling or moderating the Maladaptive Coping and Dysfunctional Parent modes. During the course of treatment, patients internalize the therapist's behavior as part of their own Healthy Adult mode. Initially, the therapist serves as the Healthy Adult whenever the patient is incapable of doing so. Gradually the patient takes over the Healthy Adult role.

We have developed seven general steps in schema mode work: (1) identify and label the patient's modes; (2) explore the origin and (when relevant) adaptive value of the mode in childhood or adolescence; (3) link maladaptive modes to current problems and symptoms; (4) demonstrate the advantages of modifying or giving up one mode if it is interfering with access to another mode; (5) access the Vulnerable Child through imagery; (6) conduct dialogues among the modes; (7) help the patient generalize mode work to life situations outside therapy sessions.

In the next chapter, we apply modes to the assessment and treatment of borderline personality disorder.

Chapter 9

SCHEMA THERAPY FOR BORDERLINE PERSONALITY DISORDER

SCHEMA CONCEPTUALIZATION OF BORDERLINE PERSONALITY DISORDER

Early Maladaptive Schemas are the memories, emotions, bodily sensations, and cognitions associated with the destructive aspects of the individual's childhood experience, organized into patterns that repeat through life. For both characterological and healthier patients, the core themes are the same: They are themes such as Abandonment, Abuse, Emotional Deprivation, Defectiveness, and Subjugation. Characterological patients may have *more* schemas and their schemas may be more *severe*, but they do not generally have *different* schemas. It is not the presence of schemas that differentiates characterological patients from healthier patients but rather the extreme coping styles they employ to deal with these schemas and the modes that crystallize out of these coping styles.

As we have explained, our concept of modes grew largely out of our clinical experience with patients with BPD. When we attempted to apply the schema model to these patients, we consistently encountered two problems. First, patients with BPD usually have almost all of the 18 schemas (especially Abandonment, Mistrust/Abuse, Emotional Deprivation, Defectiveness, Insufficient Self-Control, Subjugation, and Punitiveness). To work with so many schemas simultaneously utilizing our original schema approach proved unwieldy. We needed a more workable unit of analysis. Second, in our work with patients with BPD, we (like many other clinicians) were struck by the tendency of these patients to shift rapidly from one intense affective state to another. One moment these patients are angry, the next moment they are terrified, then fragile, then impulsive—to the point at which it became it is almost like dealing with different people. Schemas, which are essentially traits, did not explain this rapid flipping from state to state. We developed the concept of modes to capture the shifting affective states of our patients with BPD.

The patient with BPD switches continually from mode to mode in response to life events. Whereas healthier patients usually have fewer and less extreme modes and spend longer periods of time in each one, patients with BPD have a greater number of more extreme modes and switch modes from moment to moment. Moreover, when a patient with BPD switches into a mode, the other modes seem to vanish. Unlike healthier patients, who can experience two or more modes simultaneously, so that one mode moderates the intensity of the other, patients with BPD who are in one mode seem to have virtually no access to the other modes. The modes are almost completely dissociated.

Schema Modes in the Patient with BPD

We have identified five main modes that characterize the patient with BPD:

1. Abandoned Child
2. Angry and Impulsive Child
3. Punitive Parent
4. Detached Protector
5. Healthy Adult

We summarize the modes briefly to provide an overview, then describe each one more fully.

The *Abandoned Child* mode is the suffering inner child. It is the part of the patient that feels the pain and terror associated with most of the schemas, including Abandonment, Abuse, Deprivation, Defectiveness, and Subjugation. The *Angry and Impulsive Child* mode is predominant when the patient is enraged or behaves impulsively, because her[1] basic emotional needs are not being met. The same schemas may be triggered as in the Abandoned Child mode, but the emotion experienced is usually anger. The *Punitive Parent* mode is the internalized voice of the parent, criticizing and punishing the patient. When the Punitive Parent mode is activated, the patient becomes a cruel persecutor, usually of herself. In the *Detached Protector* mode, the patient shuts off all emotions, disconnects from others,

---

[1]Throughout the chapter, we use "she" and "her" to refer to patients with BPD since the majority of these patients are female.

and functions in an almost robotic manner. The *Healthy Adult* mode is extremely weak and undeveloped in most patients with BPD, especially at the beginning of treatment. In a sense this is the primary problem: patients with BPD have no soothing parental mode to calm and care for them. This contributes significantly to their inability to tolerate separation.

The therapist models the Healthy Adult for the patient, until the patient eventually internalizes the therapist's attitudes, emotions, reactions, and behaviors as her own Healthy Adult mode. The major goal of treatment is to build up the patient's Healthy Adult mode in order to nurture and protect the Abandoned Child, to teach the Angry and Impulsive Child more appropriate ways of expressing anger and getting needs met, to defeat and expel the Punitive Parent, and to gradually replace the Detached Protector.

The simplest way to recognize a mode is by its feeling tone. Each mode has its own characteristic affect. The Abandoned Child mode has the affect of a lost child: sad, frightened, vulnerable, defenseless. The Angry and Impulsive Child mode has the affect of an enraged or uncontrollable child—screaming and attacking the caretaker who is frustrating the child's core needs or acting impulsively to get those needs met. The tone of the Punitive Parent mode is harsh, critical, and unforgiving. The Detached Protector has a flat, emotionless, mechanical affect. Finally, the Healthy Adult mode has the affect of a strong and loving parent. The therapist can usually differentiate the modes by listening to the tone of the patient's voice and observing the manner in which the patient is speaking. The schema therapist becomes adept at identifying the patient's mode at any given moment and responding accordingly, with strategies designed specifically for working with that mode.

We now describe each of the modes in greater detail: the function of the mode, the signs and symptoms, and the therapist's broad strategy in helping patients with BPD when they are in that mode.

The Abandoned Child Mode

In Chapter 8, we introduced the Vulnerable Child mode. As we noted, we believe this mode is innate and universal. The Abandoned Child is the version of the Vulnerable Child common to patients with BPD, in this case specifically characterized by the patient's focus on abandonment. In the Abandoned Child mode, patients appear fragile and childlike. They seem sorrowful, frantic, frightened, unloved, lost. They feel helpless and utterly alone and are obsessed with finding a parent figure who will take care of them. In this mode, patients seem like very young children, innocent and dependent. They idealize nurturers and have fantasies of being rescued by them. They engage in desperate efforts to prevent caretakers from abandoning them, and at times their perceptions of abandonment approach delusional proportions.

The very young age at which the patient's Vulnerable Child typically functions explains much about these patients' cognitive styles. Healthier patients have Vulnerable Child modes that are older (typically 4 years or older), whereas patients with BPD have Vulnerable Child modes that are younger (usually less than 3 years old). In the Abandoned Child mode, patients with BPD usually lack object permanence. They cannot summon a soothing mental image of the caretaker unless the caretaker is present. The Abandoned Child lives in an eternal present, without clear concepts of past and future, increasing the patient's sense of urgency and impulsivity. What is happening now is all that there is, was, or ever will be. The Abandoned Child mode is largely preverbal and expresses emotions through actions rather than words. Emotions are unmodulated and pure.

The four individual modes can function at different ages in patients with BPD. For example, the Detached Protector is often an adult, whereas the Vulnerable Child and Angry Child modes are childlike. The patient often attributes to the Punitive Parent the power and knowledge young children ascribe to their parents.

The Abandoned Child mode "carries" the patient's core schemas. The therapist comforts the child in the grip of these schemas and provides a partial antidote through the limited reparenting of the therapy relationship. When patients with BPD are in the Abandoned Child mode, the therapist's broad strategy is to help them identify, accept, and satisfy their basic emotional needs for secure attachment, love, empathy, genuine self-expression, and spontaneity.

The Angry and Impulsive Child Mode

This is the mode that mental health professionals most frequently seem to associate with patients with BPD, even though it is the one that, in our experience, typical patients experience least often. Most patients with BPD who are seen in outpatient settings spend a majority of their time in the Detached Protector mode—this is their "default" mode. Frequently they flip into the Punitive Parent or Abandoned Child modes. Much less often, when they cannot hold back anymore, they flip into the Angry Child mode, venting the fury they have contained and impulsively acting to get their needs met.

The Detached Protector and Punitive Parent modes operate to keep most of the patient's needs and feelings suppressed, effectively blocking the needs and feelings of the Abandoned Child mode. After a while, these needs and feelings accumulate, and the patient feels a growing sense of inner pressure. The patient may say something like, "I feel something building up inside me." (The patient may start dreaming about impending disasters, such as tidal waves or storms.) The pressure builds, some "last-straw" event occurs (perhaps a problematic interaction with the therapist or a partner), and the patient flips into the Angry Child mode. The patient suddenly feels irate.

When patients are in this mode, they vent their anger in inappropriate ways. They may appear enraged, demanding, devaluing, controlling, or abusive. They act impulsively to meet their needs, and they may appear manipulative or reckless. They may make suicidal threats and engage in parasuicidal behavior. A patient might, for example, claim she is going to kill or cut herself unless the person does what she wants. (One patient, reacting to feelings of abandonment triggered by the ending of a session, flipped into the Angry Child mode and walked out saying, "I'm on my way to the bathroom to cut my ankles.") In the Angry Child mode, patients may make demands that seem entitled or spoiled and that alienate others. However, their demands do not really reflect entitlement but rather are desperate attempts to meet their basic emotional needs.

When patients are in this mode, the therapist's broad strategy is to set limits and to teach them more appropriate ways of dealing with their anger and meeting their needs.

The Punitive Parent Mode

The function of this mode is to punish the patient for doing something "wrong," such as expressing needs or feelings. The mode is an internalization of one or both parents' rage, hatred, loathing, abuse, or subjugation of the patient as a child. Signs and symptoms include self-loathing, self-criticism, self-denial, self-mutilation, suicidal fantasies, and self-destructive behavior. Patients in this mode become their own punitive, rejecting parent. They become angry at themselves for having or showing normal needs that their parents did not allow them to express. They punish themselves—for example, by cutting or starving themselves—and speak about themselves in mean, harsh tones, saying such things as that they are "evil," "bad," or "dirty."

When patients are in the Punitive Parent mode, the therapist's broad strategy is to help them reject punitive parental messages and build self-esteem. The therapist supports the needs and rights of the Abandoned Child and attempts to overthrow and supplant the Punitive Parent.

The Detached Protector Mode

Except for severe cases, patients with BPD typically spend most of their time in the Detached Protector mode. The function of this mode is to cut off emotional needs, disconnect from others, and behave submissively in order to avoid punishment.

When patients with BPD are in the Detached Protector mode, they often appear normal. They are "good patients." They do everything they are supposed to do and act appropriately. They arrive at their sessions on time, do their homework, and pay promptly. They do not act out nor lose control of their emotions. In fact, many therapists mistakenly reinforce this mode. The problem is that, when patients are in this mode, they are cut off from their own needs and feelings. Rather than being true to themselves, they are basing their identity on gaining the therapist's approval. They are doing what the therapist wants them to do, but they are not really connecting to the therapist. Sometimes therapists spend whole treatment sessions with a patient without realizing that the patient has been in the Detached Protector mode nearly the entire time. The patient does not make significant progress but just floats from session to session.

Signs and symptoms of the Detached Protector mode include depersonalization, emptiness, boredom, substance abuse, bingeing, self-mutilation, psychosomatic complaints, "blankness," and robot-like compliance. Patients often switch into the Detached Protector mode when their feelings are stirred up in sessions in order to cut the feelings off. When patients are in the Detached Protector mode, the therapist's broad strategy is to help them experience emotions as they arise without blocking, to connect to others, and to express their needs.

It is important to realize that one mode can activate another mode. For example, a patient might express a need in the Abandoned Child mode, flip into the Punitive Parent mode to punish herself for expressing the need, and then flip into the Detached Protector mode to escape the pain of the punishment. Patients with BPD often get trapped in these vicious cycles, with one mode triggering another in a self-perpetuating loop.

If we were to rank order the modes in terms of psychological health across a wide range of patients with BPD, the Healthy Adult and the Vulnerable Child are the most healthy; then the Angry Child, who experiences genuine emotions and desires; then the Detached Protector, who maintains control over the patient's behavior. Finally, the Punitive Parent has no redeeming features whatsoever. The Punitive Parent is the most destructive to the patient over the long term.

Hypothesized Origins of Borderline Personality Disorder

Biological Factors

In our observation, the majority of patients with BPD have an emotionally intense, labile temperament. This hypothesized temperament may serve as a biological predisposition to developing the disorder.

Three-fourths of patients diagnosed with BPD are female (Gunderson, Zanarini, & Kisiel, 1991). This might be partially the result of temperamental differences: Perhaps women are more likely than men to have intense, labile temperaments. However, the gender difference might also be due to environmental factors. Girls are more often sexually abused, a frequent feature of the childhood histories of patients with BPD (Herman, Perry, & van de Kolk, 1989). Girls are more often subjugated and discouraged from expressing anger. It is also possible that men with BPD are an underdiagnosed group. Men manifest the disorder differently than women do. Men tend to have more aggressive temperaments and are more likely to be domineering rather than compliant and to act out against others rather than against themselves. Hence, they are probably more likely to be diagnosed with narcissistic or antisocial personality disorders (Gabbard, 1994), even when the underlying modes and schemas are similar.

Environmental Factors

We have identified four factors in the family environment that we believe interact with this hypothesized biological predisposition to lead to the development of BPD.

1. *The family environment is unsafe and unstable.* The lack of safety almost always arises from abuse or abandonment. The majority of patients with BPD experienced physical, sexual, or verbal abuse as children. If there was no actual abuse to the patient, then there was usually the threat of explosive anger or violence; or the patient may have observed another family member being abused. In addition, the child was frequently abandoned. The child may have been left alone for long periods without a caretaker or left with an abusive caretaker (for instance, one parent may abuse the child while the other denies and enables the abuse). Alternatively, the child's primary caretaker may have been unreliable or inconsistent, such as happens with a parent who has extreme mood swings or is a substance abuser. Instead of feeling secure, the attachment to the parent often feels unstable or terrifying.

2. *The family environment is depriving.* Early object relations are often impoverished. Parental nurturing—physical warmth, empathy, emotional closeness and support, guidance, protection—is typically absent or deficient. One or both parents (but especially the primary caretaker) may be emotionally unavailable and provide minimal empathy. Emotionally, the patient feels alone.

3. *The family environment is harshly punitive and rejecting.* Patients with BPD do not grow up in families that are accepting, forgiving, and loving toward them. Rather, they grow up in families that are critical and rejecting of them, harshly punitive when they make mistakes, and unforgiving. The punitiveness is extreme: As children, these patients were made to feel worthless, evil, bad, or dirty, not as though they were just normal children misbehaving.

4. *The family environment is subjugating.* The family environment suppresses the needs and feelings of the child. Usually there are implicit rules about what the child can and cannot say and feel. The child gets the message: "Don't show what you feel. Don't cry when you're hurt. Don't get angry when someone mistreats you. Don't ask for what you want. Don't be

vulnerable or real. Just be who we want you to be." Expressions by the child of emotional pain—particularly sadness and anger—often make the parent angry and lead to punishment or withdrawal.

DSM-IV BPD Diagnostic Criteria and Schema Modes

Table 9.1 lists DSM-IV diagnostic criteria for BPD matched to the relevant schema mode(s). We include four modes: the Abandoned Child, the Angry Child, the Punitive Parent, and the Detached Protector.

When a patient with BPD is suicidal or parasuicidal, the therapist must recognize which mode is experiencing the urge. Is the urge coming from the Punitive Parent mode and designed to punish the patient? Or is the urge coming from the Abandoned Child mode as a wish to end the pain of unbearable loneliness? Is it coming from the Detached Protector mode in an effort to distract from emotional pain through physical pain or to pierce the numbness and feel something? Or is it coming from the Angry Child mode in a desire to get revenge or hurt another person? The patient has a different reason for wanting to attempt suicide in each of the modes, and the therapist addresses the suicidal urge in accord with the particular mode that is generating it.

Case Illustration

Presenting Problem

Kate is a 27-year-old patient with BPD. The following excerpts are from an interview Dr. Young conducted with her as part of a consultation. (The patient had recently begun therapy with another schema therapist.)

Kate saw her first therapist at the age of 17. This excerpt illustrates the characteristic vagueness of her presenting problem at that time.

THERAPIST: What was it that brought you into therapy when you first came into treatment?

KATE: That was about 10 years ago. I was just very, very unhappy. I was just extremely depressed and confused and angry, and I was just having a very difficult time functioning—getting up in the morning and talking to people, and just walking down the street. I was just very upset and angry and sad.

THERAPIST: Had anything happened at that time to trigger that reaction?

KATE: No, it was just a bunch of things sort of building up.

THERAPIST: Do you remember what things were building up?

KATE: Just problems at home. Problems with myself and my identity. Not fitting in anywhere. Just general negative feelings.

TABLE 9.1. DSM-IV Diagnostic Criteria for Borderline Personality Disorder and Relevant Schema Modes

DSM-IV diagnostic criteria	Relevant schema modes
1. Frantic efforts to avoid real or imagined abandonment.	Abandoned Child mode.
2. A pattern of unstable and intense interpersonal relationships characterized by alternating between extremes of idealization and devaluation.	All modes. (It is the rapid flipping from mode to mode that creates the instability and intensity. For example, the Abandoned Child idealizes nurturers, and the Angry Child devalues and reproaches them.)
3. Identity disturbance: markedly and persistently unstable self-image or sense of self.	a. Detached Protector mode. (Because these patients must please others and are not allowed to be themselves, they cannot develop a secure identity.)
	b. Constantly switching from one nonintegrated mode to another, each with its own view of the self, also leads to an unstable self-image.
4. Impulsivity (e.g., spending money, promiscuous sex, substance abuse, reckless driving, binge eating).	a. Angry and Impulsive Child mode (to express anger or get needs met).
	b. Detached Protector mode (to self-soothe or break through numbness).
5. Recurrent suicidal behavior, gestures, threats, or self-mutilating behavior.	All four modes.
6. Affective instability due to a marked reactivity of mood (e.g., intense episodic dysphoria, irritability, or anxiety).	a. Hypothesized intense, labile biological temperament.
	b. Rapid flipping of modes, each with its own distinctive affect.
7. Chronic feelings of emptiness.	Detached Protector mode. (The cutting off of emotions and disconnection from others leads to feelings of emptiness.)
8. Inappropriate, intense anger or difficulty controlling anger.	Angry Child mode.
9. Transient, stress-related paranoid ideation or severe dissociative symptoms.	Any of the four modes (when affect becomes unbearable or overwhelming).

THERAPIST: But nothing had happened, like someone died or someone left you?

KATE: No.

The sense of identity diffusion that Kate reports is linked to her Detached Protector mode: Patients with BPD feel confused about who they are while in the Detached Protector mode. When patients with BPD are in this mode, they do not know what they are feeling. They are almost completely focused on complying with other people to avoid abandonment or punishment and to block out their own desires and emotions. Because they do not follow their natural inclinations, they cannot develop a distinct identity of their own. Rather, they feel empty, bored, restless, foggy, or confused.

Characteristically, Kate has experienced an array of Axis I disorders, including depression, bulimia, and substance abuse.

THERAPIST: Are there other symptoms that you have?

KATE: Yeah, I feel just worthless, and just not really a whole person, whatever a whole person is, I don't even know. I just know that I look at other people, and I just don't see myself equal to anybody.

THERAPIST: And do you ever do things to punish yourself, that kind of thing?

KATE: Yeah, I used to.

THERAPIST: What things did you do?

KATE: Well, I used to cut myself a lot. I was bulimic for about nine years. Just self-destructive things.

THERAPIST: Do you ever have impulses to do any of those things now?

KATE: Yes.

THERAPIST: Do you act on any of them anymore?

KATE: I haven't in a while. Sometimes I drink a bit much, but I haven't done drugs in a while, in a few months.

History of the Current Illness

Kate's current course of treatment began 2 years ago when she was hospitalized following a suicide attempt. In the next excerpt, the therapist asks Kate to describe the series of events leading up to that hospitalization:

THERAPIST: What was going on at that time?

KATE: I had a drug overdose.

THERAPIST: What drug was it?

KATE: Klonopin.

THERAPIST: That was intentional then?

KATE: Yes.

THERAPIST: Do you remember why you took it at the time? Did something happen then?

KATE: Yes, well, I was married. I was doing well, I was happy, but he met somebody else. And he wanted me just to be out of his life. He said he met somebody else, and just wanted me out of the house, and just wanted me away from him. At first, when it happened, I guess I was in shock, and then I just became so depressed and I just didn't want to live anymore.

THERAPIST: Do you remember what the feeling was that was making you feel so depressed?

KATE: (*speaking passionately*) I just felt that I was no good, that I was worthless, and that he finally realized it, and he was doing right by himself, and I was just *nobody*.

Kate expresses that her suicide attempt arose from her Abandoned Child mode, in which she was flooded with the pain of her Abandonment and Defectiveness schemas. Abandonment by a significant other is a common trigger for this mode.

Childhood History

When we turn to Kate's history, we see that her childhood was marked by all four of the predisposing environmental factors we named earlier: Her family environment was unsafe, emotionally depriving, harshly punitive, and subjugating of her feelings.

The following excerpt (a continuation of the previous one) illustrates Kate's childhood deprivation. She had no one who nurtured her, empathized with her, protected her, or guided her.

THERAPIST: Do you know where those feelings came from or started, the feelings of being no good or worthless?

KATE: I've just always felt them, just from my family life, just not really feeling that I was important, or like I made a difference, or that I was significant in my family.

THERAPIST: How did they let you know that you weren't important, that you didn't make a difference?

KATE: Oh, they just never listened to me, never acknowledged me. I could do whatever I wanted, whenever I wanted.

THERAPIST: So you had complete freedom.

KATE: Right.

THERAPIST: But no one paid any attention.

KATE: Right.

THERAPIST: So you were ignored.

KATE: Right.

THERAPIST: Like no one cared enough . . .

KATE: (*finishing the sentence*) . . . to say anything, to implement any discipline or direction, or anything of that sort, ever.

Kate's childhood environment was also unsafe. Her older brother was diagnosed with attention deficit disorder and frequently abused her physically and sexually. Neither parent protected her. They were emotionally removed, and both parents blamed her for her brother's misbehavior.

KATE: Well, my brother was hyperactive. I guess my parents just spent so much time watching him and fearing him. He wasn't taking medication, so he was out of control.

THERAPIST: He got all the attention because he was sick?

KATE: Yes.

THERAPIST: And there wasn't anything left for you?

KATE: Yes, for the most part. I think my father was off in his own world. He wasn't really home a lot. He was very depressed. He always was, and I think it was just a bit much for him.

THERAPIST: So that's mainly what your father was like? Off in his own world?

KATE: Yes. All the time.

THERAPIST: So it felt like you were all alone?

KATE: Yes.

Kate's childhood environment was also punitive and rejecting. Her mother was especially critical of her and intolerant of her emotions.

THERAPIST: And how about your mother?

KATE: She and I didn't get along. I was just very unhappy, and that really bothered her. So there was a lot of tension. She didn't appreciate the fact that I wasn't just a happy-go-lucky person, she couldn't understand why. She figured that something was wrong with me, and she didn't know what to do with me, and she didn't like me very much.

THERAPIST: Was she rejecting or critical?

KATE: Yeah, she was very critical, especially as I got older. We were always fighting. She told me she didn't like me, that I was just hopeless, that I was just so miserable she couldn't stand it. (*Cries.*)

THERAPIST: How did it make you feel when she used to talk to you that way?

KATE: Oh, I just believed it, because it was true.

THERAPIST: What was the essence of her statement? What do you feel her main criticism of you was?

KATE: Just that I was so unhappy, and that I was nasty to her, and that I was bitchy.

THERAPIST: And you felt she was right?

KATE: Yes.

Kate's childhood environment was subjugating. Even though she was experiencing serious neglect and abuse, she was not allowed to be sad or angry about what was happening to her. Such manifestations of emotion infuriated her parents and triggered her brother's abuse of her.

One way Kate tries to suppress her feelings is by flipping into the Punitive Parent mode whenever she becomes angry with others.

THERAPIST: The angry side, the part that feels that she was mistreated, people weren't there for her, do you ever feel that side?

KATE: Yes. I feel that, but then I feel that I just deserved it, that people had a right to treat me that way. And then I get angry 'cause I think that, but . . . (pause).

THERAPIST: Could it be that you then become the Punitive Parent and punish the little child for being angry? Does that feel like what you are doing? Like you're saying, "You're bad, who are you to think that you have any rights?"

KATE: Yes. That's what prevents me from sticking up for myself and taking care of myself, because I just don't feel like I have the right. And I don't think that anyone has the right to want to take care of me, because I don't deserve it.

The Four Modes in Patients with BPD

In the course of the interview, Kate experiences all four modes. We provide examples of each one.

The Detached Protector Mode

Kate starts the interview in the Detached Protector mode. In this segment, which takes place near the beginning of the interview, Kate stops herself from crying. When the therapist comments, Kate answers in the Detached Protector mode.

THERAPIST: Do you feel like crying?

KATE: Yes, but I'm not going to.

THERAPIST: Why are you afraid to cry in here? Are you embarrassed?

KATE: Yes. I know I'm just supposed to be myself, but this is just really hard for me.

THERAPIST: You mentioned that your mother criticized you for being unhappy. Is there any feeling that if you show that side that it's a bad side? Is that part of it?

KATE: Yeah, just sort of like being what you want me to be. I don't want to be crying here in front of you.

THERAPIST: What do you feel that I want you to be?

KATE: I don't know, just very intelligent and articulate.

THERAPIST: Without too many emotions?

KATE: Yes. Like helping you achieve your goals (*laughs*), even though I don't know you very well. Just helping, making things easier for you. Making you feel comfortable. Like, I don't know, I think that's your drink over there. I was going to offer it to you.

THERAPIST: So your whole focus is really on doing what I want you to do and being what I want you to be.

KATE: Yes. Because I don't know what it is that I am. I think I'm just a miserable person deep down. That's just what I think.

THERAPIST: So, since you feel you're miserable deep down, the best way to overcome that is to be what other people want you to be. What will that do for you? Why would you want to do that?

KATE: It sort of gets me out of myself, I start to emulate people, and just sort of like change myself, and I can be whoever and whatever I want. But what I've found is that it's just made me feel worse, more empty.

THERAPIST: You mean to be what other people want you to be?

KATE: Yes, because I don't know what I expect. I don't know what I want. I don't know what's important to *me*. I don't know. I'm 27 years old and I have no clue.

Kate expresses the sense of identity diffusion characteristic of the Detached Protector mode. Cut off from her needs and emotions, she does not know who she is. She is whoever other people want her to be.

Kate discusses a prior therapy in which she had been in the Detached Protector mode almost the entire time.

KATE: I remember the first therapist I saw. I saw him for about five years, and he helped me with some things. But, I don't know, I was just too busy trying to please him. I really wanted him to just like me, and I was so scared that he was judging me. He said he wasn't, but I *believed* he was judging me. I just wanted him to accept me.

THERAPIST: So in a sense you were doing with him what you've done with other people in your life, which is to not share what you really feel and who you really are.

KATE: Yes.

This segment illustrates how important it is for the therapist to distinguish the Detached Protector from the Healthy Adult mode. Many therapists, like the one Kate described, mistakenly believe that the patient is improving or healthy when, in fact, the patient has shifted into the Detached Protector mode.

When patients are in the Healthy Adult mode, they can experience and express needs and feelings. When they are in the Detached Protector mode, they are disconnected from their needs and feelings. They may behave appropriately, but it is without affect and it is without regard to their own needs. Patients with BPD are not able to engage in authentic intimate relationships when they are in the Detached Protector mode. They might be in a relationship, as Kate was with her prior therapist, but they are not acting in an intimate, vulnerable way. The body is present, but the soul is gone.

The Abandoned Child Mode

Kate describes how, in the month before her suicide attempt, she had alternated between the Detached Protector and Abandoned Child modes: "I kept detaching myself, and getting involved in other things, but then I just couldn't do it anymore. I just used up all my resources." She could not escape her feelings of desolation and worthlessness.

KATE: Right before I swallowed the pills, I went to see my husband at work. I used to go there and, sort of like, bother him. He was just like, "It's over, that's it." Then I just felt so alone, more alone than I've ever, ever felt. And I just said, I'd just rather be dead than feel this way. And I'd rather feel dead than hurt, and I can't take the hurt anymore. I knew that I didn't know what was going to happen, I took a lot of pills, and I figured it would probably hurt, the way that I would die. But I figured that it would be *over*, instead of every day just living with pain. *Every day*. I couldn't take it anymore.

Patients with BPD sometimes want the comfort of knowing that they could commit suicide if the pain became too great, that they would have some release from their suffering. The therapist does not have to take this comfort away from the patient. The patient can think about committing suicide and talk about committing suicide as much as she needs to do. But she must agree to reach her therapist and discuss her feelings thoroughly before making an attempt.

The Angry Child Mode

Most patients with BPD cannot easily discuss or remember their Angry Child mode. Therefore, we often utilize imagery techniques to access it. The therapist asks Kate to generate an image of her Angry Child.

THERAPIST: Would it be too scary to get an image of Angry Kate as a child and see what she looks like?

KATE: No, I have an image.

THERAPIST: And what does Angry Kate look like?

KATE: Just destroying my room.

THERAPIST: And why is she destroying it?

KATE: Because she's just so mad. She's mad at everybody.

THERAPIST: Can you get an image of the people she's mad at?

KATE: Her father and her brother.

THERAPIST: Can you be her now and have her express her anger out loud to them, as they're standing there? Have her tell them why she's so mad at them?

KATE: No.

It is the Punitive Parent mode that stops Kate from expressing her anger. She flips into the Punitive Parent mode to prohibit anger or to punish the Angry Child for expressing anger.

The Punitive Parent Mode

This mode contains the patient's "identification" with the punitive aspects of her parents, now internalized and usually self-directed. In the following segment, Dr. Young helps Kate link the voice of her Punitive Parent mode to her father's voice. This segment is the continuation of the previous one.

THERAPIST: Why is it hard to express your anger, do you think?

KATE: Because I just don't have the right to do it.

THERAPIST: Can you have them now saying that to you? Which one would say that to you? Your father or your brother?

KATE: My father. (Cries.)

THERAPIST: Then be your father now, and have him say that to you, that you don't have the right to be angry. Say it so I can hear what he says.

KATE: He just says, "You always provoke your brother and you make him angry. You know he's sick, but you get him mad. I just want you to just sit up in your room and be *quiet*."

Kate does not have the right to express her anger. In a later segment, when Kate is in the Punitive Parent mode, she says, "I'm just bad, I'm just evil, I'm just dirty." This is the essential message of this mode.

TREATMENT OF PATIENTS WITH BPD

Philosophy of Treatment

Mental health professionals tend to have a negative view of patients with BPD, and to speak about them in pejorative terms. Professionals often regard these patients as manipulative, selfish people. This negative view of patients with BPD is destructive to their treatment. As soon as the therapist views the patient negatively, the therapist feeds into one of the patient's dysfunctional schema modes. Often the therapist becomes the Punitive Parent, angry at the patient, critical and rejecting. Needless to say, this has a damaging effect on the patient. Rather than building up the patient's Healthy Adult and healing the Abandoned Child, the therapist further reinforces the patient's Punitive Parent mode.

Working with patients with BPD is tumultuous and intense. Often the therapist's own schemas are triggered. Later in this chapter we discuss how therapists can work with their own schemas when treating patients with BPD.

The Patient with BPD as Vulnerable Child

In our view, the most constructive way to view patients with BPD is as vulnerable children. They may look like adults, but psychologically they are abandoned children searching for their parents. They behave inappropriately because they are desperate, not because they are selfish: They are "needy, not greedy." They are doing what all young children do when they have no one who takes care of them and makes sure they are safe. Most patients with BPD were lonely and mistreated as children. There was no one who comforted or protected them. Often they had no one to turn to except the very people who were hurting them. Lacking a Healthy Adult they could internalize, as adults they lack the internal resources to sustain themselves; when they are alone, they feel panicked.

When therapists become confused in their treatment of patients with

BPD, we sometimes find that mentally superimposing the image of a small child over the patient can help the therapist understand the patient better and figure out what to do. This strategy seems to counteract negative reactions to the patient's behavior, reminding the therapist that—whether the patient is angry, detached, or punitive—underneath she is an abandoned child.

Balancing the Rights of the Therapist and the Rights of the Patient with BPD

Patients with BPD almost always need more than the therapist can provide. This does not mean that the therapist should attempt to give these patients everything they need. On the contrary, therapists have rights, too. Therapists have the right to maintain a private life, to be treated respectfully, and to set limits when patients infringe on these rights. This does not mean that therapists have to get angry when patients infringe on their rights, however. Patients with BPD do not infringe on therapists' rights in order to torment them, but because they are desperate.

The therapy relationship exists between two people, both of whom have legitimate rights and needs. The patient with BPD has the rights and needs of a very young child. The patient needs a parent. Because the therapist can only provide the patient with "limited reparenting," it is inevitable that there will be a gulf between what the patient wants and what the therapist can give. No one is to blame for this. It is not that the borderline patient wants too much and that the schema therapist gives too little; it is simply that therapy is not an ideal way to reparent. Thus there is certain to be conflict in the therapist–patient relationship. Conflict is inherent in the fact that the patient with BPD will always have greater needs than the therapist can meet. The patient will predictably become frustrated with the therapist. Patients with BPD are thus apt to view professional boundaries as cold, uncaring, unfair, selfish, or even cruel.

At some point in therapy, many patients with BPD have the fantasy that they will live with the therapist—perhaps the therapist will adopt them, marry them, or move in with them. This is not usually primarily a sexual fantasy. Rather, what the patient wants is a parent who is always available. Patients with BPD look for a parent in almost every person they meet—and in every therapist. They want their therapist to be their substitute parent. As soon as the therapist tries to be something other than this parent, patients often flip modes and become angry, withdraw, or leave. We believe the therapist must accept this parental role to some degree. This is our challenge as therapists: to balance the patient's rights and needs with our own, finding a way to become the patient's substitute parent for a period of time, while still maintaining the sanctity of our private lives and without becoming victims of burnout.

Limited Reparenting for the Patient with BPD

The patient's progress in treatment in some respects parallels child development. Psychologically, the patient grows up in therapy. The patient begins as an infant or very young child and—under the influence of the therapist's reparenting—gradually matures into a healthy adult. This is the reason that effective treatment of the patient with BPD at a deep level cannot be brief. To treat this disorder fully requires relatively long-term treatment (at least 2 years and often longer). Many patients with BPD stay in treatment indefinitely. Even though they improve dramatically, as long as circumstances permit, they continue to attend therapy. Most patients can only terminate once they have established a stable, healthy relationship with a partner. Even when the patient stops therapy, the therapist is likely to retain the role of parent figure, and there is a good chance that someday the patient will contact the therapist again.

Therapists frequently become frustrated when treating patients with BPD. As we have noted, no matter how much the therapist gives, it still falls short of what the patient requires. If the patient becomes demanding or hostile, there is a risk that the therapist might retaliate or withdraw and thus contribute to a vicious cycle with the potential to destroy therapy. As noted, when therapists become frustrated in this way, we suggest that they try to regain empathy by looking through the patient's adult exterior to the Abandoned Child at the core.

To be effective, the relationship between the therapist and the patient must be characterized by mutual respect and genuineness. The therapist must truly care about the patient for therapy to work. If the therapist does not truly care about the patient, the patient will realize it and act out or leave. The therapist must be real, not an actor playing the role of a therapist. Patients with BPD are frequently very intuitive and immediately detect any falseness on the part of the therapist.

Overall Treatment Objectives

Modes

Stated in terms of modes, the overall goal of treatment is to help the patient *incorporate the Healthy Adult mode, modeled after the therapist,* in order to:

1. Empathize with and protect the Abandoned Child.
2. Help the Abandoned Child to give and receive love.
3. Fight against, and expunge, the Punitive Parent.
4. Set limits on the behavior of the Angry and Impulsive Child and help patients in this mode to express emotions and needs appropriately.

5. Reassure, and gradually replace, the Detached Protector with the Healthy Adult.

Tracking Modes. This is the heart of the treatment: The therapist tracks the patient's modes from moment to moment in the session, selectively using the strategies that fit each one of the modes. For example, if the patient is in the Punitive Parent mode, the therapist uses the strategies designed specifically to handle the Punitive Parent; if the patient is in the Detached Protector mode, the therapist uses the strategies designed specifically for the Detached Protector. (We discuss the strategies for each mode below.) The therapist learns to recognize the modes and to respond appropriately to each one. In tracking and modulating the patient's modes, the therapist serves as the "good parent." The patient gradually identifies with and internalizes the therapist's reparenting as her own Healthy Adult mode.

Overview of Treatment

In order to give readers an overview of schema therapy for the patient with BPD, we will briefly describe the entire course of treatment over time. In this section, we present the elements of the treatment roughly in the order in which we introduce them to the patient. In the next section, we present a more detailed description of the steps involved in treatment.

Mirroring early child development, the treatment has three main stages: (1) the Bonding and Emotional Regulation stage, (2) the Schema Mode Change stage, and (3) the Autonomy stage.

Stage 1: Bonding and Emotional Regulation

The Therapist Bonds with the Patient, Bypasses the Detached Protector, and Becomes a Stable, Nurturing Base. The first step is for the therapist and patient to form a secure emotional attachment. The therapist starts to reparent the patient's Abandoned Child, providing safety and emotional holding (Winnicott, 1965). The therapist begins by asking the patient about current feelings and problems. As much as possible, the therapist encourages the patient to stay in the Abandoned Child mode. One reason for this is that keeping the patient in the Abandoned Child mode helps the therapist develop feelings of sympathy and warmth for the patient and to bond with her. Later, when the other modes start emerging and the patient becomes angry or punitive, the therapist will have the caring and patience to endure it. Keeping the patient in the Abandoned Child mode also helps the patient bond with the therapist. This bond keeps the patient from leaving therapy prematurely and gives the therapist leverage to confront the patient's other, more problematic modes.

In order to bond with the Abandoned Child, the therapist must first bypass the Detached Protector. This can be a difficult process, because, usually, the Detached Protector does not trust anybody. In a pilot treatment outcome study in the Netherlands that compared schema therapy with psychoanalytic therapy for outpatients with BPD, it was our observation that most schema therapists found that the first year of treatment was typically devoted to overcoming the Detached Protector mode so that they could reparent the Abandoned Child.

The Therapist Encourages Expression of Needs and Emotions in Sessions. A silent, reflective therapeutic stance is generally not suitable for patients with BPD. These patients often interpret silence as a lack of caring or as a withholding of support. The therapeutic alliance is better served by more active participation on the part of the therapist. The therapist asks open-ended questions that encourage patients to express their needs and emotions. For example, the therapist might ask, "Do you have any other thoughts about that?"; "What are you feeling as you talk about that?"; "What did you want to do when that happened?"; "What did you want to say?" The therapist provides continual understanding and validation of the patient's feelings. As the patient begins to bond with the therapist, the therapist makes special efforts to encourage her to express her anger. The therapist is careful not to criticize the patient for expressing anger (within reasonable limits). The goal is for the therapist to create an environment that is a partial antidote to the one the patient knew as a child—one that is safe, nurturing, protective, forgiving, and encouraging of self-expression.

As Kate does in the previous interview, the patient will spontaneously hold back needs and feelings, thinking the therapist just wants her to be "nice" and polite. However, this is not what the therapist wants. The therapist wants the patient to be herself, to say what she feels and ask for what she needs—and the therapist tries to convince the patient of this fact. This is a message the patient probably never got from a parent. In this way, the schema therapist tries to break the cycle of subjugation and detachment in which the patient is caught.

When the therapist encourages the patient to express emotions and needs, these emotions and needs generally arise from the Abandoned Child mode. Keeping the patient in the Abandoned Child mode and nurturing the patient is stabilizing to the patient's life. The patient flips less often from mode to mode, and the modes become less extreme. If the patient is able to express her emotions and needs in the Abandoned Child mode, then she will not have to flip into the Angry and Impulsive Child mode to express them. She will not have to flip into the Detached Protector mode to shut off her feelings. And she will not have to flip into the Punitive Parent mode, because, in accepting her, the therapist replaces the Punitive Parent with a parent figure who allows self-expression. Thus, as the therapist encourages the patient to express needs and feelings and thus reparents her, gradually the patient's dysfunctional modes drop away.

The Therapist Teaches the Patient Coping Techniques to Manage Moods and Soothe Abandonment Distress. The therapist teaches the patient coping techniques to contain and regulate affect as early as possible in therapy. The more severe the patient's symptoms are (especially suicidal and parasuicidal behaviors), the sooner the therapist introduces these techniques. Many of the skills elucidated by Linehan (1993) as part of dialectical behavior therapy (DBT)—such as mindfulness meditation and distress tolerance—can be helpful in reducing these destructive behaviors.

However, we have found that the majority of patients with BPD cannot accept and benefit from cognitive-behavioral techniques until they trust both the therapist and the stability of the reparenting bond. If the therapist introduces these techniques too early, they tend not to be effective. Early in treatment, the patient's primary focus is on the therapist–patient bond—on making sure the bond is still there—and she lacks the free attention to focus on most cognitive-behavioral techniques. Although some patients with BPD are able to use the techniques early in treatment, many more reject them as too cold or mechanical. Whenever the therapist brings up the techniques, these patients feel emotionally abandoned and say something like, "You don't really care about me. I'm not a real person to you." As patients increasingly trust the safety and stability of the therapy relationship, they become more capable of allying themselves with the therapist in the pursuit of therapeutic goals.

There is another danger in introducing cognitive techniques too early: The patient might misuse the techniques to strengthen the Detached Protector mode. Many cognitive techniques can become good strategies for detaching from emotion. In teaching the techniques to the patient, the therapist risks bolstering the Detached Protector mode. Because the overriding goal of therapy is to elicit and treat all the modes in the sessions, if the therapist teaches the patient techniques that suppress the other modes—the Abandoned Child, the Angry and Impulsive Child, and the Punitive Parent—then the therapist ultimately undermines this goal.

When we decide that the patient seems amenable to cognitive techniques, we usually begin with techniques designed to enhance the patient's self-control of moods and self-soothing. These might include safe-place imagery, self-hypnosis, relaxation, self-monitoring of automatic thoughts, flash cards, and transitional objects—whatever appeals most to the patient. The therapist also educates the patient about schemas and begins to challenge the patient's schemas using the cognitive techniques we described in Chapter 3. The patient reads *Reinventing Your Life* (Young & Klosko, 1993) as part of this educational process. Through these coping techniques, the therapist seeks to reduce schema-driven overreactions and to build the patient's self-esteem.

The Therapist and the Patient Negotiate Limits Regarding Therapist Availability, Based on Severity of Symptomatology and the Therapist's Personal Rights. Limit-setting is an important part of the early stage of treatment. Limit-setting is based foremost on safety. The therapist must do what is necessary to ensure the patient's safety and the safety of those around the patient. Once the therapist has established safety, then limits are based on a balance between the patient's needs and the therapist's personal rights. The basic principle is that therapists should not agree to anything they are likely to regret and therefore resent later.

For example, if the patient wants to leave the therapist a short message on the answering machine each evening and if the therapist feels this will not lead to resenting the patient over time, then the therapist might agree. But if the therapist believes that, eventually, these daily messages will cause resentment toward the patient, then the therapist should not agree. Because sources of resentment are personal matters, specific limits will differ from therapist to therapist.

The Therapist Deals with Crises and Sets Limits Regarding Self-Destructive Behaviors. Crises usually involve self-destructive behaviors such as suicidality, self-mutilation, and substance abuse. The therapist reparents, educates, sets limits, and draws on adjunctive resources. The therapist also helps the patient put the emotional regulation skills discussed previously into practice when crises arise.

The therapist is the primary resource for the borderline patient in crisis. Most crises occur because the patient is feeling worthless, bad, unloved, abused, or abandoned. The therapist's capacity to acknowledge these feelings and respond to them compassionately is what enables the patient to resolve the crisis. Ultimately, it is the patient's conviction that the therapist truly cares about and respects her, in contrast to the Punitive Parent, that stops the self-destructive behavior. As long as the patient is confused about whether the therapist truly cares, she will keep acting out self-destructive behaviors in response to stressful life events.

The therapist draws on adjunctive resources in the community to help manage the patient, such as 12-Step groups, groups for incest survivors, and suicide hotline numbers.

The Therapist Initiates Experiential Work Related to the Patient's Childhood. As therapy progresses and the patient stabilizes, the therapist begins imagery work based on the nontraumatic aspects of the patient's early childhood experiences. (Later, the therapist uncovers and focuses on any traumatic memories.) The primary experiential techniques are imagery and dialogues. The therapist instructs the patient to generate images of each of the modes, to name them, and to carry on dialogues. Each mode becomes a character in the patient's imagery, and the characters speak aloud to one another. The therapist, modeling the Healthy Adult, helps the other modes communicate needs and feelings effectively and negotiate with one another.

Stage 2: Schema Mode Change

The therapist models the Healthy Adult mode by reparenting the patient. The Healthy Adult acts to soothe and protect the Abandoned Child, to set limits on the Angry Child, to replace the Detached Protector, and to expunge the Punitive Parent. The patient gradually internalizes this Healthy Adult mode. This is the essence of schema therapy. In the pilot outcome study we mentioned earlier, after the bonding stage, schema therapists devoted much of the second year of treatment to combating the Punitive Parent mode, which is resistant to change. Once the Punitive Parent mode has been substantially weakened, usually change progresses rapidly.

Stage 3: Autonomy

The Therapist Advises the Patient about Appropriate Partner Choices and Helps Generalize Changes in Session to Relationships Outside of Therapy. As they move into the third stage, the therapist and patient focus intensively on the patient's intimate relationships outside of therapy. When a patient enters treatment in the midst of a destructive relationship, the therapist offers advice early on about ways of changing or leaving the relationship. However, we have observed repeatedly that, until the reparenting bond is secure, the patient is usually unable to follow the advice. The patient typically cannot let go of the destructive relationship and tolerate the feelings of abandonment.

Once the patient bonds with the therapist and the therapist becomes a stable base—and as the mode work brings about a greater sense of self-esteem and mood regulation—the patient can often let go of the destructive relationship and begin forming healthy relationships. The therapist helps the patient make better partner choices and behave more constructively in relationships. The patient learns to express affect in appropriate, modulated ways and to ask appropriately for what she needs.

The Therapist Helps the Patient Discover Her Natural Inclinations and Follow Them in Everyday Situations and Major Life Decisions. As the patient stabilizes and spends less time in the Detached Protector, Angry and Impulsive Child, and Punitive Parent modes, she gradually becomes more able to focus on self-realization. The therapist helps the patient identify life goals and the sources of fulfillment in life. The patient learns to discover and follow her natural inclinations in areas such as career choice, appearance, subculture, and leisure activities.

The Therapist Gradually Weans the Patient from Therapy by Reducing the Frequency of Sessions. On a case-by-case basis, therapist and patient address termination issues. The therapist allows the patient to initiate and set the pace for termination. The therapist permits as much independence as the patient can handle but is there as a secure base when the patient needs refueling.

A Detailed Description of Treatment

We now present a more detailed description of our treatment of the patient with BPD, emphasizing strategies for working with each of the modes.

Getting Started: Facilitating the Reparenting Bond

As we have noted, the therapist's first and primary goal is to facilitate the reparenting bond. The therapist and patient discuss the patient's current concerns and presenting problems, and the therapist seeks to provide safety, stability, empathy, and acceptance. The therapist asks the patient to describe her previous therapy experiences and what attributes she desires in a therapist. The therapist listens attentively to the patient and tries to create an open, receptive atmosphere.

Therapists can strengthen the reparenting bond in a number of ways. One is through tone of voice. Rather than speaking coldly and clinically, the therapist speaks in a warm and sympathetic manner. Therapists can strengthen the bond by truly giving of themselves emotionally. Rather than acting the role of the detached professional, the therapist is a real person who responds spontaneously, shares emotional responses, and self-discloses (when it would be helpful to the patient). Therapists can strengthen the bond by making direct statements to the patient conveying that the therapist wants to hear everything the patient has to say, understands what she is feeling, and supports her. Essentially, it is by caring about the patient that the therapist facilitates the reparenting bond.

Throughout, the therapist encourages the patient to speak freely about her needs and feelings regarding the therapist. The therapist is direct, honest, and genuine and encourages the patient to be the same.

The Therapist Outlines the Goals of Therapy

The therapist spells out the goals of therapy in a personal way, making such statements as: "I want to give you a safe place in therapy"; "I want to be there for you so you're not so alone"; "I want to help you become more aware of your own needs and feelings"; "I want to help you establish a stronger sense of identity"; "I want to help you become less self-punitive";

"I want to help you handle your emotions more constructively"; and "I want to help you improve your relationships outside therapy."

The therapist tailors the presentation of goals to the individual patient, weaving in what the patient has said so far in the therapy. The therapist explains how therapy will address the patient's presenting problems, and elicits her goals for therapy. If the patient states a goal that is countertherapeutic (such as remaining in a destructive relationship), the therapist does not agree to it but postpones focusing on the discrepancy until the reparenting bond is stronger. Eventually, the therapist discusses the goal with the patient and, through guided discovery, helps the patient recognize why the goal is self-defeating.

The Therapist and Patient Explore the Patient's Life History

The therapist asks about the patient's life, emphasizing the patient's early childhood experiences in the family and with peers. Proceeding informally, the therapist takes a history. The therapist assesses whether the four predisposing factors identified earlier in this chapter were present in the patient's early childhood environment, especially within the family: (1) abuse and lack of safety; (2) abandonment and emotional deprivation; (3) subjugation of needs and feelings; and (4) punitiveness or rejection. The therapist and patient begin to identify themes and triggers.

The Therapist and Patient Review Assessment Instruments

Patients who are willing to do so gradually complete the following assessment instruments for homework:

1. Multimodal Life History Inventory
2. Young Parenting Inventory
3. Young Schema Questionnaire (if the BPD diagnosis is unclear)

These assessment instruments were discussed in greater detail in Chapter 2.

Although completed inventories are extremely useful, the therapist's first priority is to establish the reparenting relationship. If patients with BPD resist filling out the forms, the therapist does not press the issue; and, if the patient is very fragile, we suggest that the therapist forgo the forms altogether. Completing the forms can be distressing to many patients, because doing so can trigger painful memories and emotions. Other patients with BPD find filling out questionnaires too mechanical. Many of these patients will fill out the forms later, without needing to be pushed, as they become better able to deal with their emotions and modes.

We have found that, of all the forms, the one that is usually most helpful with patients with BPD is the Young Parenting Inventory. In this questionnaire, the patient rates her mother and father on a variety of dimensions. The patient fills out the inventory for homework and brings it to the next session. The therapist uses the inventory as a starting point for a discussion about childhood origins of schemas and modes. The therapist does not "score" the inventory, but points out items with high scores and asks the patient to talk more about them. Discussing the items helps patients begin to explore their childhoods and to understand the origins of their problems. It also helps patients begin to see their parents more objectively and realistically.

The Young Schema Questionnaire is useful primarily for diagnostic purposes. Because most patients with BPD have almost every schema and because filling out the questionnaire can be upsetting to them, we administer it only when the BPD diagnosis is unclear. If the diagnosis is clear, the questionnaire does not yield much additional information.

The therapist discusses the forms with the patient in a personal way. How the therapist presents the forms in large measure determines how the patient will respond to them. If the therapist presents them in a mechanical way, most likely the patient will not accept them. If the therapist uses the forms as a way to connect emotionally to the patient, then most likely the patient will respond positively to them.

The Therapist Educates the Patient about Modes

The therapist explains the schema modes to the patient. If the therapist presents the modes in a personal way, most patients with BPD relate to them quickly and well. Here is how Dr. Young explained them to Kate (in an abbreviated form, because of time constraints imposed by the nature of the consultation):

THERAPIST: Let me tell you a little bit about the way that we view the type of problems that you have, and tell me if it fits. Let me write it down for you, and you can try to follow along. The idea is that people with the type of problems you have, have different sides of themselves, and the different sides sort of click in at different times.

One side I call the Abandoned Child. The Abandoned Child is the part that feels lost, lonely, that no one cares, alone. Can you relate to that side?

KATE: Yes. (*Cries.*) All the time.

THERAPIST: Is that what you feel most of the time?

KATE: Yes.

THERAPIST: The next side is called the Punitive Parent. And that's the side

that's down on yourself, attacking yourself, wanting to punish yourself, like "I'm bad, I'm no good." Do you relate to that side at all?

KATE: (*Nods yes and cries.*)

THERAPIST: When does that side come up? Can you think of what happens
   when you feel that side? What does it feel like?

KATE: Just that I'm bad, I'm just evil, that I'm dirty. That's what I feel.

THERAPIST: What do you usually do when you feel that side, the Punitive
   Parent side? Do you do something to distract yourself?

KATE: Yes. That's usually what I do. I try to fill my life up a lot.

THERAPIST: The third part we call the Detached Protector. The Detached
   Protector is the side that tries to keep you from feeling these other
   things. So what it does is, it tries to block feelings out, escape, drink,
   think about other things. . . .

KATE: (*Interrupts.*) Or become somebody else?

THERAPIST: Yes, or become somebody else.

THERAPIST: Then the last side, we call the Angry Child, which is the part
   that feels she was mistreated—people weren't nice to her. . . .

It is worth noting that, in practice, we speak of a mode as if it were a
person. This has been therapeutically effective, because it helps patients
distance from and observe each mode. However, we do not actually view a
mode conceptually as a separate personality.

Notice the ease with which Kate relates to the four modes. However,
some patients with BPD reject the idea of modes. When this happens, the
therapist does not insist. Rather, the therapist drops the labels and uses
some other expressions, such as "the sad side of you," "the angry side of
you," "the self-critical side of you," and "the numb side of you." It is important that the therapist label these different parts of the self in some way,
but it does not have to be with our labels.

The therapist asks the patient to read chapters in *Reinventing Your Life*
that relate to the modes (and to the particular patient). Although the book
does not mention modes directly, it describes the experience of the
schemas—how it feels to be abused, abandoned, deprived, subjugated—
and the three coping styles of surrender, escape, and counterattack. The
therapist asks the patient to read relevant chapters. It is important that the
therapist assign one chapter at a time and pace the chapters, because when
patients with BPD read *Reinventing Your Life*, they tend to see themselves
everywhere and become overwhelmed.

To reiterate, the therapist's general approach to treatment is to track
the patient's modes from moment to moment and utilize the strategies appropriate for the current mode. The therapist acts as the good parent. The

goal is to build the patient's Healthy Adult mode, modeled on the therapist, to care for the Abandoned Child, reassure and replace the Detached Protector, overthrow and banish the Punitive Parent, and teach the Angry Child appropriate ways to express emotions and needs.

The Abandoned Child Mode: Treatment

The Abandoned Child is the patient's wounded inner child. It is the child part of the patient who was—in our hypothesized, prototypical family of origin—abused, abandoned, emotionally deprived, subjugated, and harshly punished. Within the limits of the therapy relationship, the therapist attempts to furnish the opposite: a relationship that is safe, secure, nurturing, encouraging of genuine self-expression, and forgiving.

The Therapist–Patient Relationship. The therapeutic relationship is central to the treatment of the Abandoned Child mode. Through limited reparenting, the therapist seeks to provide a partial antidote to the patient's toxic childhood. The therapist works to create a "holding environment" (Winnicott, 1965) in which the patient can develop from a young child into a healthy adult. The therapist becomes a stable base upon which the patient gradually builds a sense of identity and self-acceptance. By empathizing with the abandoned-child part of the patient, the therapist tries to guide the patient into the Abandoned Child mode and keep her there, and then to nurture the patient as a parent nurtures a child.

The therapist reparents the patient within the appropriate boundaries of the therapeutic relationship. This is what we mean by "limited reparenting." There is the danger that the therapist will go too far and become enmeshed with the patient or try to become like an actual parent. The therapist stays within the appropriate limits of the therapeutic relationship. For example, the therapist does not meet with the patient outside of the office, use the patient as a confidante or caretaker, touch the patient, engage in dual relationship with the patient, or foster excessive dependence. However, we go further in reparenting than therapists from many other therapeutic modalities do.

Within these boundaries, the therapist tries to satisfy many of the patient's unmet childhood needs for safety, caring, autonomy, self-expression, and appropriate limits. When the patient is in the Abandoned Child mode, she is very vulnerable. The therapist tells the patient: "I'm here for you," "I care about you," "I won't abandon you," "I won't abuse or exploit you," "I won't reject you." These messages affirm the therapist's role as a stable, nurturing base.

The therapist uses direct praise to help build the patient's confidence. When patients are in the Abandoned Child mode, the therapist attempts to give as much direct, sincere praise as possible. Patients with BPD usually do not recognize their own assets. They need the therapist to tell them what their assets are—for example, that they are generous, loving, intelligent, sensitive, creative, empathic, passionate, or loyal. If the therapist waits for the patient to identify her assets on her own, it will probably never happen. When therapists tell patients what they admire about them, the patients almost always deny that they are worthy of admiration. The patient switches from the Abandoned Child to the Punitive Parent mode, and the Punitive Parent negates the praise. However, even though the Punitive Parent negates the praise, the Abandoned Child still hears it. Months later, the patient might bring up what the therapist has said, even though she discounted it at the time.

Through the use of reciprocity and self-disclosure, the therapist uses the therapy relationship to model for the patient how to respect the rights of others, express emotions appropriately, give and receive affection, assert needs, and be authentic. It is important for therapists to be willing to share their personal reactions with patients. We do not mean to imply that therapists should share intimate details of their personal lives. Any type of self-disclosure is helpful—it does not have to go very deep. It could be about a trivial matter, such as an interaction with a stranger on the street or an experience with a salesperson in a store. Therapists acknowledge their vulnerable side to patients. In doing so, they model how to be vulnerable, accept their feelings, and share their feelings with another human being.

Experiential Work. In imagery, the therapist nurtures, empathizes with, and protects the Abandoned Child. Gradually, patients internalize these therapist behaviors as their own Healthy Adult mode, which then replaces the therapist in the imagery.

In imagery, the therapist helps the patient work through upsetting events from childhood. The therapist enters the images and reparents the child. Later in therapy, when the therapeutic bond is secure and the patient is strong enough not to decompensate, the therapist guides the patient through traumatic images of abuse or neglect. Once again, the therapist enters the images to take care of the child. The therapist does whatever a good parent would have done: removes the child from the scene, confronts the perpetrator, stands between the perpetrator and the child, or empowers the child to handle the situation. Gradually, the patient takes over the role of the Healthy Adult, enters the image as an adult, and reparents the child.

Experiential work can also help the patient manage upsetting situations in her current life. The patient can work through her trepidations about a given situation: She can close her eyes and generate an image of the situation or act out the situation in role-plays with the therapist. Sometimes the patient plays whichever mode is active while the therapist plays the Healthy Adult. In other situations, the patient expresses, in turn, the conflicting feelings and desires she has in each mode; then, through mode dialogues, she negotiates a healthy response to the situation.

Cognitive Work. The therapist educates the patient about normal human needs. The therapist begins by teaching the patient about the developmental needs of children. Many patients with BPD have never learned what normal needs are, because their parents taught them that even normal needs were "bad." These patients do not know that it is normal for children to need safety, love, autonomy, praise, and acceptance. The early chapters of *Reinventing Your Life* are helpful in this stage of treatment, because they validate the normal developmental needs of children.

Cognitive techniques can help patients with BPD feel connected to the therapist in upsetting situations. For example, one patient with BPD who suffered from panic attacks told her therapist that reading flash cards in phobic situations was helpful because the cards made her feel connected to the therapist. To make it even more personal, the patient can talk *to* the therapist in the upsetting situation, either in her mind or with pen and paper.

Behavioral Work. The therapist helps the patient learn assertiveness techniques. The patient practices these techniques both during sessions, in imagery or role-play exercises, and between sessions, in homework assignments. The goal is for the patient to learn to manage affect in productive ways and to develop intimate relationships with appropriate significant others in which she is able to be vulnerable without overwhelming the other person.

We discuss cognitive-behavioral coping skills for patients with BPD further in the section on helping the Angry Child and the Abandoned Child to cope.

Dangers in Working with the Abandoned Child Mode. The first danger is that the patient might become overwhelmed. She might leave the session in the Abandoned Child mode and become depressed or upset. Patients with BPD cover a broad spectrum of functionality, and what one patient can handle, another cannot. It is best for the therapist to observe the patient closely and come to know what she can manage. The therapist is careful not to overwhelm patients when they have opened themselves up, as opening up can be so difficult for many patients with BPD to do. The therapist starts with simple strategies and gradually moves to those that are more emotionally charged.

A second danger is that the therapist might inadvertently act in a way that causes the patient to shut off the Abandoned Child mode. For example, if the therapist responds to the patient when she is in this mode by trying to solve a problem, the patient might flip into the Detached Protector mode. The patient might interpret the therapist's behavior to mean that the therapist wants her to be objective and rational rather than subjective and emotional. Similarly, if the therapist treats the patient too much like an adult and ignores the patient's childlike side, the patient might switch into the Detached Protector because the child feels unwanted. All their lives, most patients with BPD have been given the message that their Vulnerable Child mode is not welcome in interpersonal interactions.

A third danger is that the therapist might become irritated with the patient's "childish" behavior and poor problem-solving when she is in the Abandoned Child mode. Any display of anger or irritation on the therapist's part will immediately shut off the Abandoned Child. The patient will flip into the Punitive Parent mode, to punish herself for making the therapist angry. The therapist can use the technique of superimposing the image of a young child over the patient to maintain empathy. This will help the therapist to regard the patient as in a more developmentally appropriate stage and thus to have more reasonable expectations.

The Detached Protector Mode: Treatment

The Detached Protector mode serves to cut off the patient's emotions and needs in order to protect the patient from pain and to keep the patient from harm by appeasing and mollifying others. This mode is an empty shell of the patient, which acts to please automatically and mechanically. The Detached Protector does this because, in this mode, the patient feels that it is not safe to be truly vulnerable with the therapist (or with other people). The Detached Protector exists to protect the Abandoned Child.

The Therapist–Patient Relationship. The therapist reassures the Detached Protector that it is safe to let the patient be vulnerable with the therapist. The therapist consistently protects the patient so that the Detached Protector does not have to do it. This can be accomplished in several ways. The therapist helps the patient contain overwhelming affect by soothing the patient so that it is safe for the Detached Protector to let the patient experience her feelings. The therapist allows the patient to express all her feelings (within appropriate limits), including feelings of anger at the therapist, without punishing the patient. When necessary, the therapist increases the frequency of contact with the patient so that the patient feels nurtured. By reparenting the patient, the therapist ensures that the patient feels safe.

Bypassing the Detached Protector. There are several steps to bypassing the Detached Protector. The therapist begins by labeling the Detached Protector mode, helping the patient to recognize the mode and to identify the cues that trigger it. Next, the therapist analyzes the development of the mode in the patient's childhood and highlights its adaptive value. The therapist helps the patient observe events preceding activation of the mode in her outside life and the consequences of detaching. Together, the therapist and patient review the advantages and disadvantages of detaching in the present as an adult. It is important for the therapist to be forceful in insisting that the patient agree to fight the Detached Protector and experience other modes in therapy because no real progress can occur as long as the patient remains in the Detached Protector mode. As the Healthy Adult, the therapist challenges and negotiates with the Detached Protector. When all these steps have been navigated successfully and the therapist has bypassed the Detached Protector, then the patient is ready to do imagery work.

Here is an example with Kate. Dr. Young begins by pointing out to the patient that she is in the Detached Protector mode and, reminding her of why the mode is there, asks her to generate an image of her Abandoned Child mode.

THERAPIST: Close your eyes. (*Pause.*) Remember I talked about the Abandoned Child? You know, Little Kate, the little girl who wants to be loved. Picture yourself as a little girl. (*Pause.*) Can you picture yourself? Can you get an image of Little Kate?

KATE: Yes, I have a photograph of me, and that's what I'm looking at.

THERAPIST: And what do you look like in the photo? Can you see what Little Kate feels?

KATE: In that picture I was happy, and I was four.

THERAPIST: So that's a happy image of little Kate. Can you get an image of Little Kate where she's not so happy? Picture her where she's sad or alone. Maybe she's in the house and nobody's paying attention to her, maybe her father's off in his own world. Can you get any image like that?

KATE: Yeah, a little bit. I guess. I don't know.

THERAPIST: Is it that you really know, but you're afraid to say it, or is it that you don't want to look at it?

KATE: I guess I don't want to look at it. But I forget things, too. It's just hard for me.

THERAPIST: This is what I call the Detached Protector mode. That's the side of you that's trying to protect you from these feelings, and it's jumping in right now and saying, "Kate, don't let yourself think about these things or look at these things, because it's going to hurt you too much." Is it possible that's what's happening?

KATE: (*Cries and nods yes.*)

The therapist asks the patient to call up an image of the Detached Protector and begins a dialogue with the mode. The Detached Protector becomes a character in the image. In conducting the dialogue, the therapist's goal is to convince the Detached Protector to step aside and allow the therapist to interact with the Vulnerable Child and other child modes. The therapist approaches the Detached Protector with an attitude of empathic confrontation.

THERAPIST: Could you say something to this detached side of yourself, to say that you need to let yourself look at some of these things?

KATE: It's just hard. It's just really hard. It's just painful. And the more I try to think, the more I forget. The more I try to concentrate, the more I can't.

THERAPIST: Again, it's the struggle between this little child part and the detached part. Can you get a picture of the part of you that's afraid to let you do this? Can you picture a side of you that's sort of saying, "Kate, don't feel these things"?

KATE: Yes.

THERAPIST: Can you talk to her and ask her, "Why don't you want to let me look at these things? Why do you confuse me like this?" What does she say?

KATE: I think she's just trying to take care of herself.

THERAPIST: Let me talk to her. "Kate, what are you afraid is going to happen if you let these feelings out and you remember these things?"

KATE: Then I'm just gonna be so *angry* and mad, just so angry that I won't know what to do.

THERAPIST: Are you afraid that the feelings are going to go out of control or that the anger will hurt somebody?

KATE: Yes.

THERAPIST: Would it be too scary to get an image of Angry Kate and see what she looks like?

At this point the therapist and Kate are finally able to break through the Detached Protector to the Angry Child already activated beneath.

Experiential Work. Once the therapist has bypassed the Detached Protector, the imagery work can begin. From this point on in the treatment, the therapist can usually utilize imagery work to bypass the Detached Protector. We find that the best single strategy for getting a patient with BPD out of the Detached Protector mode is imagery work, particularly imagery work utilizing modes. When we ask patients with BPD to close their eyes and picture their Vulnerable Child, quite often they can immediately access the feelings underlying their affectively blank persona.

We describe the imagery work in more detail in discussing the treatment of the other modes.

Cognitive Work. Education about the Detached Protector mode is useful. The therapist highlights the advantages of experiencing emotions and connecting to other people. To live in the Detached Protector mode is to live as one who is emotionally dead. True emotional fulfillment is available only to those who are willing to feel and to want.

Beyond educating the patient in this way, there is something inherently paradoxical about doing cognitive work with the Detached Protector. By emphasizing rationality and objectivity, the process of doing cognitive work itself reinforces the mode. For this reason, we do not recommend focusing on cognitive work with the Detached Protector (other than educational work). Once the patient recognizes intellectually that there are important advantages to supplanting the Detached Protector with better forms of coping, the therapist moves on to the experiential work.

Biological Work. If the patient is overwhelmed by intense affect whenever she switches out of the Detached Protector mode, then the therapist can consider referring the patient to a psychopharmacologist for a medication evaluation. Medication sometimes helps the patient better tolerate coming out of the Detached Protector mode into the other modes. Medications such as mood stabilizers or antidepressants can place a container around the patient's emotions so that she does not become so overwhelmed. As we have noted, it is only in the other modes that real progress can be made in treatment. If the patient cannot stay in the other modes in therapy and remains frozen in the Detached Protector mode, then little progress is possible.

Behavioral Work. Distancing from people is an important aspect of this mode. The Detached Protector is extremely reluctant to open up to people emotionally. In behavioral work, the patient attempts to open up—gradually and incrementally—despite this reluctance. The patient practices shifting out of the Detached Protector mode and into the Abandoned Child and Healthy Adult modes with appropriate significant others.

The patient can practice imagery or role-plays with the therapist in sessions and then carry out homework assignments. For example, a patient might have the goal of sharing more of her feelings about a certain topic with one of her close friends. She might practice expressing her feelings to this friend in role-plays with the therapist and then actually do so with this friend in the week following as a homework assignment.

In addition, the patient can join a self-help group (Alcoholics Anonymous, Adult Children of Alcoholics, etc.). The patient can then practice moving out of the Detached Protector and into the Abandoned Child and Healthy Adult modes in the context of a supportive group.

It is important for the therapist to be consistently confrontational in fighting the Detached Protector. In Chapter 8 we presented a transcript of a session conducted by Dr. Young that demonstrates this process in greater detail.

Dangers in Treating the Detached Protector Mode. The first danger is that the therapist might mistake the Detached Protector for the Healthy Adult. The therapist believes the patient is doing well, but the patient has merely shut down and is behaving in a compliant manner, like a "good child" who is passive and obedient. The key distinguishing factor is whether the patient is experiencing any emotions. The therapist can say, "What are you feeling right now?" The patient who is in the Detached Protector mode will answer, "I'm not feeling anything," or "I feel numb." The therapist can say, "What would you like to do right now?" and the patient will answer, "I don't know," because when the patient is in the Detached Protector mode, she does not have a sense of her own wishes. The therapist can say, "What are you feeling toward me right now?" and the patient in the Detached Protector mode will respond, "Nothing." The patient can experience emotion in the other modes, but not in the Detached Protector mode.

A second danger is that the therapist might become drawn by the Detached Protector into problem-solving without addressing the underlying mode. Many therapists fall into the trap of trying to solve the problems of their patients with BPD, especially in the early stages of treatment. Often the patient does not want solutions—she wants caring and protection. She wants the therapist to empathize with the mode underlying the Detached Protector, with the hidden Abandoned Child and Angry Child modes.

A third danger is that the patient might become angry and the therapist fail to recognize it. The Detached Protector cuts off the patient's anger at the therapist. If the therapist does not break through the Detached Protector and help the patient express her anger, then the patient's anger will build up, and eventually the patient will act out or leave. For example, the patient might go home and cut herself, drive recklessly, engage in substance abuse, have an impulsive, unsafe sexual encounter, or abruptly terminate therapy.

The Punitive Parent Mode: Treatment

The Punitive Parent is the patient's identification with and internalization of the parent (and others) who devalued and rejected the patient in childhood. This mode punishes the patient for being "bad"—which can mean almost anything, but especially expressing genuine feelings or having emotional needs. The goal of treatment is to defeat and cast out the Punitive Parent. Unlike the other modes, the Punitive Parent serves no useful purpose. The therapist battles the Punitive Parent, and the patient gradually identifies with and internalizes the therapist as her own Healthy Adult mode and then battles the Punitive Parent herself.

The Therapist–Patient Relationship. By modeling the opposite of punitiveness—an attitude of acceptance and forgiveness towards the patient—the therapist proves the Punitive Parent false. Rather than criticizing and blaming the patient, the therapist acknowledges the patient when she expresses her genuine feelings and needs and forgives the patient when she does something "wrong." The patient is a good person who is allowed to make mistakes.

By making the self-punitive part of the patient into a mode, the therapist helps the patient undo the identification and internalization process that created that mode in early childhood. The self-punitive part becomes ego-dystonic and external. The therapist then allies with the patient against the Punitive Parent.

In joining with the patient to fight the Punitive Parent, the therapist assumes a stance of empathic confrontation. The therapist empathizes with how difficult it is for the patient, even while pushing the patient to fight the punitive voice. Staying focused on providing empathy helps prevent the therapist from inadvertently identifying with the Punitive Parent and coming across as critical or harsh.

Experiential Work. The therapist helps the patient fight the Punitive Parent mode in imagery. The therapist begins by helping the patient identify which parent (or other person) the mode actually represents. From then on, instead of calling the mode the Punitive Parent, the therapist calls the mode by name (i.e., "your Punitive Father"). Sometimes the mode represents both parents, but more often the mode is the internalized voice of one parent. Labeling the mode in this way helps the patient externalize the voice of the Punitive Parent: It is the parent's voice, and not the patient's own voice. The patient becomes more able to distance from the punitive voice of the mode and more able to fight back.

Here is an example from Dr. Young's interview with Kate. In this segment, Kate flips from the Angry Child to the Punitive Parent mode: The Punitive Parent attempts to punish the Angry Child for getting angry. Kate identifies the Punitive Parent as her father.

THERAPIST: Now I want you to try to be Angry Kate. Talk back to your father, and tell him, "I'm sick of my brother getting all the attention. I deserve some, too."

KATE: (*to father in image*) I'm just tired of him taking everything out on me, and beating me, and having you yell at me.

THERAPIST: (*coaching Kate*) "It's not fair."

KATE: (*Repeats.*) It's not fair.

THERAPIST: (*still coaching*) "And that's why I want to destroy my room. Because I'm so angry at you for doing this."

KATE: I just want you all to die.

THERAPIST: OK, that's good that you said that, Kate. Now, are you feeling bad about yourself for saying it, or does it feel like a relief?

KATE: No. (*Cries.*) It's wrong.

THERAPIST: Can you be the part of you that feels that's wrong right now? Is that your father now, telling you that?

KATE: (*Nods yes.*)

THERAPIST: Can you be your father now, telling you that's wrong?

KATE: (*as father*) "It's wrong for you to think those things and to feel those things, and to be angry, and to want me dead, to want us dead. We take care of you."

The therapist then enters the image to fight the Punitive Parent.

THERAPIST: Can you bring me into the image and let me talk to your father for a second, to protect you a little bit from him? Can we do that? Can you picture me there in the image with your father and you?

KATE: (*Nods yes.*)

THERAPIST: Now I'm going to speak up for you to the Punitive Father: "Look, it's not wrong for Kate to be angry with you. You don't give her the normal amount of attention and caring that a father gives, and your wife is no better. She doesn't give her the attention, either. No wonder she's angry. No wonder she hates all of you. What do you do to make her care about you? What do you do to make your daughter love you and feel close to you? All you do is get angry with her and blame her for things. Even when her brother beats her, you still blame her. Do you expect her to love you for that and be happy? Is that fair?" What are you feeling as I say these things for you?

KATE: I feel guilty.

THERAPIST: Do you feel like hurting yourself, like you deserve to get punished?

KATE: Like, after you leave, I'm going to get beat up.

THERAPIST: Who's going to beat you up?

KATE: My brother. (*Cries.*)

Kate has lost track momentarily of the line between imagery and reality: The imagery has taken on the quality of a flashback for her. Her statement that, after the therapist leaves, she is going to get beat up by her brother blends the present and the past. She has shifted into the Abandoned Child mode. The therapist acts to protect her and to remind her that this is only an image.

THERAPIST: But he's not in your life now, right?

KATE: (*Nods yes.*)

THERAPIST: So this is only in the image now that you are seeing that? Is that what happens in the image? It feels like he's going to beat you up for saying it?

KATE: (*Nods yes.*) For sticking up for myself.

THERAPIST: Can you in the image now imagine giving yourself some kind of wall or something to protect yourself from him in the image? What could you give yourself?

This segment with Kate demonstrates the rapidity with which patients with BPD flip modes. Kate flips from the Angry Child to the Punitive Parent (to punish the Angry Child) to the Abandoned Child (who is afraid her brother will retaliate for her anger). For patients with BPD, this kind of rapid flipping of modes does not occur only in imagery. This is how most of these patients live their lives—with the same rapid flipping of modes.

The previous segment illustrates the strategy of locating the punitive voice in the character of the parent in the image. Whenever the patient switches into the Punitive Parent mode, the therapist identifies the mode with the parent who modeled it. The therapist says, "Be your father saying that to you." It is no longer the patient's voice, it is the parent's voice. Now the therapist can join with the patient in fighting the parent.

As in the preceding segment, most patients with BPD need the therapist to step in and fight the Punitive Parent. Early in the treatment, most patients are too intimidated and afraid of the Punitive Parent to fight back in imagery. Later, as patients internalize the voice of the therapist and develop a stronger Healthy Adult mode, they become more able to fight the Punitive Parent on their own. Earlier in the treatment, the patient is essentially an observer of the battle between the Punitive Parent and the therapist. The therapist uses whatever means necessary to win this battle without overwhelming the patient. Once again, the goal is to expunge the Punitive Parent as completely as possible, not to integrate it with the other modes.

Therapists do not conduct imagery dialogues in which patients picture *themselves* as the punitive one; rather, patients always picture one of their parents. If they picture themselves instead of the parent, the therapist's attacks against the punitive voice would seem to be attacks against the patient, and the patient would not be able to distinguish between attacks on the parent and attacks on the patient. Identifying the punitive voice with the parent solves the problem of how to fight the Punitive Parent without seeming to fight the patient. Once the voice is labeled as belonging to the parent, it is no longer a debate between the therapist and the patient; it is now a debate between the therapist and the parent. In this debate, the therapist verbalizes what the Angry Child has been feeling all along. The therapist finally says what the patient feels underneath but has been unable to express because the Punitive Parent is so tyrannical.

The therapist models setting limits with the Punitive Parent rather than debating the mode or becoming defensive. The patient learns not to defend herself against the Punitive Parent but to fight the parent. The patient does not have to defend herself to prove her rights and worthiness. Rather, the patient tells the Punitive Parent, "I won't let you talk to me like that." The patient learns to set consequences when the Punitive Parent violates the patient's limits.

The therapist can use other experiential techniques. For example, the therapist can use the Gestalt "two-chair" method. The therapist asks the patient to conduct dialogues between the Healthy Adult and the Punitive Parent modes, switching chairs as she switches modes. Ideally, the therapist serves as coach, but not as either mode. This locates the conflict within the patient where it belongs, not between the therapist and the patient. In addition, patients can write letters to the people who have been punitive toward them in the past, stating their feelings and asserting their needs. The patient can write these letters as homework assignments, then read them aloud to the therapist in subsequent sessions.

Cognitive Work. The therapist educates the patient about normal human needs and feelings. It is not "bad" to have them. Due to their emotional deprivation and subjugation, most patients with BPD believe that they are wrong to express their needs and feelings and deserve punishment when they do. In addition, the therapist teaches the patient that punishment is not an effective strategy for self-improvement. The therapist does not support the idea of punishment as a value. When the patients make mistakes in their lives, the therapist teaches them to replace self-punishment with a more constructive response involving forgiveness, understanding, and growth. The goal is for the patients to look honestly at what they did wrong, experience appropriate remorse, make restitution to anyone who might have been negatively affected, explore more productive ways of behaving in the future, and, most important, forgive themselves. In this way, the patients can take responsibility for their mistakes without punishing themselves.

The therapist works to reattribute the parent's condemnation of the patient to the parent's own problems. Here is an example from Dr. Young's interview with Kate. Kate is describing how much her mother disliked her for being "unhappy" and "bitchy."

THERAPIST: Do you still think your mother was right?

KATE: Yes. But there was a reason *why* I was acting that way, maybe it just wasn't something that came from me. I'm starting to realize that now; this has been a long time coming, these feelings. Instead of just internalizing it, maybe it just wasn't me.

THERAPIST: But you've always felt, until recently, that the reason your family treated you this way was because there was something wrong with you. You have basically believed what they said.

KATE: I still believe it.

THERAPIST: But you're trying not to.

KATE: Yes.

THERAPIST: But it's a struggle.

KATE: Yes.

It can often take a year or more to conquer the Punitive Parent, as Kate is trying to do, and it is a crucial step in the treatment of patients with BPD. Over time, somehow the therapist must convince patients that their parents' mistreatment of them occurred not because they were bad children but because their parents had problems of their own or because the family system was dysfunctional. Patients with BPD cannot overcome their feelings of worthlessness until they can make this reattribution. They were good children and did not deserve mistreatment; in fact, no child deserves the mistreatment they experienced.

Together, the therapist and patient go through a process of understanding why the parent mistreated the patient. Perhaps the parent mistreated all the children (in which case the parent had a psychological problem); or the parent was jealous of the patient (in which case the parent had low self-esteem and felt threatened by the patient); or the parent was not able to understand the patient (in which case the patient was different from the parent, but not "bad"). Once patients understand the parent's reasons for mistreating them, they are more able to break the emotional tie between their parent's treatment of them and their self-esteem. They learn that, even though their parent mistreated them, they were worthy of love and respect.

The patient struggling to make this reattribution faces a dilemma. In blaming and getting angry at the parent, the patient risks losing the parent, either psychologically or in reality. This dilemma highlights once again the importance of the reparenting relationship. As the therapist becomes the (limited) substitute parent, the patient is no longer so dependent on the real parent and is more willing to blame and get angry at the parent. By becoming a stable, nurturing base, the therapist gives the patient the stability to let go of or stand up to a dysfunctional parent.

In general, it is much better for patients with BPD not to live with or have frequent contact with their families of origin, especially in the early stages of treatment. The family is very likely to continue reinforcing the very schemas and modes the therapist is fighting to overcome. If a patient is living with her family of origin and the family is still treating her in harmful ways, the therapist makes it a priority to help her find a way to move out.

Another way in which therapists can fight the Punitive Parent is by elaborating the patient's positive qualities. The therapist and patient can keep an ongoing list, periodically adding to it or reviewing it. Patients can gather data about their positive qualities for homework assignments (for example, by asking close friends) and set up experiments to counteract their negativity (for example, by sharing more genuine needs or feelings with select significant others and observing what happens). The therapist and patient can summarize this work on flash cards.

Repetition is a vital aspect of the cognitive work. Patients need to hear the arguments against the Punitive Parent over and over again. The Punitive Parent mode has developed over a long time through countless repetitions. Each time patients fight the Punitive Parent mode with self-love, they weaken the Punitive Parent mode a little bit more. Repetition slowly wears down the Punitive Parent.

Finally, it is important that the therapist and patient acknowledge the parent's good qualities. Often the parent gave the patient some love or acknowledgment, held all the more precious by the patient because it was so rare. However, the therapist insists that the parent's positive attributes do not justify or excuse the parent's harmful behavior.

Behavioral Work. Patients with BPD expect other people to treat them the same way their parents treated them. (This is part of the Punitiveness schema.) Their implicit hypothesis is that almost everyone is, or will become, the Punitive Parent. The therapist sets up experiments to test this hypothesis. The purpose is to demonstrate to the patient that expressing needs and emotions appropriately will usually not lead to rejection or retaliation by healthy people. For example, a patient might have the assignment of asking her partner or close friend to listen to her when she is distressed about work. The therapist and patient role-play the interaction until the patient feels comfortable enough to attempt it, and then the patient carries it out as a homework assignment. If the therapist and patient have chosen the significant other wisely, then the patient will be rewarded for her efforts with a positive response.

Dangers in Treating the Punitive Parent Mode. One danger in helping patients fight the Punitive Parent mode is that the Punitive Parent might fight back by punishing the patient. After the session, the patient might flip into the Punitive Parent mode and punish herself with parasuicidal behaviors, such as cutting or starving herself. It is important for the therapist to keep monitoring the patient for this possibility and to take steps to prevent its occurrence. The therapist instructs the patient not to punish herself and provides alternative activities for the patient when she experiences urges to do so. These activities include reading flash cards or mindfulness meditation.

Another danger is that the therapist might underestimate how frightened the patient is of the Punitive Parent and fail to provide enough protection during the experiential exercises. Often the punitive parent was also an abusive parent. The patient usually needs a great deal of protection to oppose the Punitive Parent. The therapist provides this protection by confronting the Punitive Parent and setting limits on the Punitive Parent's treatment of the patient in the imagery.

Similarly, the therapist might not take an active enough role in fighting the Punitive Parent. The therapist might be too passive or too calmly rational and not aggressive enough. The therapist has to fight the Punitive Parent aggressively. The therapist has to say, "You're wrong," to the Punitive Parent; the therapist has to say, "I don't want to hear you criticize her anymore. I don't want to hear your mean voice. I'm not going to let you punish her anymore." Dealing with the Punitive Parent is like dealing with a person who has neither good will nor empathy. One does not reason with such a person; one does not make appeals to empathy. These approaches do not work with the Punitive Parent mode. The method that works most often is standing up to the Punitive Parent mode and fighting back.

Another danger in doing the experiential work is that the therapist might never teach the patient how to face the Punitive Parent on her own. The therapist steps in and fights the Punitive Parent only as a transitional measure. Eventually the patient must learn to fight the Punitive Parent alone. The therapist gradually withdraws from the imagery sessions, allowing the patient to assume an increasing level of responsibility for fighting the Punitive Parent.

A final danger is that the patient might feel disloyal for criticizing the Punitive Parent. The therapist assures the patient that, later, she can choose to forgive the parent, but for now it is important to look at the truth.

The Angry Child Mode: Treatment

The Angry Child mode expresses rage about the mistreatment and unmet emotional needs that originally formed her schemas—the abuse, abandonment, deprivation, subjugation, rejection, and punishment. Although the rage is usually justified in regard to childhood, in adult life this mode of expression is self-defeating. The patient's anger overwhelms and alienates other people and thus makes it even more unlikely that the patient's emotional needs will finally be met. The therapist reparents the Angry Child by setting limits on angry behavior, while at the same time validating the patient's underlying needs and teaching her more effective ways of expressing anger and getting her emotional needs met.

The Therapist–Patient Relationship. What is the therapist's strategy when the patient with BPD flips into the Angry Child mode and becomes angry at the therapist? Anger at the therapist is common with these patients and, for many therapists, is the most frustrating aspect of treatment. The therapist often feels exhausted trying to meet the patient's needs. Thus, when the patient turns against the therapist and says, "You don't care about me. I hate you," the therapist naturally feels angry and unappreciated. Patients with BPD can sometimes be abusive. They can be manipulative and try to coerce the therapist into giving them what they want. They engage in many behaviors that anger the therapist and tempt the therapist to retaliate. Patients do these things not to hurt the therapist but out of desperation. When therapists feel anger toward patients with BPD, their first priority is to attend to their own schemas. What schemas, if any, are being triggered in the therapist by the patient's behavior? How can the therapist respond to these schemas so as to maintain a therapeutic stance toward the patient? We discuss the issue of the therapist's own schemas later in the chapter.

The next step is to set limits if the patient's anger is abusive. There is a line patients can cross from simply venting anger, which is healthy, to being abusive toward the therapist. Patients cross this line when they call the therapist demeaning names, attack the therapist personally, swear at the therapist, yell loudly enough to disturb others, try to physically dominate the therapist, or threaten the therapist or the therapist's possessions.

The therapist does not tolerate any of these behaviors and responds with a statement such as, "No, I can't let you do that. You have to stop yelling at me. It's OK for you to be angry, but it's not OK for you to scream at me." If the patient still does not stop behaving abusively, then the therapist imposes a consequence: "I would like you to go out into the waiting room for a few minutes until you can calm down. When you're calm, then you can come back in and resume telling me about your anger, but without screaming at me." The therapist gives the patient two messages: The first is that the therapist wants to hear the patient's anger; the second is that the patient has to express the anger within appropriate limits. We further discuss limit-setting later in the chapter.

In fact, most patients with BPD do not behave abusively toward the therapist, although their anger can be very intense. When the patient is in the Angry Child mode and not behaving abusively, then the therapist responds by following these four steps in order: (1) ventilate; (2) empathize; (3) reality-test; and (4) rehearse. We describe these steps one by one.

1. *Ventilate*. First, the therapist allows the patient to express the anger fully. This helps the patient feel calm enough to settle down and be receptive to the second step. The therapist says, "Tell me more about that. Explain why you're angry at me." The therapist allows the patient broad latitude in venting anger, even if the intensity seems unwarranted or exaggerated. If the therapist shows empathy at this stage, it usually neutralizes the anger. Because this is not the initial goal, it is important for the therapist to use a flat or neutral tone, not a nurturing one, and simply repeat: "And what else are you angry at me about?"

2. *Empathize*. Second, the therapist empathizes with the patient's underlying schemas. Underneath the patient's anger is usually a sense of abandonment, deprivation, or abuse. The Angry Child is a response to the unmet needs of the Vulnerable Child.

The therapist says something like, "I know that you're angry at me right now, but I think that underneath what you're feeling is hurt. You're feeling that I don't care about you. Underneath, you're feeling abandoned by me." The therapist tries to label what is happening in schema terms for the patient.

The goal of empathizing is to shift the patient from the Angry Child into the Abandoned Child mode. Then the therapist can reparent the Abandoned Child and remedy the source of the anger.

3. *Reality-test*. Third, the therapist helps the patient engage in reality-testing related to the source of the anger and its intensity. Was the patient's anger really justified, or was it based on a misunderstanding? Are there alternative explanations? Is the anger in proportion to the situation? After they have vented and they feel that the therapist understands, most patients are willing to test reality in this way.

The therapist is neither defensive nor punitive and acknowledges any realistic components of the patient's accusation. There is a fine line between reality-testing and becoming defensive. If there is any truth in what the patient is saying, the therapist admits it and apologizes. The therapist says, "You're right," and "I'm sorry."

Then, the therapist confronts the distorted, exaggerated aspects of the patient's anger, usually through personal self-disclosure: "On the other hand, when you say I don't care about you at all, that's where I feel you're going too far." The therapist shares what it is like to hear the patient say this: "When you say I don't care at all, it makes me feel that all the ways I've tried to show I care mean nothing to you." The therapist also shares what it feels like to experience the patient's anger when it is expressed inappropriately: "When you yell like that, I can't listen to what you're saying. All I can hear is that you're yelling at me and I want you to stop."

4. *Rehearsal of appropriate assertiveness.* If the patient's anger has diminished considerably after the first three steps, therapist and patient move to the final step, which is practicing appropriate assertion. The therapist asks the patient, "If you could do it over again, how would you express your anger to me? How could you express what you need and feel in a way so that I, or other people, can listen and not become defensive?" If necessary, the therapist models the behavior, and then the patient practices it. The therapist helps the patient learn how to express anger in more appropriate, assertive ways.

Experiential Work. In the experiential work, patients vent anger fully toward the significant others in their childhood, adolescence, or adult life who mistreated them. The therapist encourages them to vent in any way they like, even to imagine attacking the people who hurt them. (The exception, of course, is the previously violent patient: Therapists should not encourage patients who have a history of violent behavior to imagine violent fantasies.)

However, most patients with BPD do not have a history of violent behavior; most have a history of victimization. Rather than harming others, they have been harmed. It helps these patients to express their anger in imagery—to imagine fighting back against the people in their early lives who victimized them. By doing so, they feel empowered rather than helpless. Venting anger helps them release strangulated affect and place the current situation in perspective. Patients can do role-plays with the therapist in which they practice venting anger, and they can write angry letters addressed to people in their lives who have harmed them (although they usually do not send the letters). Patients can also use physical outlets to release their anger while doing experiential work, such as pounding a pillow or soft piece of furniture.

Patients practice healthier ways to express anger in their current lives. They utilize imagery or role-plays with the therapist to work out constructive ways to behave in problematic situations. Doing mode work, they conduct negotiations between the Angry Child and Healthy Adult and other modes to find compromises. Usually the compromise is that the patient can express anger or assert her needs, but she must do it in an appropriate manner. For example, the patient cannot yell at her boyfriend, but she can quietly tell him why she is upset.

Cognitive Work. As we pointed out, education about normal human emotions is an important part of the treatment of patients wih BPD. It is especially important to teach patients about the value of anger. Patients with BPD tend to think of anger as all "bad." The therapist reassures them that all anger is not bad: feeling angry and expressing it appropriately is normal and healthy. It is not that their anger is inherently bad; rather, their way of expressing anger is problematic. What they need to learn to do is to express their anger more constructively and effectively. Rather than flipping from passivity to aggression, they need to find a middle ground utilizing assertiveness skills.

The therapist teaches patients reality-testing techniques so that they can formulate more realistic expectations of other people. Patients come to recognize their "black and white thinking" and to stop themselves from impulsively overreacting to emotional slights. Patients can use flash cards to help themselves maintain self-control. When patients feel angry, they take a time-out and read the flash card *before* responding behaviorally. Rather than lashing out or withdrawing, they think through how they want to express their anger.

For example, one patient named Dominique, who frequently paged her boyfriend, Alan, became furious whenever he failed to call her back immediately. With the therapist's help, she composed the following flash card:

> Right now I'm angry because I just paged Alan and he isn't calling me back right away. I'm upset because I need him and he's not there for me. If he could do this to me, I believe that he doesn't care about me anymore. I feel scared that he's going to break up with me. I want to keep paging him over and over again until he answers me. I want to tell him off.
>
> However, I know that this is my Abandonment schema getting triggered. It's my Abandonment schema that's making me think Alan's going to leave me. The evidence that the schema is wrong is that I've thought Alan was going to leave me a million times before and I've always been wrong. Instead of paging him over and over or telling him off, I'm going to give him the benefit of the doubt and trust that he's got a good reason for not calling me back right away and that he's going to call me back when he can. When he finally reaches me, I am going to answer him in a calm and loving way.

Asking the patient to generate alternative explanations for the behavior of others can also be helpful. For example, the patient just described might generate a list of alternative explanations for her boyfriend not calling her back immediately, including such items as: "He's busy at work," "He's in a situation in which there's no privacy to call me," and "He's waiting for a good time to call."

Behavioral Work. The patient practices anger management and assertiveness techniques, both in imagery and role-plays during sessions and in homework practices between sessions.

We discuss these and other cognitive-behavioral techniques further, in the next section, "Helping the Abandoned Child and the Angry Child Cope."

Dangers in Treating the Angry Child. When patients are in the Angry Child mode, there is a particularly high risk that the therapist will behave countertherapeutically. One danger, already mentioned, is that the therapist might become too defensive and deny the realistic components of the patient's complaint. Therapists need to work on their own schemas so that they are prepared to respond therapeutically when their schemas are triggered by the Angry Child.

A more serious danger is that the therapist might counterattack. If the therapist retaliates by attacking the patient, this will trigger the patient's Punitive Parent mode, and the patient will join with the therapist in the attack.

Another danger is that the therapist might withdraw psychologically. When patients with BPD are in the Angry Child mode, therapists often shut down emotionally, retreating into their own "detached protector" modes. Psychological withdrawal on the part of the therapist is problematic because it gives the patient the message that the therapist cannot contain the patient's anger. In addition, withdrawal is likely to trigger the patient's Abandonment schema, as the therapist is emotionally disconnecting from the patient.

At the other extreme, the therapist may allow the patient to go too far in expressing anger, to the point at which the patient actually becomes abusive. Such behavior on the part of the therapist reinforces the patient's Angry Child in unhealthy ways. The therapist gives the patient permission to carry her anger to abusive extremes and fails to set appropriate limits. If the patient leaves the session feeling that her anger was totally justified, then the therapist has probably not done enough reality-testing or limit-setting.

Another risk is that the patient might flip into the Punitive Parent mode after the session to punish herself for getting angry at the therapist. It is important for the patient to hear that she is not "bad" for having gotten angry, that the therapist does not want her to punish herself afterward, and that the therapist wants to help her. The therapist says: "You're not bad for getting angry at me, so I don't want you to punish yourself after the session. If your Punitive Parent starts to punish you, you need to stop him [or her]; and, if you can't, you need to call me so that I can stop him [or her]. I don't want you hurt in any way because of what happened in our session today."

A final danger is that the patient might discontinue therapy because she is angry at the therapist. However, we have found that, in most cases, if the therapist allows the patient to vent fully within appropriate limits and expresses empathy, the patient does not leave therapy. The patient feels validated and accepted, and therefore stays.

Helping the Angry and Abandoned Child Cope

We describe various cognitive-behavioral techniques for helping patients cope when they are in the Angry Child or the Abandoned Child modes or under assault by the Punitive Parent. Although these techniques can be introduced at any point during the treatment at which the patient is receptive to trying them out, we usually try to teach them to patients early on, during the first stage.

Mindfulness Meditation

Mindfulness meditation is a particular type of meditation that helps patients calm themselves and regulate their emotions (Linehan, 1993). Rather than shutting down or becoming overwhelmed by emotions, the patient observes the emotions but does not act on them. The patient focuses on the present moment, attending to the sensory aspects of current experience. Patients are instructed to stay focused on mindfulness meditation until they are calm and can think through the situation rationally. This way, when they act, it will be in a thoughtful, rather than impulsive, way.

For example, the patient might practice using mindfulness meditation as a coping technique for self-soothing. When faced with an upsetting situation, she uses meditation as a tool to calm down enough to think through the situation. She focuses on the present moment, observes her emotions without acting on them, and watches her thoughts. Feeling upset is the cue that alerts the patient to do the meditation exercise.

Pleasurable Activities for Self-Nurturing

The therapist encourages the patient to nurture her Abandoned Child by engaging in pleasurable activities. These vary from patient to patient, depending on what that person finds pleasurable. Some examples might include taking a bubble bath, buying oneself a small gift, getting a massage, or cuddling with a lover. These activities counter the patient's feelings of deprivation and worthlessness. The therapist can assign them to patients as homework assignments.

Cognitive Coping Techniques

Flash Cards. Flash cards are the single most helpful coping strategy for many of our patients with BPD. Patients carry these cards around with them and read them whenever they feel upset and one of their modes has been activated. The therapist composes the flash cards with the patient's help. The cards can be in the therapist's handwriting, or the patient can write them. Therapists usually compose different cards for different trigger situations—such as when the patient gets angry, a friend disappoints her, her boss is angry with her, or her partner needs some space apart from her. In addition, we have one or more cards for each of the four modes.

In order to help therapists compose flash cards, we provide a template (see Figure 3.1). What follows is a sample flash card, written using the template as a guide, for a patient to read when her therapist is away on vacation. The therapist personalizes the flash card for the individual patient.

> Right now I feel scared and angry because my therapist is away on vacation. I feel like cutting or burning myself. However, I know that these feelings are my Abandoned Child mode, which I developed from having parents who were alcoholic and left me alone for long stretches of time. When I'm in this Abandoned Child mode, I usually exaggerate the degree to which people will never return and don't really care about me.
>
> Even though I believe that my therapist will not come back, will not want to see me again, or will die, the reality is that he will come back, will be safe, and will want to see me again. The evidence in my life supporting this healthy view includes the fact that every time he has gone away before, he has always come back, has always been fine, and has always still cared about me.
>
> Therefore, even though I feel like hurting myself, instead I will do something good for myself. I will call the backup therapist; spend time with people who love me; or do something enjoyable (take a walk, call a friend, listen to music, play a game). In addition, I will listen to my relaxation tape in my therapist's voice (or other transitional object) to help soothe me.

In addition to writing the flash card, the therapist can dictate it onto a tape that the patient can play at home. It can be helpful for the patient to hear the therapist's voice. However, it is important also to put the flash card into the more portable written form. That way, patients can carry the flash card around with them and take it out to read whenever they have the need. Many patients report to us that, when they have flash cards with them, they feel as though they have a piece of their therapist with them.

The Schema Diary. The Schema Diary (see sample in Figure 3.2) is a more advanced technique because, unlike the flash card, it requires patients to generate their own coping response when they are upset. The cue for filling out the Schema Diary is that the patient feels upset and is unsure how to handle it. In some ways, it is similar to the Daily Record of Dysfunctional Thoughts in cognitive therapy (Young et al., 2001, p. 279). Filling out the form helps the patient think through a problem and generate a healthy response. The form provides a medium for the Healthy Adult mode. The patient generally relies more on the Schema Diary later in the therapy process.

Assertiveness Training

It is important to provide patients with BPD with assertiveness training throughout the therapy so that they learn more acceptable ways to express their emotions and meet their needs. As we have noted, they especially need to improve their skills in expressing anger, because most tend to swing from extreme passivity to extreme aggression. Patients learn anger management in conjunction with assertiveness training: Anger management teaches patients self-control over their angry outbursts; assertiveness training teaches them appropriate ways to express anger. The therapist and patient role-play various situations in the patient's life that call on assertiveness skills. Usually, the patient plays herself and the therapist plays the other characters in the situation, although any configuration can be helpful. Once the patient develops a healthy response, the therapist and patient rehearse it until the patient feels confident enough to carry it out in real life.

Before turning the patient's attention to behavioral techniques in the session, the therapist gives the patient the opportunity to vent all her emotions about the upsetting situation and linked situations from childhood. Patients with BPD need to vent before they can apply behavioral strategies, or they will not have the ability to focus on appropriate assertiveness.

Setting Limits

Basic Guidelines

Therapists use the following basic guidelines when setting limits.

1. *Limits are based on the patient's safety and the therapist's personal rights.* When making decisions about limits, the two questions schema therapists ask themselves are: "Will the patient be safe?" and "Will I resent what I am agreeing to do?" (The therapist also inquires about the safety of others, although this is less often an issue with patients with BPD.)

The patient's safety is the first consideration. The therapist has to do whatever is necessary to make sure the patient is safe, whether the therapist will resent it or not. If the patient is actually in danger (and if the therapist has already tried other strategies), the therapist must set some limit that provides safety. Even if the patient is calling in the middle of the night or during the therapist's vacation, the therapist must take steps to save the patient (i.e., notify the police, then stay on the phone with the patient until they arrive).

However, if the patient *is* safe but asking the therapist to do something the therapist will resent doing, the therapist should not agree to do it. The therapist should express the refusal in a personal way, as we explain later.

2. *Therapists should not start doing anything they cannot continue doing for the patient unless they expressly state that they will only continue doing it for a specified time period.* For example, the therapist should not, as a matter of course, read long e-mails from the patient each day for the first 3 weeks of treatment and then abruptly announce that reading e-mails is now against the therapist's policy and will have to stop.

However, if the patient is going through a crisis, the therapist might agree to check in with the patient each day until the crisis passes, explaining to the patient that this will continue for a limited period of time. For example, the therapist might say: "For the next week, I want to check in with you every evening for a few minutes while you're going through this crisis."

It is important that therapists determine their limits ahead of time and then adhere to them. In the heat of the moment, the therapist does better to have limits already in mind than to try to figure them out on the spot.

3. *The therapist sets limits in a personal way.* Rather than using impersonal explanations of limits (i.e., "It is the policy of our center to forbid suicidal behavior"), the therapist communicates in a personal manner (i.e., "For the sake of my peace of mind, I have to know that you're safe"). The therapist uses self-disclosure of intentions and feelings whenever possible and avoids sounding punitive or rigid. The more the therapist gives personal reasons for limits, the more patients will accept them and try to abide by them. This policy is in line with our general stance of limited reparenting.

4. *The therapist introduces a rule the first time the patient violates it.* Unless the patient is extremely low functioning or hospitalized, therapists do not recite their limits ahead of time to patients, nor do they set up an explicit contract (except in unusual cases). Such a list or contract sounds too rigid and clinical in the context of limited reparenting. Rather, the therapist states and explains a limit the first time the patient oversteps it and does not impose any consequences until the next time the patient oversteps the limit. We explain this process in more detail later.

The therapist explains the rationale for imposing the limit and empathizes with the patient's difficulty in keeping to the limit. The therapist uses personal self-disclosure to emphasize the importance of the limit, sharing feelings of concern or frustration. The therapist attempts to understand the cause of the limit violation and the relevant modes.

5. *The therapist sets natural consequences for violating limits.* Whenever possible, therapists set consequences for limit violations that follow naturally from what the patient did. For example, if the patient called the

therapist more often than agreed on, then the therapist sets a period of time during which the patient cannot call. If the patient expresses anger inappropriately (for example, by shouting at the therapist) and will not desist, then the therapist leaves the office for a period of time or subtracts the time from a future session. If the patient is persistently self-destructive (for example, by abusing drugs), then the therapist insists that she take steps to ensure her safety, such as increasing her level of care.

Just knowing that the therapist is upset with the patient is usually a powerful deterrent. When the therapist says, "What you are doing upsets me," or "I feel angry about what you're doing," many times this will be enough. When it is not, the therapist imposes other repercussions. For example, if the patient keeps paging the therapist saying she is suicidal, the therapist says, "If you keep calling me too much, we'll have to agree on another procedure for you to follow if you become suicidal, such as going to an emergency room."

When treating patients with BPD, we tend to enforce limits more strictly as therapy progresses. We are less strict at the beginning of therapy, before the patient has formed a strong attachment to the therapist. Generally, the stronger the attachment to the therapist, the greater the patient's motivation to adhere to the limits the therapist has set.

The second time the limit is broken, the therapist expresses firm disapproval, follows through on the promised consequence, and explains the outcome the next time the limit is violated. This latter consequence should be more serious than the one following the patient's first violation of the limit. If the violated limit is a serious one, it may be necessary to escalate the consequences quickly. The therapist must do what is necessary to keep the patient safe, including hospitalizing the patient. Once the therapist has ensured the patient's safety, the therapist again explores the causes of the limits violation in terms of schemas and modes.

The third time the limit is broken, the therapist imposes even more serious consequences for the next violation, such as a temporary break in therapy for a defined length of time or temporary transfer to another therapist. The therapist might warn of permanent termination if the limit is violated a fourth time, with referral to another therapist.

Areas in Which Therapists Set Limits

There are four areas in which therapists frequently need to set limits for patients with BPD. In this section, we explain how the general guidelines listed here can be applied to each area.

Limiting Outside Contact. The first area is limiting outside therapist–patient contact. We believe that therapists who work with patients with

BPD must, at times, be prepared to give patients extra time outside sessions. But how much? How do our guidelines clarify this issue?

Our first guideline states that, once therapists have ensured the patient's safety, they should not agree to do anything for the patient that they will resent doing later. In other words, therapists should do what they feel comfortable doing: They should give patients as much outside contact as they can give without becoming angry. Patients can generally benefit from as much contact as therapists can give them—they are genuinely needy of a high degree of reparenting. The question therapists should ask themselves is, "How much am I willing to give to this patient without becoming resentful?" In order to answer this question, therapists must know themselves well. Limits concerning outside contact are a personal matter and vary from therapist to therapist. For example, some therapists allow patients to leave messages on their answering machines whenever they are upset. As long as patients do not abuse the privilege by frequently leaving extremely long messages, these therapists are comfortable. Other therapists would not be comfortable with this arrangement, and therefore should not agree to it.

Therapists should not initiate or permit any form of outside contact that they are not going to be able to continue giving indefinitely except for a circumscribed, explicit period of time. For example, the therapist should not begin speaking to the patient every night on the phone and then suddenly tell the patient that talking on the phone every night is too much and has to stop. If the therapist feels the need to check in with the patient frequently, then the therapist can institute this procedure for a preset period of time, such as a day or a week.

Therapists should tell patients about their limits when patients first overstep them, and they should do so in a personal way. For example, a patient may initiate more phone contact than the therapist feels comfortable giving. The therapist speaks in terms of personal feelings rather than professional rules, saying something such as:

> "If you want one extra 10-minute phone contact a week besides our sessions, I'm comfortable with that. That's fine with me, and I'll be glad to speak with you. But now you've been calling two or three times a week, and I'm not comfortable with that. I feel like it's too much for me, given my other commitments, and I don't want to start resenting you."

If possible, the therapist should set the limit in person, rather than on the phone, at the next session.

The therapist imposes natural consequences when patients violate limits. The therapist does so with empathic confrontation. As an example, consider the following scenario: a patient with BPD pages her therapist three times in one week for nonemergency situations (e.g., her boyfriend is late for a date). The therapist has asked the patient to use the pager only in cases of emergency. Before setting a consequence, the therapist empathizes with the feelings the patient must have had during the week to have used the pager so often. The therapist says, "You've been paging me a lot in the past week, and I know it's because you feel like you're in crisis, and there are a lot of upsetting things happening to you."

Next, the therapist explains in a personal way what is wrong with the patient's behavior:

> "Even though I care about you, it was too stressful for me this past week to get paged so often. It was making me annoyed with you, and I don't want to feel that way. If you keep paging me too often [here the therapist specifies the acceptable amount], I'm going to stop answering your pages, and we're going to have to set up another way for you to handle emergencies, such as going to the emergency room. I don't want this to happen. I want to be the one who's there for you in an emergency. Can you understand how I'm feeling?"

Patients with BPD are usually empathic and can understand the therapist's point of view when it is presented in a personal manner. The therapist helps the patient find a replacement for the problematic behavior: "Are there any other arrangements we could make to help you when you're in crisis, such as leaving me a message on my answering machine or calling a crisis hot line?"

In addition to setting a limit and modeling appropriate assertion, the therapist is conveying to the patient a lesson about the nature of anger. This helps the patient understand her own pattern—that her own unexpressed anger builds until she flips into the Angry Child mode—and how to overcome the pattern by addressing sources of annoyance assertively, before they have a chance to build to anger.

Contacting the Therapist When Suicidal or Parasuicidal. The therapist asks patients to agree that they will not make a suicide attempt without contacting the therapist first. This agreement is a condition of therapy. The therapist brings up the condition the first time patients say that they are suicidal or have been suicidal in the past. Patients must agree to the rule if they want to continue therapy. Patients with BPD can express the wish to commit suicide as much as they need to do in therapy sessions, but they cannot act on this wish: Patients must speak to the therapist directly before they act, so that the therapist has an opportunity stop them.

We have found that requiring patients with BPD to agree that they will not commit suicide does not work, because they experience suicide attempts as beyond their control and often cannot bear to give up the coping mechanism of preserving suicide as a backup. Thus many patients with

BPD refuse to agree not to commit suicide. Rather than exclude them from treatment, we modified the requirement, asking these patients to agree to call and reach the therapist before making an attempt. Patients with BPD tend to see this requirement as caring and agree to it readily.

The therapist provides the patient with a home phone number or personal pager number for emergency access. We believe that therapists who treat patients with BPD should be willing to offer this kind of access as a vital component of the limited-reparenting relationship. A "surrogate," such as a colleague or doctor-on-call, is not an adequate replacement, except when the therapist is unreachable; in that case, the therapist provides someone else for the patient to access instead. The therapist explains that home or pager access is for life-or-death emergencies only and sets limits if the rule is violated.

Following Specific Rules When Suicidal or Parasuicidal. In order to continue in therapy, patients must agree not only to contact the therapist before attempting suicide but also to follow the hierarchy of rules that the therapist sets down for dealing with suicidal crises. We discuss what these rules are in the section, "Handling Suicidal Crises." The point we want to make here is that the therapist sets the following limit: Whenever the patient is suicidal, the patient must agree to follow a specific sequence of steps. It is up to the therapist, not the patient, to determine what these steps are. The therapist is the ultimate authority about what steps the patient must take in order to be safe.

The therapist brings up the limit the first time the patient expresses suicidal ideation. If the patient refuses to adhere to the limit, even after being warned, the therapist sees the patient through the current suicidal crisis and then terminates with the patient. The therapist warns the patient in advance that this is what will happen if the patient refuses to adhere to the limit and gives the patient a chance to reconsider and follow the limit. The therapist says: "I respect your rights, and you have to respect mine. I can't live my life with you as my patient knowing that, when you become suicidal, you won't follow the rules I think you must follow in order to be safe. It's just too anxiety-provoking for me, and I can't work that way."

Limiting Impulsive Self-Destructive Behaviors. Patients with BPD can become so inundated with unbearable affect that impulsive, self-destructive behaviors such as cutting themselves or abusing drugs seem the only viable forms of release. Teaching patients coping skills, such as those we described previously, can help these patients learn to tolerate distress, but sometimes they become too overwhelmed to benefit from their coping skills. Until the reparenting bond is firmly established, the therapist will probably not be able to get the patient to completely stop all self-destructive behaviors. The therapist attempts to set firm limits but realizes that, at the beginning of therapy, it will be necessary to tolerate some of these behaviors because the patient is not stable enough to stop doing them completely. The therapist expects, though, that within approximately 6 months of therapy, the patient will no longer be exhibiting these behaviors with significant frequency.

Once patients with BPD connect to the therapist as a stable, nurturing base, and once they are able to express anger toward the therapist and others directly during sessions, then the impulsive self-destructive behaviors tend to reduce significantly in all but the most extreme environmental circumstances, such as the loss of a long-term relationship.

This behavior can derive from any of the four schema modes, although the Angry and Impulsive Child mode may be the most common. Many of these behaviors occur because the patient is angry at someone and cannot express it directly. The patient's anger builds, eventually coming out in the form of impulsive self-destructive behaviors. Other impulsive behaviors come from the Abandoned Child, Punitive Parent, or Detached Protector modes. As we have noted, when patients with BPD cut themselves, they may be in the Abandoned Child mode and attempting to use physical pain as a distraction from emotional pain; or they may be in the Punitive Parent mode and punishing themselves; or they may be in the Detached Protector mode and trying to break through the numbness to feel that they exist. The therapist sets limits in accordance with which mode is generating the self-destructive behavior.

The therapist does not tolerate any destructive behaviors toward others. If the patient is a threat to other people, then the therapist sets the following limit: If the patient does anything that is in any way abusive or destructive to other people, such as hitting, stalking, or sexual abuse, then the therapist will have to notify the endangered person and/or call the police, depending on the severity of the behavior. The therapist says something such as, "If I know that you're about to harm someone, I must step in to stop you. I will not let you abuse or hurt other people."

Limiting Absences and Breaks. The therapist does not allow patients with BPD to miss sessions habitually. Missed sessions are primarily an expression of the Detached Protector mode. For example, if a patient flips into a mode that distresses her during a session—such as the Abandoned Child or the Angry Child—she might miss the next session in order to avoid a recurrence. Alternatively, if a patient is angry at her therapist and afraid of flipping into the Angry Child mode, she might miss a session. Therapy cannot proceed this way, because the therapist needs to work with patients when they are actively in these modes in order to make progress. Patients must agree to come to therapy sessions regularly and only to miss sessions in extreme situations (e.g., illness, the funeral of someone close to them, a snowstorm shutting down the city).

If patients persist in missing sessions, the therapist imposes a consequence for missing any more sessions. For example, the therapist might say: "If you miss another session, I'm going to discontinue contact with you outside of our sessions for a week," "If you miss again, we're going to have to take a break from therapy for a week," or, "If you miss a session, the entire next session will be focused *only* on why you missed it."

The therapist imposes the limit in a way that sounds caring rather than punitive. The therapist says, "I'm not doing this to punish you or because I think you're 'bad.' I'm doing it because the only way I can help you is if you come to our sessions, even when you're upset. If you don't come to our sessions, I can't help you. So I have to impose a limit on you to get you to come even when you really don't want to be here."

Their noncompliance of patients with BPD is usually not part of the Abandoned Child mode. The exception is contacting the therapist too frequently because the patient feels separation anxiety. The Abandoned Child is dependent on the therapist and relies on the therapist for guidance and therefore is likely to be compliant. The noncompliance usually comes from one of the other modes—the Detached Protector, the Punitive Parent, or the Angry and Impulsive Child. In order to overcome the patient's noncompliance, the therapist works with these modes until the patient abides by the limits.

For example, the therapist might ask the patient to conduct a dialogue between the noncompliant mode (such as the Detached Protector) and the Healthy Adult. The therapist might ask the Angry Child to vent anger at the therapist about the limit, then empathize and reality-test. The therapist might ask the patient to enact each mode in turn, expressing feelings about the limit.

Ultimately, the therapist's ability to set limits rests on the strength of the reparenting bond. This bond is the therapist's leverage in persuading patients to follow the rules. The patient usually agrees to follow rules out of respect for the therapist's feelings, even if she cannot always comprehend the reason for the rules.

Handling Suicidal Crises

Therapists follow a hierarchy of steps whenever a borderline patient is suicidal or parasuicidal.

Increase the Frequency of Contact with Patient

This is the first step and very important; usually therapist contact is the most effective antidote to the patient's suicidality. If the therapist checks in with the patient a few minutes each day until the crisis has passed, it is often sufficient. The suicidal crisis passes, and the therapist does not have to go any higher on the hierarchy.

The therapist assesses which mode is generating the patient's suicidality and uses the strategies appropriate to that mode. If it is the
Abandoned Child mode, the therapist nurtures and protects the patient.
If it is the Angry Child, the therapist allows the patient to vent, empathizes, then reality tests. If it is the Punitive Parent, the therapist defends
the patient and fights the punitive voice. When the Punitive Parent is
generating the urge, then the therapist sets limits on parasuicidal behavior as well, as the patient might resort to parasuicidal behavior in order
to numb herself.

Assess Suicidality at Each Contact

When a patient is in a suicidal crisis, the therapist assesses suicidality each
time he or she talks to the patient. The therapist says, "What is the actual
risk that you are going to hurt yourself between now and the next time we
talk?" The therapist can ask the patient to rate the risk on a scale of "high,"
"medium," and "low." If the level of suicidality is high, then the therapist
goes to the next step on the hierarchy, which is obtaining permission to
contact significant others.

Obtain Permission to Contact Significant Others

The therapist says,

> "We only have a few options right now, because you are so acutely sui-
> cidal. Either you have to go to a hospital, or we have to find someone
> who can stay with you, a friend or family member who will watch over
> you and keep you company until the crisis has passed. Is there anybody
> you can stay with temporarily or who can stay with you? If you do not
> want to go into the hospital, then you're going to have to let me talk to
> somebody close to you, because I don't feel secure that you can go from
> now until our next contact without hurting yourself."

(*Note*: The family of origin should be used only as a last resort if the family
environment was what largely formed the patient's schemas.)

Arrange a Consultation with a Cotherapist

Concurrently, the therapist arranges a consultation with a cotherapist.
This person shares the burden of the patient's suicidality, so that the therapist does not have to carry it alone, and helps ensure that the therapist
handles the suicidality optimally. The therapist shares the patient with the
cotherapist, who serves as a backup to the principal therapist. If the patient cannot reach the principal therapist, or if the patient and therapist are
having a conflict that they cannot resolve themselves, then the cotherapist

can intercede. Therapists who treat patients with BPD can work together and support one another by serving as cotherapists for each other.

Initiate Psychotropic Medication

If the therapist is not a psychiatrist, the therapist arranges a consultation with a psychiatrist. The psychiatrist can handle issues of medication and hospitalization. Many patients with BPD respond well to psychotropic medication. Medication can significantly reduce their terror and pain and allow them to function at higher levels.

Consider Adjunctive Treatments

The therapist considers adjunctive treatments that might provide the patient with additional support. Some examples include: day hospitals, group therapy, telephone crisis lines, incest survivor support groups, and 12-Step groups.

Arrange Voluntary Hospitalization, If Necessary

Both the intensity and frequency of suicidal crises determine whether patients require hospitalization. If a patient is extremely suicidal, or suicidal too much of the time, then the patient requires hospitalization. The therapist says, "If you're chronically in a life-or-death situation, then you should be in the hospital where you'll be safe."

If the patient refuses to go into the hospital and suicide seems imminent, then the therapist hospitalizes the patient involuntarily. The therapist does whatever is necessary to keep the patient alive, including calling the police to take her against her will. The therapist says, "If you refuse to go into the hospital voluntarily, then I will have no choice but to hospitalize you involuntarily. I want you to know that, if I have to do that, I will no longer be your therapist when you come out." The therapist imposes a consequence for the patient's refusal to cooperate and gives her a chance to relent: "If you go to the hospital voluntarily, I'll remain your therapist, and I'll resume treatment with you when you come out of the hospital. If you will not go voluntarily, I will have to arrange for an involuntary admission. I cannot be your therapist if you will not accept my limits."

Working Through Traumatic Childhood Memories of Abuse or Abandonment

Working through traumatic childhood memories is the last and most difficult stage of the experiential work. With the therapist acting as guide, the patient recalls and relives traumatic memories of abuse or abandonment in imagery (or other traumatic memories).

The therapist does not begin traumatic imagery work until certain conditions are met. The first is that the patient is stable and functioning at a high enough level to withstand the process without becoming overwhelmed or suicidal. The therapist and patient can decide together whether the patient is ready. Second, the therapist does not begin traumatic imagery work until the therapist and patient have discussed the patient's trauma at length in earlier sessions. In other words, the therapist and patient work through the trauma on a cognitive level before attempting the experiential work. Third, we believe that therapists should obtain advanced training in working with trauma before applying imagery techniques to traumatic material.

The defining characteristics of trauma are fear, helplessness, and horror (DSM-IV; American Psychiatric Association, 1994). The emotions connected with traumatic memories are not ordinary emotions, but extreme ones. They overwhelm the ordinary human capacity to endure emotion. Trauma that is human-made, occurs early in life, and is repeated over an extended period of time is especially devastating, characteristics that are unfortunately often true of childhood abuse and neglect.

The therapist helps the patient contain the emotions associated with the trauma within the context of the therapeutic relationship, so that the patient does not have to experience them alone. Ultimately it is the security of the therapist–patient bond that enables the patient to bear the emotions and live through the trauma again. The therapist–patient bond counteracts the meaning the patient has typically attributed to the original trauma: that she is worthless, helpless, and alone. In contrast, the therapy bond allows the patient to feel valued, sheltered, and connected to other human beings, despite the traumatic experience.

Presenting the Rationale

Because memories of abuse can evoke painful emotions, it is important to give patients a convincing rationale for reliving them. Without the context of a good rationale, reliving the abuse in imagery can be retraumatizing rather than healing. It can hurt rather than help the patient.

The therapist presents the rationale in the form of "empathic reality-testing." The therapist empathizes with the patient's pain in remembering the abuse, expresses understanding of her wish to avoid it, but confronts the reality of the situation. The more the patient avoids remembering the abuse, the more the abuse will dominate the patient's life; whereas the more the patient processes the abuse, the less power the abuse will have over her life. As long as the patient continues to dissociate the memories, the memories will continue to overwhelm the patient's life in the form of symptoms and self-destructive behaviors; whereas if the patient can recall and integrate the memories, the patient will eventually become free of symptoms.

The therapist explains the purpose of reliving the abuse. The patient will first experience the emotions and memories of the trauma without blocking them; and then, with the therapist's help, she will fight back against the abuser. This will help the patient feel empowered in the future, both against the abuser and against any other individual who attempts to abuse her. It will also weaken the trauma's hold on her life as she explores what happened and gives it a new meaning in her life. If the patient can create something "good" out of the abuse, then she can feel victorious over it.

The therapist reassures the patient of the therapist's steady presence during the imagery. The therapist says, "I'll be here with you. I'll help you bear the painful feelings." The goal is to get to the point at which the memories of abuse are no longer so devastating to the patient.

Conducting Imagery of Traumatic Events

Once the patient has understood and accepted the rationale, the therapist is ready to begin the imagery. In order to increase the patient's sense of control, the therapist begins by explaining what is going to happen. The therapist says,

> "I'm going to ask you to close your eyes and picture an image of the abuse (or abandonment) you told me about earlier. When the image comes, I want you to tell me what's happening in as much detail as you can. Talk in the present tense, as though it's happening right now. If you become frightened and want to run away from the image, I'll help you to stay with it, but, if you want to stop at any time, raise your hand, and we'll stop. Afterward, I'll help you to make the transition back from the imagery to the present moment, so that we can talk about what happened in the image. We can talk about it for as long as you like."

The therapist asks if the patient has any questions.

In working with traumatic memories, the therapist conducts very short imagery exercises and often allows a couple of weeks to pass before resuming the procedure. During this time, the therapist and patient discuss the imagery thoroughly. The process is one of gradual exposure, not flooding. Patients are often reluctant to engage fully in traumatic imagery, especially the most harrowing parts. The therapist helps the patient by approaching the feared images gradually.

The first time the patient describes the image, the therapist says very little, speaking only when the patient becomes stuck in order to encourage the patient to go on. Otherwise, the therapist remains quiet and listens. Over successive imagery sessions, the therapist gradually becomes more active. When patients start to block images, the therapist helps them persist. When patients relive memories, the therapist helps them experience the memories vividly. The aim is increasing the patient's emotional involvement with the imagery. The therapist slows the action down by asking questions and encourages the patient to put more of the story into words. What is the patient seeing, hearing, touching, tasting, smelling? What are the patient's bodily sensations? What is the patient thinking? What are all the patient's feelings? Can the patient express all her feelings aloud?

When dealing with traumatic memories, often the patient is able to generate only disconnected images of what happened. She is able to get only "flashes" of images or is unable to see the whole image. Most survivors of child abuse have certain moments they cannot bear to remember. As they approach these moments in the imagery, the narrative breaks down. They may see only a series of frozen images. Often when they remember these moments, they are flooded with emotion. They may shake in fear, experience waves of nausea, raise their hands to ward off the images, or turn their heads away. The therapist helps patients assemble these fragments into a coherent narrative that integrates most of the traumatic images. The goal is that, by the end, as little of the memory will remain dissociated as possible. The therapist must be especially careful not to "suggest" elements of the memory and thus create a "false memory." (This issue was discussed more fully in Chapter 4, "Experiential Strategies.")

The therapist encourages patients to do or say things in the image that they could not in their childhood, such as fighting back against the abuser. The therapist enters the image in order to help the patient. In our opinion, fighting back against the abuser in imagery is central to the treatment of childhood abuse. Until the patient can fight back against the abuser—and thus against her own Punitive Parent mode—she will not be able to heal from the abuse. We allow patients to fight back in any way they choose, including aggressive behaviors, with one important exception. We do not help patients elaborate fantasy images of committing violence if they have a history of violent behavior.

After ending an imagery exercise, the therapist leads the patient through some kind of relaxation procedure. This could be any of the self-soothing skills the patient has learned thus far in treatment, such as mindfulness meditation, progressive muscle relaxation, safe-place imagery, or positive suggestions. The therapist continues the relaxation procedure until the patient is calm. Once the patient is calm, the therapist takes a few moments to ground the patient in the present moment. The therapist draws the patient's attention to the immediate surroundings; for example, the therapist asks the patient to look at something in the office, gives the patient a drink of water, or talks quietly with the patient about mundane matters.

Once the patient is calm, the therapist thoroughly discusses the imagery session with the patient. The therapist encourages the patient to fully express all of her reactions to reliving the abuse and praises the patient for having the strength to endure it. The therapist is careful to leave enough time for the patient to recover (at least 20 minutes). The therapist does not let the patient leave the session extremely upset about the imagery work. If necessary, the therapist allows the patient to remain in the waiting room after the session or asks the patient to call later in the day or evening to check in.

Promoting Intimacy and Individuation

As treatment progresses, the therapist fosters generalization from the therapy relationship to appropriate significant others outside of therapy. The therapist helps the patient select stable partners and friends and then encourages the patient to develop genuine intimacy with them.

When the patient resists engaging in this process, the therapist responds with empathic confrontation: The therapist expresses understanding of how difficult it is for the patient to risk intimacy but acknowledges that only through such measured risks will the patient experience meaningful intimate relationships with others. When the patient avoids intimacy, the therapist conducts mode work with the avoidant part of the patient; the therapist makes the "resistant" part a character in the patient's imagery and then carries on dialogues with that mode. The therapist also empathically confronts self-defeating social behaviors, such as clinging, withdrawal, and excessive anger.

In addition, once the patient has stabilized, the therapist helps her individuate by discovering her "natural inclinations." She learns to act on the basis of her genuine needs and emotions rather than in order to please others. In Dr. Young's interview with Kate, she poignantly expressed the importance of this part of treatment:

KATE: I can say I have a strong conviction or I feel really strongly about something, but, in the next minute, it's just gone. It's weird, but a couple of months ago I figured out what my favorite color was, and I was so excited (*laughs*). Because I had a favorite color. And it was something that I actually pointed to.

THERAPIST: And you knew it was *you*.

KATE: Yes. (*Cries.*) I was 27 years old and that was it. This is the color that I really like, not because somebody says it's the color I should like, or somebody that I want to be like likes it, it's just—to *me*—it's very pleasing. So I was real proud of myself (*laughs*).

THERAPIST: That's wonderful. So you were able to find the part of yourself that's real, as opposed to the part that's trying to be what everyone else wants you to be.

KATE: Yes.

THERAPIST: And that's something you haven't been able to do for much of your life.

KATE: And it's funny, but, whenever I see that color, I just want to hang on to it, because it's something that I know that I like and it's important to me. Because there are so few things that I know that I like and that I want.

The final step is for the therapist to encourage gradual independence from therapy by slowly reducing the frequency of sessions. As we have noted, we have found that, in most cases, successfully treated patients with BPD never completely terminate. Even if long periods pass between contacts, most of these patients eventually call the therapist again. The patient views the therapist as a substitute parent and continues to maintain contact.

Therapist Pitfalls

Because their modes are continually shifting, patients with BPD do not have a stable internal image of the therapist. Instead, their image of the therapist shifts along with their modes. In the Abandoned Child mode, the therapist is an idealized nurturer who might suddenly disappear or who might engulf the patient. In the Angry Child mode, the therapist is a devalued depriver. In the Punitive Parent mode, the therapist is a hostile critic. In the Detached Protector mode, the therapist is a distant, remote figure. The patient's perceptions of the therapist are thus perpetually changing. These shifts can be highly disconcerting for the therapist. Therapists who are the object of these shifting appraisals are prone to a variety of intense countertransference reactions, including guilt feelings, rescue fantasies, angry desires to retaliate, boundary transgressions, and profound feelings of helplessness.

We briefly list some of the dangers that therapists most often face when treating patients with BPD. The dangers are tied to the therapist's own particular schemas and coping styles.

The Therapist's Subjugation Schema

Therapists who have Subjugation schemas and who use surrender or avoidance as coping styles face the danger of becoming too passive with their patients. They may avoid confrontation and fail to set appropriate limits. The consequences can be negative for both the therapist and the patient: The therapist becomes increasingly angry over time, and the patient feels increasingly anxious about the lack of limits and may engage in impulsive or self-destructive behavior.

Therapists who have Subjugation schemas must make conscious and determined efforts to confront patients whenever it is indicated—through empathic confrontation—and to set and enforce appropriate limits.

The Therapist's Self-Sacrifice Schema

A danger for therapists with Self-Sacrifice schemas (and almost all therapists have this schema, in our experience) is that they permit too much outside contact with patients and then become resentful. Underlying most therapists' Self-Sacrifice is an underlying sense of Emotional Deprivation—many therapists give to patients what they wish they had been given themselves as children. The therapist gives too much, resentment builds, and eventually the therapist withdraws or punishes the patient.

The best way for therapists with this schema to manage the situation is to know their own limits ahead of time and to adhere to them faithfully.

The Therapist's Defectiveness, Unrelenting Standards, or Failure Schema

Therapists with any of these schemas risk feeling inadequate when the patient with BPD fails to progress, relapses, or criticizes the therapist. It is important for therapists with these schemas to remember that the course of treatment with a patient with BPD is characterized by discouraging periods, relapses, and conflicts, even under the best of circumstances with the best of therapists. Having a cotherapist and good supervision can help therapists maintain a clear vision of what is realistic to achieve in what time period.

Schema Overcompensation by Therapists

This pitfall is extremely dangerous and can destroy the therapy relationship. If the therapist tends to be a schema overcompensator—that is, tends to counterattack—then the therapist may become angry and blame or punish the patient. Therapists who tend to be schema overcompensators are at high risk for damaging patients with BPD rather than helping them and should be closely supervised when they treat these patients.

Schema Avoidance by Therapists

Therapists who are schema avoiders may inadvertently discourage the patient's expression of intense needs and emotions. When the patient expresses strong affect, these therapists feel uncomfortable and withdraw or otherwise express dismay. Patients with BPD often detect these reactions and misinterpret them as rejections or criticisms. Therapists sometimes encourage termination prematurely to avoid the intense affect of these patients.

In order to be an effective therapist for patients with BPD, schema avoiders must learn to tolerate their own and their patients' emotions.

The Therapist's Emotional Inhibition Schema

Therapists who have the Emotional Inhibition schema often come across to patients with BPD as aloof, rigid, or impersonal. This is a serious danger. Therapists who are extremely emotionally inhibited may cause harm to patients with BPD and probably should not work with them. The patient with BPD needs to be nurtured and reparented. An outwardly cold therapist is probably not going to be able to give the patient the nurturing she needs in a manner that she can recognize and accept.

If the therapist chooses to try to heal the schema, there is the possibility of overcoming the emotional inhibition through therapy.

CONCLUSION

Therapy with a patient with BPD is a long-term process. For a patient to achieve individuation and intimacy with others, 2 or 3 years of treatment are often required, perhaps longer. But patients generally show significant improvement all along the way.

We feel a sense of optimism and hope about utilizing schema therapy with patients with BPD. Although treatment is often slow and difficult for both the patient and the therapist, the rewards are great. We have found that most patients with BPD make significant progress. In our opinion, the essential curative elements of schema therapy for these patients are the "limited reparenting" the therapist provides, mode work, and progressing through therapy in the stages we have described.

Chapter 10

SCHEMA THERAPY FOR NARCISSISTIC PERSONALITY DISORDER

In our experience, it is patients with borderline or narcissistic personality disorder who present the most consistent difficulty for therapists. In a sense, these two groups of patients pose opposite dilemmas to therapists: Patients with BPD, are too needy and oversensitive for many therapists, whereas patients with narcissistic personality disorder are often not vulnerable or sensitive enough. Both groups are ambivalent about the process of therapy. As with our treatment of patients with BPD, our approach to patients with narcissistic personality disorder utilizes a mode-based approach. It was largely in order to treat these two types of patients more successfully that we developed the concept of modes. The mode approach allows us to build a therapeutic alliance with the parts of the patient that strive for health, while simultaneously fighting the maladaptive parts—those that move toward isolation, self-destruction, and harming others.

SCHEMA MODES IN THE PATIENT WITH NARCISSISTIC PERSONALITY DISORDER

We have observed three primary modes that characterize most patients with narcissistic personality disorder (in addition to the Healthy Adult mode, which the therapist tries to augment):

1. The Lonely Child
2. The Self-Aggrandizer
3. The Detached Self-Soother

Not all patients with narcissistic personality disorder have all three modes, and some have other modes. However, these three modes are by far the most common ones. As we discuss the three modes, we link them to the schemas and coping styles that we theorize constitute narcissism.

In our experience, these patients are generally unable to give and receive genuine love (with the occasional exception of their own children). The core schemas of narcissism are Emotional Deprivation and Defectiveness, which are part of the Lonely Child mode. The Entitlement schema is an overcompensation for the other two schemas and is part of the Self-Aggrandizer mode. Because most patients with narcissistic personality disorder are not able to experience genuine love, they are likely to perpetuate their Emotional Deprivation and Defectiveness schemas throughout their lives. They ensure through their own behavior that they remain unable to love or be loved—unless they undergo therapy or engage in some other healing relationship.

The Lonely Child almost always has an Emotional Deprivation schema with a coping style of Overcompensation. To compensate for the schema, patients come to feel entitled. They demand much from, and give little to, the people closest to them. Because they expect to be deprived, they behave in a demanding way to ensure that their needs are met. It is their Emotional Deprivation schema that causes these patients to exaggerate how much they are neglected and misunderstood.

The Defectiveness schema is usually present in narcissism. Most patients with narcissistic personality disorder feel defective. For this reason they do not let other people get too close to them. Patients with narcissistic personality disorder are ambivalent about intimacy: They simultaneously long for it and feel uncomfortable and ward it off when they begin to receive it. (One might consider this the tension between their Emotional Deprivation and Defectiveness schemas. Their sense of deprivation motivates them to get closer to others, but their sense of defectiveness motivates them to pull away.) They believe that the exposure of any flaw is humiliating and will ultimately lead to rejection. Whenever they publicly fail to meet high standards, they collapse from grandiosity into inferiority and feel shame. Such failures often produce depression or other Axis I symptoms such as anxiety or psychosomatic disorders. In addition, failures usually precipitate renewed efforts to overcompensate.

In actual practice, we often fine-tune or alter the names of the modes to better fit each individual patient. For example, we might name the Lonely Child the "Rejected Child," the "Ignored Child," or the "Inadequate Child"; we might name the Self-Aggrandizer the "Competitor" or the "Critic"; we might name the Detached Self-Soother the "Excitement Junkie" or the "Speculator." We use whatever name best captures the mode for that patient.

Other Schemas

Emotional Deprivation, Defectiveness, and Entitlement are the most prominent schemas in patients with narcissistic personality disorder, but there are often others. We frequently observe some of the following schemas as well.

    Mistrust/Abuse
    Social Isolation/Alienation
    Failure
    Insufficient Self-Control/Self Discipline
    Subjugation
    Approval-Seeking/Recognition-Seeking
    Unrelenting Standards/Hypercriticalness
    Punitiveness

Because they use overcompensation and avoidance as coping styles, patients with narcissistic personality disorder are largely unaware of their schemas most of the time.

The Lonely Child Mode

This mode is the version of the Vulnerable Child mode found in patients with narcissistic personality disorder. At the core, most of these patients feel like lonely children who are valued only insofar as they can aggrandize their parents. The patient, however, usually has little awareness of this core feeling. Because the most important emotional needs of the child have generally not been met, the patient usually feels empty and alone. The therapist forms the deepest bond with the patient's Lonely Child mode.

In this mode, patients with narcissistic personality disorder often feel undeserving of love. The Lonely Child feels unloved and unlovable. Many patients with narcissistic personality disorder believe that they have somehow been able to succeed at a level far beyond their true capacity. Somehow they have tricked everybody or have been incredibly lucky. Thus they usually feel underneath that they cannot live up to the expectations that other people have set for them and that they seem on the surface to be meeting. They feel that they will not be able to keep meeting these expectations for much longer. Much of the time, these patients have the underlying sense that the areas of life in which they overcompensate to gain recognition and value are on the verge of collapse.

For these patients, the opposite of feeling "special" is feeling "average." Average is one of the worst feelings for most patients with narcissistic personality disorder, because their self-image is split: either they are the center of attention and wonderful or they are nothing. There is no middle ground. This is a result of the conditional approval these patients received as children. To be average is to be ignored and unacceptable. If they are not special, no one will love them, no one will spend time with them. They will be alone.

The Lonely Child mode is usually triggered in patients with narcissistic personality disorder by the loss of some source of validation or special status: Their businesses fail; they are fired from their jobs; their spouses or partners leave them; they lose a competition; someone else achieves more success or acclaim; someone they respect criticizes them; or they get sick and are unable to work. Once these patients flip into the Lonely Child mode, they try to flip as quickly as possible back into one of the other modes (the Self-Aggrandizer or the Detached Self-Soother). Most patients stay in the Lonely Child mode for as short a time as possible, because experiencing the Lonely Child is intensely painful: The Lonely Child feels sad, unloved, humiliated, and (usually) inflicted with self-loathing. At some point in their lives—as a result of defeat, failure, or rejection—most patients with narcissistic personality disorder have spent some time in the Lonely Child mode. However, they usually do not remember it clearly, resist thinking about it, and will do almost anything to avoid feeling vulnerable again.

The Self-Aggrandizer Mode

The Self-Aggrandizer mode is an overcompensation for the patient's feelings of emotional deprivation and defectiveness. When patients are in this mode, they behave in entitled, competitive, grandiose, abusive, or status-seeking ways. Typically, this is their "default" or automatic mode, especially around other people: It is the mode patients with narcissistic personality disorder experience most of the time. They generally flip into the Detached Self-Soother mode when they are by themselves for extended periods, and only rarely do they flip into the Lonely Child mode.

Because the Lonely Child (usually) feels defective, the Self-Aggrandizer tries to demonstrate superiority. In this mode, patients often crave admiration and become critical of others. They are prone to such competitive behaviors as speaking in a condescending tone, retaliating with anger to perceived slights, one-upmanship, and always having to be right. These behaviors are compensatory: Underneath, these patients are feeling inferior and insulted. The schema also manifests in such intimacy-avoiding behaviors as expressing anger whenever they feel vulnerable and controlling the flow of conversation away from emotionally revealing material (as Carl, the case example we present later in this chapter, tries to do).

It is the Entitlement schema that leads to the patient's self-centeredness, lack of concern for other people's needs and rights, and sense of "specialness." In the Self-Aggrandizer mode, patients with narcissistic personality disorder tend to behave in insensitive ways. They insist on doing and having whatever they want, regardless of the cost to others. They are almost completely self-absorbed, and show little empathy for the needs and feelings of others. They try to direct the behavior of others in accordance with their own desires. They expect to be treated as special and do not believe they should have to follow the rules that apply to everyone else.

As noted, the therapist often changes the name of the Self-Aggrandizer mode to more accurately fit the individual patient. We might call this mode the "Entitled Side" or the "Status-Seeker." The therapist can use the most salient feature of the patient's coping style to help name the mode.

In our experience, the most common coping styles of patients with narcissistic personality disorder when they are in the Self-Aggrandizer mode are as follows:

Aggression and Hostility
Dominance and Excessive Self-Assertion
Recognition and Status-Seeking
Manipulation and Exploitation

These coping styles represent extremes. It is important to remember that narcissism presents in many forms. Not all patients show such extreme coping styles. There is a "spectrum of narcissism" from relatively benign to malignant. At one extreme, patients are sociopathic; at the other extreme, they are self-absorbed but capable of empathy and warmth with some people. (See Kernberg's [1984] discussion of "malignant" narcissism.) Therapy patients span the whole range. All of them, we believe, have a Vulnerable Child underneath.

When patients with narcissistic personality disorder use the coping style of Aggression and Hostility, they lash out in anger when others fail to meet their needs or challenge one of their compensations. These patients believe the saying, "The best defense is a good offense." Feeling threatened, they attack. In the extreme, this coping style manifests itself as violence toward others. The function of the coping style is to force other people to meet their emotional needs (countering underlying feelings of emotional deprivation) or to preserve a mask of superiority (countering feelings of defectiveness).

Another coping style, Dominance and Excessive Self-Assertion, is the tendency to bully others in order to maintain control over situations. Patients who use this coping strategy can behave like tyrants. They often attempt to tower over others physically or psychologically in order to intimidate them. They attempt to be the "alpha"—and thus to get their emotional needs met or establish their superiority. They do this whenever one of their underlying schemas is triggered (usually Emotional Deprivation or Defectiveness).

Recognition- and Status-Seeking is a strong desire to obtain admiration from others, and is a dominant component of almost every patient with narcissistic personality disorder. Patients place an exaggerated importance on the outward signs of success, such as social status, high achievement, physical appearance, and wealth. They almost always do this to cope with underlying feelings of defectiveness. Because they feel "one down," they attest that they are "better than." In the Self-Aggrandizer mode, most patients with narcissistic personality disorder are envious of other people's successes, including those of the people closest to them—and they frequently seek to destroy or diminish the accomplishments of others.

The coping style of Manipulation and Exploitation is the tendency to use others for one's own gratification. At the extreme, patients who adopt this coping style are ruthless. They will do anything to get what they want, whatever the cost to others. They have little empathy and view other people as objects to use for their own satisfaction rather than as individuals in their own right. They feel entitled in order to overcompensate for their feelings of emotional deprivation. (In fact, several schemas are narcissistic overcompensations: Entitlement, Unrelenting Standards, Recognition-Seeking.)

Some patients are "closet narcissists." They have the same three modes, but the Self-Aggrandizer mode exists in fantasy rather than reality. Like the meek title character in James Thurber's "The Secret Life of Walter Mitty," it is not obvious to the outside world that they see themselves as special or fantasize about another life. To the outside world, closet narcissists may appear unassuming or even people-pleasing. However, in their fantasy lives, they are superior to most people. These patients have very similar personality structures to those of more overly narcissistic individuals, but they do not openly display the Self-Aggrandizer mode around other people.

The Detached Self-Soother Mode

While they are with other people, patients with narcissistic personality disorder are usually in the Self-Aggrandizer mode. When they are alone, cut off from the admiration they derive from interacting with others, they usually flip into the Detached Self-Soother mode. In this mode they shut off their emotions by engaging in activities that will somehow soothe or distract them from feeling. Patients flip into the Detached Self-Soother mode when they are alone because, without other people to boost them up, they shift into the Lonely Child mode. They begin to feel empty, bored, and depressed. In the absence of external sources of validation, the Lonely Child starts to surface; the Detached Self-Soother mode is a way to avoid the pain of the Lonely Child.

The Detached Self-Soother can take many forms, all representing mechanisms of schema avoidance. Patients often engage in a variety of activities to stimulate themselves. These behaviors are usually undertaken in an addictive or compulsive way. With some patients, the mode takes the form of workaholism; with others, it takes the form of behaviors such as gambling, speculative stock investing, dangerous sports such as car racing or rock climbing, promiscuous sex, pornography or cybersex, or drugs such as cocaine. These activities provide stimulation and excitement.

Another group of patients compulsively engage in solitary interests that are more self-soothing than self-stimulating, such as playing computer games, overeating, watching television, or fantasizing. These compulsive interests focus their attention away from the pain of their Emotional Deprivation and Defectiveness schemas—away from the Lonely Child mode. The activities are all basically ways of avoiding feelings of emptiness and worthlessness.

DSM-IV CRITERIA FOR NARCISSISTIC PERSONALITY DISORDER

The DSM-IV diagnostic criteria for narcissistic personality disorder are listed her. Note that all of them focus on just one of the three modes, the Self-Aggrandizer.

- Has a grandiose sense of self-importance (e.g., exaggerates achievements and talents, expects to be recognized as superior without commensurate achievements).
- Is preoccupied with fantasies of unlimited success, power, brilliance, beauty, or ideal love.
- Believes that he or she is "special" and unique and can only be understood by, or should associate with, other special or high-status people (or institutions).
- Requires excessive admiration.
- Has a sense of entitlement, i.e., unreasonable expectations of especially favorable treatment or automatic compliance with his or her expectations.
- Is interpersonally exploitative, i.e., takes advantage of others to achieve his or her own ends.
- Lacks empathy: is unwilling to recognize or identify with the feelings and needs of others.
- Is often envious of others or believes that others are envious of him or her.
- Shows arrogant, haughty behaviors or attitudes.

We are critical of these DSM-IV criteria because they focus almost exclusively on the outward, compensatory behaviors of patients and do not focus on the other modes that we believe are central to the problems of these patients. Furthermore, by focusing solely on the Self-Aggrandizer mode, DSM-IV leads many clinicians to hold an unsympathetic view of patients with narcissistic personality disorder rather than one of empathy and concern for the deeper level of pain that most of these individuals share. Finally, we believe that the diagnostic criteria for narcissistic personality disorder—as with many other Axis II disorders—do not lead to effective treatments. The criteria describe only the patient's coping styles and do not guide clinicians to understand the relevant underlying themes or schemas, which we are convinced must change for Axis II patients to achieve lasting improvement.

NARCISSISTIC PERSONALITY DISORDER VERSUS PURE ENTITLEMENT

It is important to distinguish the narcissistic personality we are describing from pure entitlement—that is, from cases in which the person has the Entitlement schema in its pure form, without the underlying Emotional Deprivation and Defectiveness schemas.

The Entitlement schema can develop in two ways. In the pure form, the child is simply spoiled. The parents set too few limits and do not require the child to respect the feelings and rights of others. The child fails to learn the principle of reciprocity in relationships. However, the child is neither emotionally deprived nor rejected, so the Entitlement schema is not compensatory.

Alternatively, the Entitlement schema can develop as an overcompensation for feelings of emotional deprivation and defectiveness. Unlike the "spoiled" patients who display pure Entitlement schemas, these are the "fragile" patients. Their sense of entitlement is fragile because underneath they know what it is like to be ignored and devalued. There is always the risk that their compensations could fall down around them, leaving them vulnerable and exposed.

Like the "spoiled" patients, "fragile" patients with narcissistic personality disorder also behave in demanding and superior ways. However, patients with pure Entitlement schemas do not have a Lonely Child mode at the core. Deep inside there is no sad, lost, vulnerable, defective child. At the core of the pure "spoiled" patient is an impulsive, undisciplined child. Although spoiled patients and fragile patients with narcissistic personality disorder might look similar from the outside, their inner worlds are very different.

Actually, most patients with narcissistic personality disorder that we treat show a combination of spoiled and fragile entitlement. Their sense of entitlement is partially learned and partially compensatory—in part they were spoiled and indulged as children, and in part the entitlement is a way of making up for underlying feelings of emotional deprivation and defectiveness. Therefore, most patients need some combination of limit-setting and mode work. However, most patients with narcissistic personality disorder who seek treatment have a significant fragile component; they have come in because one of their overcompensations has collapsed and they are depressed. Most of these patients require the major focus of treatment to be mode work. Limit-setting is part of treatment, but it is not a primary part.

When experts on narcissism write about patients with narcissistic personality disorder, typically they are referring to more fragile, compensated patients rather than to those who have pure Entitlement schemas. We address this chapter to the treatment of fragile patients. There is no point in doing the mode work we describe in this chapter with patients who have pure Entitlement schemas because there are no maladaptive underlying modes to reach. There is just the Entitlement schema, and the therapist's role is to teach the patient proper limits and reciprocity. (This can be done with a simpler form of mode work: conducting dialogues between the "Spoiled Child" and the "Healthy Adult.")

THE CHILDHOOD ORIGINS OF NARCISSISM

We have found four factors that often characterize the childhood environments of patients with narcissistic personality disorder:

1. Loneliness and isolation
2. Insufficient limits
3. History of being used or manipulated
4. Conditional approval

Loneliness and Isolation

Most patients with narcissistic personality disorder were lonely as children. They were unloved in some significant way. Most endured significant emotional deprivation. The mother (or other main caretaking figure) may have paid a lot of attention to them but was not often physically affectionate or demonstrative. There was a lack of empathy and attunement on the part of the mother, as well as an absence of genuine love and emotional attachment. In addition, many patients felt rejected by or different from peers. Patients with narcissistic personality disorder have childhood histories that include such schemas as Emotional Deprivation, Defectiveness, and Social Isolation. Typically patients are unaware (or only vaguely aware) of these schemas.

Insufficient Limits

Most patients with narcissistic personality disorder were not given sufficient limits as children and were usually indulged. However, they were not indulged emotionally; rather, they were indulged in material ways or permitted to behave as they wanted without regard to the feelings of others. Perhaps they were allowed to mistreat others or were given their way whenever they had "temper tantrums." They may have been largely unsupervised—except in regard to sources of narcissistic gratification for their parents—in activities such as household chores or curfews. A feeling of "specialness" served as a substitute for love: It was the best the child got. These patients have childhood histories that include such schemas as Entitlement and Insufficient Self-Control/Self-Discipline.

History of Being Used or Manipulated

Most patients were used or manipulated in some way as children, usually by one of their parents. For example, a parent might have used them sexually, manipulated them to fill the role of a substitute spouse, or pushed them to vicariously fill the parent's need for achievement, success, status, or recognition. As children many of these patients were used to overcompensate for a parent's schemas—to fill the parent's unmet needs for sexual gratification, emotional support (the Emotional Deprivation schema), or feelings of inadequacy (the Defectiveness schema).

Typically this happened largely out of the child's awareness. Patients often begin treatment saying, "I had a great childhood; both of my parents were wonderful." They do not consciously realize that something was wrong. However, when the therapist looks more closely at the childhoods of such patients, the therapist finds parents who did not understand the needs of their children but were gratifying their own needs through their children. Often, the therapist finds parents with a narcissistic personality disorder.

As children, most of these patients experienced a confusing situation. They received attention, praise, and admiration; and all of these felt good, so they believe they were loved. But typically they lacked basic nurturing: They were not touched, they were not kissed, they were not hugged. They were not mirrored nor understood—they were not "seen" and they were not "heard." Thus they got approval but did not experience genuine love: They were used, in the sense that they were given attention only when they performed up to certain standards. Their childhood histories often include such schemas as Mistrust/Abuse and Subjugation. In these cases, someone, usually a parent, used or dominated them, as though they were objects meant only for the parent's gratification.

Conditional Approval

Most patients were given conditional approval as children, rather than genuine, unselfish love. (It is hard to say whether the parent "loved" the child—whether the parent's feelings actually constituted love. As one patient put it, "Yes, my father loved me, like the wolf loves the lamb.") As children, they felt special when they met some high standard imposed by the parent; otherwise, they were ignored or devalued by that parent. The parent emphasized "appearances" at the expense of true happiness and intimacy. The child tried to be perfect in order to be worthy of the parent's approval and to ward off the parent's criticisms and demands. The child was unable to develop a stable sense of self-esteem; rather, the child's self-esteem became dependent on the approval of others. When others approved, the child felt momentarily worthwhile; when others disapproved, the child felt worthless. Patients with narcissistic personality disorder have childhood histories that include such schemas as Defectiveness, Unrelenting Standards, and Approval-Seeking.

Typical Childhood Histories

We describe some typical childhood histories of patients narcissistic personality disorder. These are common patterns but not universal ones in narcissism. A large number of patients had one doting parent in childhood who treated them preferentially, as if they were "special," and set few limits. Usually this parent was the mother, but sometimes it was the father. The mother spoiled and indulged them, but her behavior was based on her own needs, not their needs. The mother sought to meet her own needs for status and recognition through them. She idealized them and set very high expectations for them to meet. In order to keep them in line with her desires, she could be manipulative and controlling. She lacked empathy for their needs and feelings and did not give them physical affection (except perhaps in front of others, for show, or when *she* wanted it). The other parent also played an important role. For most of these patients, the other parent was at the opposite extreme. They had fathers who were absent, passive, distant, rejecting, critical, or abusive. Thus, as children, these patients often received two distinctly opposite messages from their parents: One parent inflated their value, whereas the other parent ignored or devalued them.

Many patients with narcissistic personality disorder were gifted in some way as children: They were brilliant, beautiful, athletic, or artistic.

Typically, one or both parents pushed them hard to gain accolades through this talent. When they excelled in their achievements or appearance in a way that reflected positively on the parent, they were showered with adoration and attention; otherwise, they were given little or nothing—they were ignored or devalued. They labored to keep displaying their gift for the sake of the parent's approval, because they were afraid that, if they stopped, the parent would abruptly withdraw attention or criticize them. There was a discrepancy between their specialness in one situation—when they were displaying their gift—and their worthlessness in another situation—when they were ordinary children.

Similarly, some patients with narcissistic personality disorder grew up in families that others viewed as special. Perhaps the family was wealthier than other families, one parent was famous or highly successful, or the family was in some other way higher in status. As children, these patients learned, "I'm special because my family is special." However, inside the family it was different—inside the family they were ignored or rejected. Inside the family, they learned that the children who got praise and attention were the ones who excelled. Children who were average were invisible. Again, there was a tension between their high value in one situation—outside the family—and their low value in another situation—inside the family.

Another common childhood origin of narcissism is social rejection or alienation. Some patients were loved and valued within the home, but outside the family they were rejected by peers or felt different in some significant way. Perhaps they were unattractive to the opposite sex, unathletic, or not as rich as the children around them. As adolescents, they were not popular or part of the "in crowd."

THE PATIENT WITH NARCISSISTIC PERSONALITY DISORDER IN INTIMATE RELATIONSHIPS

In treating patients with narcissistic personality disorder, the therapist's overarching goal is to help them learn how to get their core emotional needs met, both in therapy and in the outside world. The goal is to help the Lonely Child. Stated in terms of modes, the goal of treatment is to help the patient incorporate the Healthy Adult mode, modeled on the therapist, in order to recognize and nurture the Lonely Child, help the Lonely Child give and receive love, and reassure, and gradually replace, the Detached Self-Soother and the Self-Aggrandizer modes. In order to do this, the therapist must explore what patients do in their intimate relationships to cause their own core needs and their partner's core needs to go unmet. The patient's intimate relationships are a thus central focus of treatment.

We describe some characteristics often displayed by patients with narcissistic personality disorder in intimate relationships. Individual patients may have some or all of these characteristics.

Patients with Narcissistic Personality Disorder Are Unable to Absorb Love

Genuine love is so foreign to patients with narcissistic personality disorder that they are unable to absorb it. When someone tries to express empathy or nurture them, they simply cannot take it in. They can take in approval, they can take in admiration, they can take in attention, but they cannot take in love. This inability to absorb love perpetuates their Emotional Deprivation and Defectiveness schemas.

Relationships as Sources of Approval and Validation

In even the patient's most intimate relationships with romantic partners and spouses, admiration becomes the substitute for genuine love. This is one of the primary reasons that patients with narcissistic personality disorder are often so unhappy: Their core needs for love are not met, even in their most intimate relationships.

Many of these patients select partners who are themselves emotionally distant and have difficulty giving love. This is schema perpetuation—they are drawn to partners who are like the parent who emotionally deprived them. They feel comfortable not being loved and are willing to tolerate it (usually because they are unaware of what they are missing). Other patients select partners who are warm and giving and proceed to take everything and give nothing back. These patients do not set limits on how much they take; if the partner does not set limits, they will take endlessly, without reciprocating.

Limited Empathy

Largely because of the deprivation of empathy that they endured as children, many patients are unempathic, especially toward the people who are closest to them. Because they received so little empathy themselves, they do not know how to feel or express empathy for significant others.

Interestingly, when these patients are in the Lonely Child mode, they can often be quite empathic. It is when they are in the other two modes— the Self-Aggrandizer and the Detached Self-Soother—that these patients are most unempathic. It seems that most patients are capable of empathy but that when they are overcompensating for or avoiding their underlying schemas, they lose their capacity for empathy. Thus patients with narcissistic personality disorder often present a mixed picture in regard to empathy. For example, a father with narcissistic personality disorder might watch a movie about an unloved child and become very emotional. The father might even cry. Yet that same father might treat his own child the same way the child in the movie was treated and have little or no empathy. When he watches the child in the movie, the father switches into the Lonely Child mode and can empathize; but when he is with his own child, he switches into the Self-Aggrandizer mode and cannot empathize. What he is able to do in one mode, he is unable to do in another.

Envy

Patients with narcissistic personality disorder frequently feel envious of others whom they perceive as one-up in some way. The reason for this envy is that when someone else gets approval, these patients feel as if something has been taken away from them. They feel that there is not enough nurturance, attention, or admiration to go around. If someone else gets some, then they feel as if there is less left for them. They switch into the Lonely Child mode and feel cheated, unloved, deprived, and envious. Either they become depressed or more likely they mobilize and do something to restore their position as the center of attention. That is, they flip into the Self-Aggrandizing mode.

Idealization and Devaluing of Love Objects

Patients with narcissistic personality disorder often idealize their love objects in the initial stages of the relationship as a compensation for their Defectiveness schemas. They see the love object as perfect because, by gaining the approval of a perfect partner, they feel their own value has been heightened. In this stage, patients are hypersensitive to signs of criticism or rejection from their partner. They will often go overboard and do almost anything to win over the object of their affection.

These patients often select partners who make them look good—who are attractive and whom other people admire. At first they idealize and adore this partner. However, as time goes on, they begin to devalue the partner, spotting every little flaw and imperfection. Patients almost always display this pattern of devaluing their partners over time. There are a number of reasons for this. One reason is schema perpetuation: Every flaw in the partner triggers their own sense of defectiveness. To avoid feeling this defectiveness, they compensate by feeling superior to their partners. Patients devalue their partners in order to boost their own self-esteem. They make themselves feel better by putting the partner below them. They also devalue their partners because they can maintain control over the partners by keeping them in a lower position. Devaluing the partner makes it less likely that the partner will feel worthwhile enough to look for someone better and thus leave the patient. Each time one of the partner's imperfections is exposed, the patient becomes critical or contemptuous. Some patients become sadistic and humiliate their partners. Eventually they diminish the partners until the partners have little or no value to them. At this point the partners are no longer valuable as a source of approval.

If the partner responds to this treatment by trying harder to please the patient—as often happens—the strategy usually backfires. The more the partner tries to please the patient, the more the patient devalues the partner. The more the partner tries to appease, empathize with, or make excuses for the patient, the more devalued the partner becomes. In general, patients with narcissistic personality disorder only respect people who stand up to them and fight back. The more the partner fights back, the more the patient will value the partner, and the more the patient will value the partner's approval.

Entitlement in Relationships

These patients' Entitlement schema is usually a direct result of having been indulged as a child by one parent. It also serves as an additional source of validation. The patient reasons, "If I'm treated as special by my partner, then I have value. The more special I'm treated, the more value I have." Patients demand that almost every aspect of the relationship serve to satisfy them. They attempt to exert control over the environment and over the partners' behavior in order to gratify their own needs and desires (just as a parent often did to them in childhood).

The Detached Self-Soother in the Absence of External Validation

As these patients devalue their partners over time, they begin to distance from their partners and become more involved in solitary self-soothing behaviors. As the partners lose the capacity to serve the aggrandizing function, these patients increasingly isolate themselves from their partners by flipping into the Detached Self-Soother mode. To avoid the pain of the Lonely Child mode, patients turn to solitary addictions, compulsive behaviors, or stimulation-seeking rather than turning to their partners.

ASSESSMENT OF NARCISSISM

There are several methods for assessing narcissism. The therapist can observe the following: (1) the patient's behavior in therapy sessions; (2) the nature of the patient's presenting problem and history; (3) the patient's response to imagery exercises and questions about childhood (including the Young Parenting Inventory); and (4) the patient's Young Schema Questionnaire.

Observing the Patient's Behavior in Therapy Sessions

What are some early signs in therapy that a patient is narcissistic? In the beginning of treatment the most likely signs are behaviors that demonstrate entitlement. The patient cancels sessions at the last minute or comes late (yet expects a full session); asks detailed questions about the therapist's credentials to determine if he or she is "good enough"; tries to impress the therapist by mentioning achievements or talents; expects the therapist to return phone calls immediately; frequently makes unreasonable scheduling demands; complains about conditions in the therapist's office; requests special treatment; views the therapist as perfect (only to later devalue the therapist); interrupts the therapist when the therapist is talking or otherwise fails to listen to the therapist; constantly corrects the therapist about minor points; or refuses to adhere to the limits that the therapist has set.

Another early sign that a patient is narcissistic is a propensity to blame others. Rather than taking responsibility, these patients tend to blame other people as they discuss their own problems. As treatment progresses, the therapist sometimes becomes one of the targets of the patient's blame.

A final sign is that the patient appears to lack empathy, especially for significant others, including the therapist.

The Nature of the Patient's Presenting Problem and History

Often the presenting problem and history provide clues that the patient is narcissistic. One common reason that these patients enter treatment is that they are facing a crisis in their personal or professional lives because someone important to them—a lover, spouse, best friend, child, sibling, boss, business partner—is rejecting them or retaliating against them as a result of their own self-centered behavior. (There is a significant risk that, once the crisis resolves, the patient will prematurely leave treatment.)

Sometimes these patients come to treatment because someone is forcing them. Their partners or other family members are threatening to end the relationship unless they seek treatment. Their bosses have demanded that they either seek treatment or leave their jobs. Perhaps the criminal justice system has ordered them into treatment because they have done something illegal, such as driving while intoxicated. They have come to treatment against their will and do not believe their problems are their own fault. They frequently believe that it is other people who should change.

Another reason these patients may seek treatment is a sense of emptiness. Even though they have the outward trappings of success, their lives frequently lack a sense of inner meaning. At the center of their lives, there is a void: the unmet emotional needs of the Lonely Child. Although these patients may seem to have everything, their lives lack both intimate connections to others and true self-expression.

> We are the hollow men
> We are the stuffed men
> Leaning together
> Headpiece filled with straw. Alas!
> Our dried voices, when
> We whisper together
> Are quiet and meaningless
> As wind in dry grass
> Or rats' feet over broken glass
> In our dry cellar.
> —T. S. ELIOT, "The Hollow Men"

Some patients with narcissistic personality disorder come to treatment at moments of failure in their personal or professional lives. They have failed in some area of their lives that has served as an overcompensation, and they are now experiencing the underlying feelings of humiliation and despondency. They come for help rebuilding their overcompensations and become irritated whenever the therapist deviates from this function. (This is an important point: We do not believe that therapists should support the patient's narcissistic compensations. To do so means allying with the patient's Self-Aggrandizing mode, rather than the Lonely Child or Healthy Adult modes).

Some patients come to treatment because of problems arising from their Detached Self-Soother mode. They are gambling, abusing substances, acting out sexually in ways they later regret, or otherwise engaging in impulsive or compulsive behaviors that are self-destructive.

Finally, dissatisfaction with their marriages is another reason these patients come to therapy. For example, they might come to decide whether to leave a spouse for another person with whom they are having an affair.

Description of Childhood and Response to Imagery Exercises

Unless they are presenting "perfect" childhood memories, patients with narcissistic personality disorder are generally unable to accurately answer questions that explore deeper themes in their childhoods. They willingly discuss pleasant childhood memories, but they are unaware of painful childhood memories. These patients are usually opposed to doing imagery exercises of childhood involving any painful affect (other than anger).

They resist becoming vulnerable and switching into the Lonely Child mode.

Some patients—probably those with a better prognosis—are more willing to acknowledge the existence of the Lonely Child early in therapy. They are more willing to discuss painful childhood memories and to do imagery exercises. And when they generate childhood images, healthier patients can express and experience their feelings of loneliness or shame.

The Young Schema Questionnaire and Other Assessment Measures

We have found a consistent profile for patients with narcissistic personality disorder on the Young Schema Questionnaire. They typically score high on Entitlement, Unrelenting Standards, and Insufficient Self-Control and low on almost everything else. This profile is a testament to these patients' powers of overcompensation and avoidance. They are largely unaware of their core Emotional Deprivation and Defectiveness schemas, as well as their other schemas.

Interestingly, these patients are often able to identify many negative aspects of their parents' treatment of them as children on the Young Parenting Inventory. Even though they are unaware of their schemas, they are frequently able to report on the inventory what their parents did that was damaging to them. Patients with narcissistic personality disorder predictably score high on the Young Compensation Inventory, as they have a large number of compensatory behaviors.

CASE ILLUSTRATION

Presenting Problem and Current Clinical Picture

Carl is a 37-year-old patient with a diagnosis of narcissistic personality disorder. He first entered therapy with a schema therapist named Leah at the age of 36. We present segments of a consultation Dr. Young conducted with Carl that occurred approximately 1 year into Carl's therapy with Leah. Leah had requested this consultation with Dr. Young because she felt stuck in her therapy with Carl.

In the first segment, Dr. Young and Leah discuss the patient. (All other segments are from Dr. Young's session with the patient.) As the segment begins, Leah is describing how Carl presented when he first came to treatment and what it was like to work with him.

LEAH: Carl was very challenging. I did not believe that he would sustain therapy beyond a couple of sessions. I thought he would perhaps "try me out."

He could push my buttons almost the minute he walked through the door. He would never say my name, he was not one who would respond to nor initiate a greeting of any kind. He'd drop his jacket on the floor and sort of slump into the chair and say things like, "Did you practice those words to impress me this session? You want me to think you're smart, don't you?" So he would use very condescending language, and his very esoteric nature came right across, almost deliberately, to try to challenge me.

It felt like a game. It felt like a game from the very beginning.

DR. YOUNG: And what did that make you feel when you could see that he was making it like a game, challenging you, trying to beat you?

LEAH: Angry. I'd feel angry at him, that he was setting me up. My own schemas came up—and the temptation to want to play the game, and to win.

These are some of the typical feelings therapists experience when working with patients with narcissistic personality disorder. However, therapists should not make the mistake of trying to compete with or impress the patient. Such behavior only reinforces the patient's narcissism and prompts the patient to devalue the therapist over time.

After meeting with Leah, Dr. Young began his consultation with Carl. In the next segment, Carl tells Dr. Young his reasons for entering treatment. He is experiencing serious problems in both his marriage and his work life.

CARL: I'm 37 years old, I'm married, with two children. I grew up in Los Angeles, and I'm currently between careers.

DR. YOUNG: And are you planning to start a second career, or are you just enjoying not having one right now?

CARL: I'm certainly enjoying not having a career, and I may start a second career. This is part of what I'm doing now, trying to figure out what to do.

DR. YOUNG: I see. And what's your wife's name?

CARL: Danielle. We've been married about 9 years.

DR. YOUNG: Can you tell me what your current goals in therapy are? At this particular point, why do you think you're in treatment?

CARL: Well, right now I would say that I haven't yet been able to demonstrate any mastery whatsoever of what, in broad terms, I would call impulse control. In practical terms, I like to stay up all night and sleep during the day, in spite of the fact that I have an idea that this might not be the best way, because it interferes in a lot of ways with my life.

And so far I have been completely unable to make any meaningful progress in changing it.

DR. YOUNG: And are there any other goals you want to accomplish in therapy besides mastering this impulse control issue?

CARL: Well, that's the tangible goal. I think that I still recognize the need to continue working to discover how to be a person, and how to get along with people.

DR. YOUNG: And you feel that's something that's difficult for you? In what way is it difficult for you to get along with people?

CARL: Well, I consider myself a little bit different, unusual, or—there was one person who referred to me as a maverick; I don't know if that's really accurate. You can call me a maverick, or a nerd, or your typical maladjusted, self-centered kind of intellectual. (*Laughs.*)

DR. YOUNG: When you think about being different, does it seem like it's different and better, or different and worse, or different and comparable to other people?

CARL: Well, different and different, but also different and better. But in some contexts, different and worse.

DR. YOUNG: You also mentioned on one of your forms a "paralysis of the will." Is that still an issue, and what does that mean to you?

CARL: Well, at the time it meant that I was incapable of carrying out even the slightest act that was different from my daily routine, such as make a phone call, schedule an appointment to see a psychotherapist. I determined nearly 2 years ago that I really felt I needed help, and I didn't make a phone call about it for about 6 months.

DR. YOUNG: Because of the same paralysis.

CARL: Yeah.

DR. YOUNG: Do you have a sense now of what the paralysis was caused by, what it was about?

CARL: Well, I'm really not sure. It seems to be kind of a funk, kind of a state of depression.

It is noteworthy that Carl's tone of voice and manner of relating to the therapist are somewhat arrogant. He spoke as though he and Dr. Young were on an equal footing, not like a patient coming for help. He was detached in his manner, and his description of his problems was somewhat self-aggrandizing. An arrogant tone and manner are often the first clue that a patient is narcissistic.

Carl describes several reasons for seeking treatment. The first is his lack of impulse control. This is his Insufficient Self-Control/Self-Discipline schema, and it is part of the Self-Aggrandizer mode. He cannot place limits on his own behavior. The second reason is his difficulty relating to other people. This is a common problem among patients with narcissistic personality disorder—Carl is at least aware of this difficulty, unlike many other patients. The third reason is his "paralysis of the will"—the depression he feels when he is not getting enough stimulation or approval. Note that Carl does not understand this symptom, although he is aware that he is depressed. Later, the interviewer will try to connect his depression to his Lonely Child mode.

In the next segment, Carl discusses the reasons he is having trouble getting along with people. He begins by explaining why he thinks people might find him boring. The segment shows he has some insight into his behavior.

DR. YOUNG: Why do you think people would see you as boring?

CARL: Well, if I had to guess, I would say I'm the kind of person who starts every sentence with the word "I" (*laughs*).

DR. YOUNG: So you're boring because you're self-absorbed? That's what you're saying?

CARL: Yes. I think so.

DR. YOUNG: And do you have any sense of why you're self-absorbed? Why do you think you are so focused on yourself during conversations?

CARL: Oh, well, do you want me to talk to you about my mother? (*Laughs sarcastically.*)

DR. YOUNG: (*Laughs also.*) No, I wasn't thinking so much historically, more just at a gut level. What do you think that it is inside of you that keeps the focus on you, particularly when you now seem to have an awareness that this might turn some people off?

CARL: Well, that's the point, I don't really have the awareness. I don't go into a social interaction with the kind of mindfulness that theoretically one would think that one would be capable of. That's very hard for me. And it's not just a self-absorption, I think there's a kind of shyness or fear.

Carl has the capacity to recognize that he is too self-centered in social situations, but only when he is in the mode he is in at this point in the interview. This is a detached mode. Getting him out of this detached mode is the focus of the interview. When Carl is actually in social situations, his Self-Aggrandizer mode is dominant, and he loses his awareness that he is too self-centered.

Carl shows some awareness of the shyness that is underneath his Self-Aggrandizer mode, which is a good prognostic sign. However, he seems blasé about the fact that he is self-centered—he does not appear to be troubled by it. This is typical of patients with narcissistic personality disorder. Even when they show some insight into their self-centered behavior, they do not seem particularly disturbed by it. In their *belle indifférence,* they are not upset to discover that they have alienated other people or been unfair.

In this next segment, Carl describes his feelings toward his wife. He exhibits the devaluing of the partner that we mentioned earlier as characteristic of patients with narcissistic personality disorder at later stages of relationships.

DR. YOUNG: How about with your wife? How do you feel with her? One of the things you said on here (*points to questionnaires*) was that one of your wishes would be to "trade in your wife."

CARL: Yes.

DR. YOUNG: So there must be some negative feelings about the relationship, some disappointment. . . .

CARL: She's doing a little better now. We're doing a little better. I've more or less moved past that.

DR. YOUNG: What was the disappointment in her? In what ways was she disappointing?

CARL: Well, she was disappointing in her level of integrity, her level of commitment to truth, her level of commitment to self-awareness, and her intellectual capacity.

As one might deduce from the unsympathetic way that criticisms of his wife roll off his tongue here, Carl's narcissism is not fully healed yet.

In the next segment, Carl describes his wife's self-absorption. The segment shows that, even though he denigrates her, he still has some insight into her realistic limitations.

DR. YOUNG: How do you treat Danielle?

CARL: Well, sometimes I've been in the past very cold, very distant. Sometimes she doesn't even notice it. In her own way she's more self-absorbed than I am. She'll obsess on her problems to the extent that she really blocks out the world, and, if I have trouble getting in touch with *my* emotions, I would say that she has more trouble getting in touch with *her* emotions.

DR. YOUNG: What drew you to her in the first place?

CARL: Well, originally I saw this kind of kindred spirit, because I think that we have a lot of things in common in terms of our dysfunctionality.

As often happens with patients with narcissistic personality disorder, Carl chose a woman to marry who reinforced his childhood sense of emotional deprivation.

TREATMENT OF NARCISSISM

Primary Goal of Treatment

The primary goal of treatment is to build up the patient's Healthy Adult mode, modeled on the therapist, capable of reparenting the Lonely Child and fighting the Self-Aggrandizer and the Detached Self-Soother modes. The goal is increased vulnerability with less overcompensation and less avoidance.

More specifically, the goal of treatment is to help construct a Healthy Adult mode to:

1. Help the Lonely Child to feel nurtured and understood, and to nurture and empathize with others.
2. Confront the Self-Aggrandizer so that the patient gives up the excessive need for approval and treats others based on reciprocity, as the Lonely Child takes in more genuine love.
3. Help the Detached Self-Soother give up maladaptive addictive and avoidant behaviors and replace them with genuine love, self-expression, and experiencing of affect.

The therapist helps the patient establish authentic intimate relationships, first with the therapist and then with appropriate significant others. As the Lonely Child takes in more love and empathy, the patient no longer has to substitute applause or numbness for love and no longer has to act in a demeaning or self-centered manner with others. Both the Self-Aggrandizer and the Detached Self-Soother modes weaken and gradually fade.

The primary focus of treatment, therefore, is the patient's intimate relationships—both the therapy relationship and the patient's other significant relationships. As with our treatment of the patient with BPD, the primary strategy is mode work.

We present the elements of the treatment roughly in the order in which we introduce them to the patient.

The Therapist Establishes the Current Complaints as Leverage

The therapist strives to keep patients in touch with their emotional suffering because as soon as the suffering is gone, they are likely to leave treatment. The more the therapist keeps patients aware of their inner emptiness, feelings of defectiveness, and loneliness, the more the therapist has leverage for keeping them in treatment. If the patient comes into treatment in a state of emotional distress, this state can serve as leverage to keep the patient motivated to stay in treatment and try to change. The therapist also focuses on the negative consequences of the patient's narcissism, such as rejection by loved ones or setbacks in one's career.

Most patients with narcissistic personality disorder do not come to treatment with the goal of working on their underlying feelings of emotional deprivation and defectiveness. Rather, their goal is to get back some source of approval they have lost or to rid themselves of some negative consequence of their self-aggrandizing or self-soothing behaviors. They come for help bolstering their Self-Aggrandizer and Detached Self-Soothing modes. Once it becomes clear that the therapist will not serve the interests of these two modes, some patients become angry and decide to leave treatment. However, if the therapist can keep these patients aware of their emotional suffering and of the inevitable life losses and negative consequences if they do not change, then these can be reasons to stay. The emotional connection to the therapist and fear of reprisal from others are the main motivators for continuing in therapy. If the therapist can keep the patient in the Lonely Child mode and nurture the patient, then the patient is likely to stay in treatment, even though, in the other modes, the patient does not want to stay.

The Therapist Bonds with the Lonely Child

Within the therapy relationship, the therapist tries to create a place in which the patient feels cared about and valued, without having to be perfect or special, and in which the patient cares about and values the therapist, without the therapist having to be perfect or special. The therapist establishes a bond with the Lonely Child. The therapist values the patient for expressing vulnerability and gives the patient "unconditional positive regard" (Rogers, 1951).

Patients with narcissistic personality disorder often do not know that they have trouble experiencing intimacy. They may never have experienced true intimacy. Through the therapy relationship, they begin to realize how difficult it is for them to get emotionally close to other human beings. The therapist reframes the goal of therapy as helping patients to stay in the Lonely Child mode and try to get their basic emotional needs met. In contrast to the parent, who was there for the Self-Aggrandizer, the therapist is there for the Lonely Child. The therapist helps the patient tolerate the pain of being in the Lonely Child mode without switching into one of the other modes. The therapist nurtures the patient in the Lonely Child mode, promoting schema healing. Through "limited reparenting," the therapist provides a partial antidote to the patient's Emotional Deprivation and Defectiveness schemas, as well as to the patient's other schemas.

The therapist confronts the patient's approval-seeking behavior without devaluing the patient. The therapist always gives the same message: "It's you I care about, not your performance or appearance." Similarly, the therapist confronts the patient's entitled behavior without devaluing the patient. Emphasizing the principle of reciprocity, the therapist sets limits. The therapist gives the message: "I care about you, but I also care about myself and others. We all deserve caring equally."

When the patient becomes inappropriately angry at the therapist, the therapist empathically confronts the patient. The therapist expresses sympathy and understanding of the patient's point of view but corrects any of the patient's distorted ideas that the therapist is selfish, depriving, devaluing, or controlling. If the patient notes a valid criticism, but in a demeaning way, then the therapist asserts the right to be valued nonetheless. The therapist gives the message, "We all deserve caring, even when we are imperfect." The therapist points out how the devaluing behavior makes the therapist feel and what its impact would be on other people outside therapy. The therapist also helps the patient rise above the incident in order to understand in mode terms, why the patient is engaging in the behavior.

The Therapist Tactfully Confronts the Patient's Condescending or Challenging Style

Sooner or later, most patients with narcissistic personality disorder begin to treat their therapists the same way they treat everybody else—in a condescending or challenging manner. The patient begins to devalue the therapist. It is important for the therapist to stand up to the patient when this happens, or else the therapist will lose the patient's respect.

Confronting these patients is often difficult for therapists, especially because, in our experience, so many therapists have Self-Sacrifice or Subjugation schemas. These schemas tend to make assertiveness in the face of narcissism a formidable task. If these patients resemble one of the therapist's parents in an important way—for example, if they are demanding, critical, or controlling—then the therapist is at risk of resuming maladaptive childhood coping behaviors rather than doing what is best for the patient. For example, therapists may give in to unreasonable requests or tolerate entitled behavior.

Therapists must be alert to the activation of their own schemas in their treatment of patients with narcissistic personality disorder. The triggering of the therapist's schemas can lead to counterproductive responses, such as retaliating or competing, that damage rather than help patients. Therapists with Self-Sacrifice or Subjugation schemas generally had a parent who was cold, needy, or controlling, so that the behaviors of patients with narcissistic personality disorder often replicate what that parent did that was hurtful when they were children. These therapists are thus at risk to revert to their childhood coping strategies with these patients, rather than reparenting the patient.

It is important that the therapist stand up to the patient, but through empathic confrontation. The therapist can make statements such as the following:

> "I know that you don't mean to hurt me, but, when you speak to me that way, it *feels* like you're trying to hurt me."

> "When you talk to me in that tone of voice, I feel distant from you, even though I know you're upset and need me to be here for you."

> "When you speak to me in such a demeaning way, it causes me to pull away from you, and makes it harder for me to give you what you need."

> "Even though underneath you want to be close to people, if you speak that way to them, they are not going to want to be close to you."

The therapist points out the patient's devaluing behavior, showing understanding of why the patient is behaving in this manner, yet still letting the patient know the negative consequences of the behavior in relationships—with the therapist and with other people in the patient's life.

In the following segment, Dr. Young begins to confront Carl's Self-Aggrandizing and Detached Self-Soother modes. In the context of a discussion about Carl's early relationship with his wife Danielle, Dr. Young points out that Carl is behaving in a devaluing way toward him.

DR. YOUNG: What did Danielle look like at that time? Was she beautiful? Was she your ideal?

CARL: She was beautiful. But don't forget, I was drunk, I was sitting down, she was sitting down (*laughs*). I always tell the joke that I would never have fallen in love with someone so short, except I was drunk and we were sitting down.
     She had the right body type, she had the right hair color.

DR. YOUNG: So she met all these objective criteria.

CARL: (*annoyed*) They're not objective criteria. These are the felt, somewhat ineffable criteria that we have, that we don't know where they come from.

DR. YOUNG: But she seemed to fit all these things that intuitively connect you . . .

CARL: (*Interrupts.*) Well, she fit *close enough*. And she was interested in me, and I was ready. I mean, there's a confluence of factors here.

DR. YOUNG: (*pause*) One thing that it feels like as we talk, Carl, is that when I say something that is slightly off base, maybe like one degree off base from what you feel, you pick up on it and sort of fight back as if we were in an argument. Do you know what I mean? Rather than saying, "Yeah, you're right, that's right, but it's not quite it," you say, "That's completely off."

CARL: (*annoyed*) I don't see it as one degree off. I wouldn't say *one* degree off, but I would say *five* degrees off—I see it as being different. I'm very picky that way, aren't I?

The therapist confronts Carl gently, then Carl responds in a challenging manner. The therapist continues to speak empathically, while Carl continues to devalue the therapist's observations. However, this does not deter the therapist, who continues to confront Carl without becoming angry or punitive toward him; instead, the therapist repeatedly points out the consequences of Carl's behavior in his relationships with the therapist and with other people in his life. The therapist tries to rise above the immediate incident, calmly observe the patient, express empathy, and provide objective feedback and education.

DR. YOUNG: What is the effect on the other person you're talking to of your doing that, of your making those corrections?

CARL: I don't know (*laughs softly*).

DR. YOUNG: What would you guess? You mentioned that you're a sensitive person . . .

CARL: (*Interrupts.*) I'm sensitive normally to how people are reacting. Right now, it seems to bother you. It seems to make you upset, that kind of correction.

DR. YOUNG: Well, I think it would upset other people to be corrected every time they said something. I'm a psychologist, and I understand that, with the kind of issues you have, being perfectionistic and getting everything right on target is very important, so I'm able to say, "Well, from his perspective, the task of getting everything right is crucial and important."

CARL: (*Interrupts.*) It only seems to be crucial or important to me in a conversation.

DR. YOUNG: Yes, but what I'm saying is, with somebody who isn't a psychologist trying to understand your makeup, if you do the same thing, the person is going to experience it, I think, as a kind of criticism, that what they said was not intelligent enough, it wasn't living up to your expectations for a conversation.

CARL: Or as an unnecessary addendum to a subject that requires no more continuation.

DR. YOUNG: Yes, but I'm not so concerned about that as the part where their feelings are hurt, though.

Carl tries to shift the focus away from the idea of hurting other people: He tries to keep the discussion at an intellectual level and to justify what he is doing as not very serious. However, the therapist does not allow him to get away with this. The therapist keeps gently but firmly reasserting that Carl's behavior is hurtful to others. In the next segment, Carl begins to demonstrate some insight into his behavior in the session.

CARL: So what you're pointing out to me, which I think is a useful observation, is that I have a tendency to contextualize all interactions as this kind of game—you could call it a game—where the object is a kind of intellectualization. So it's a very narrow context for whatever interaction is going on.

DR. YOUNG: What it does is that it has the effect of cutting off feelings. Whatever feelings I'm having about you, or that you might be having about me, sort of get lost in the verbiage. It's sort of like reading a book that is so much about the words that there's not enough emotion.

CARL: Perhaps it's my pattern. Perhaps it's my pattern to cut off the emotion.

Carl acknowledges the truth of what the therapist is saying—that he intellectualizes and criticizes to avoid his feelings—which is a sign of progress on his part. However, he soon goes back to deriding the therapist. Dr. Young brings up Carl's current therapist, Leah.

DR. YOUNG: One of the things Leah had mentioned was this "dance of domination"—that's one of your themes.

CARL: (*Laughs mockingly.*) I thought it was just something *you* picked up on. I don't know if it's one of my themes. It's a catchy phrase.

DR. YOUNG: Yes, she mentioned it, but it seems like it might be relevant in this context. It might be that in intellectual conversations, there's a subtext of two people competing on an intellectual level to see who's smarter, or to see who is more precise.

CARL: (*challenging*) Yeah, yeah. And if you'll notice, that it *takes two to tango*.

DR. YOUNG: (*in disbelief*) And you're saying that I enjoyed it, too?

This kind of jousting back and forth is intrinsic to the treatment of patients with narcissistic personality disorder. The patient keeps debating with or devaluing the therapist, and the therapist keeps responding by pointing out the effects of this behavior, both on the therapist and on other important people in the patient's life.

As the interview between the therapist and Carl progresses, Carl gradually begins to acknowledge the truth of what the therapist is saying. Even though there is a part of Carl that keeps fighting the therapist—the self-aggrandizing, detached mode that does not want to feel diminished and refuses to give up—there is also a healthy part of him that becomes more receptive to the therapist and more aware of what he is doing. It is the goal of treatment to help Carl elaborate this Healthy Adult mode

The Therapist Tactfully Expresses His or Her Rights Whenever the Patient Violates Them

The therapist is appropriately assertive with the patient each time the patient behaves in a devaluing manner. The therapist sets limits for the patient in the same way that a parent does for a child. Just as a good parent does not permit behaviors inside the home that would be unacceptable outside of the home—such as bullying or speaking in a demeaning manner—the therapist does not allow the patient to act toward the therapist in ways that would be unacceptable with people outside of therapy. The therapist sets limits when the patient misbehaves.

Here are some guidelines that therapists can follow when setting limits with patients with narcissistic personality disorder.

1. *Therapists empathize with the narcissistic point of view and are tactful in confronting entitlement.* The therapist empathizes with why it feels "right" for the patient with narcissistic personality disorder to act selfishly, while at the same time letting the patient know how this behavior affects others. The therapist must strike just the right balance between empathy and confrontation.

If the therapist does not express enough empathy, then the patient will feel misunderstood and denigrated and will not listen to what the therapist is saying. If the therapist does not confront the patient enough, then the patient will feel as though the therapist has given implicit permission for the entitled behavior.

2. *Therapists neither defend themselves nor attack back when patients devalue them.* The therapist does not get lost in the content of the patient's attacks. The therapist rises above the specific content and does not take it personally, focusing not on the content but on the interpersonal aspects of the discussion. The therapist who argues about the content of what the patient is saying is usually making a mistake. As soon as the therapist be-

comes defensive or attacks back, then the therapist is playing the patient's "game," and the patient is controlling the session. Rather, the therapist stays focused on the *process* of what is happening—that the patient is devaluing the therapist to avoid his own emotions—and keeps empathically confronting the patient about the consequences of this behavior.

3. *Therapists assert their rights nonpunitively.* When patients violate the therapist's rights, the therapist, again using empathic confrontation, points it out. The therapist says something like: "I know that you're probably not intending to hurt me, and deep down what you're feeling is misunderstood, but I'm not comfortable with the way you're speaking to me right now."

4. *Therapists do not let themselves be bullied by patients into doing things they do not want to do.* Rather, therapists set clear limits based on what feels comfortable and fair to them, regardless of the pressures the patient brings to bear. For example, therapists do not allow patients to persuade them to constantly reschedule, run over the session time, analyze potential lovers or rivals to help patients manipulate them or win power struggles, or otherwise exceed the boundaries of the therapeutic relationship. In addition, therapists do not try to bully their patients back.

5. *Therapists establish that the therapy relationship is mutual, based on reciprocity, not on a master–slave principle.* When the patient treats the therapist in an entitled way, the therapist points it out. The therapist says something like: "I know you're afraid and you need me to help you right now, but I feel like you're treating me like a servant, and that's pushing me away" or "You're treating me disrespectfully, and it's making it hard for me to be there for you in the way I want to be there, since I know you're suffering underneath."

Often the patient will respond, "I'm paying you." The therapist can respond: "You're paying for my time, not for the right to treat me disrespectfully." The therapist communicates that the only acceptable terms for the relationship are those of equals. The fact that the patient is paying the therapist does not entitle the patient to mistreat the therapist, nor does it obligate the therapist to fulfill all of the patient's demands.

6. *Therapists look for evidence of underlying vulnerability and point it out each time it occurs.* The therapist looks for the Lonely Child in the patient and draws the patient's attention to the mode whenever it surfaces. Such signs include expressions of anxiety, sadness, or shame; admissions of weakness; and acknowledgment of unmet needs. The therapist encourages the patient to stay in the Lonely Child mode as much as possible and reparents the patient.

7. *Therapists rise above specific incidents and ask the patient to explore the motivation behind entitled, self-aggrandizing, devaluing, or avoidant state-*

ments. Therapists do not get caught up in the content of arguments. Rather, they address the *way* the patient is behaving and the *effect* this behavior has on other people. The therapist realizes that the patient is feeling vulnerable underneath. When patients behave in a devaluing manner, many times they are trying to make the therapist feel the way the therapist made them feel, and the content of the argument reveals more about how the patient felt denigrated than about the patient's perceptions of the therapist's flaws.

To avoid sounding accusatory, the therapist asks questions. The therapist says, "Why are you doing this right now? Why are you being condescending? Why are you pushing me away? Why don't you want to talk about this? Why are you angry with me?"

Often patients with narcissistic personality disorder are very bright and are able to outsmart the therapist and win arguments. However, even when they are winning arguments, they are still wrong if they are treating the therapist in a devaluing or uncaring way. They may not be wrong in the content of the argument, but they are certainly wrong in the process and style. By rising above incidents, the therapist can avoid most arguments.

8. *Therapists look for common narcissistic themes and point them out to the patient.* Examples of common narcissistic themes are (a) condescending, one-up, competitive behavior; (b) judgmental, critical, and evaluative comments, positive or negative; and (c) status-seeking statements or those that reflect an emphasis on external appearances or performance instead of internal qualities such as love and fulfillment.

Once again, in order to be supportive rather than critical, the therapist can point out the themes in the form of questions. The therapist says: "Why do you think you might be acting in a condescending way right now?" or "Why are you pushing me away?" or "Why do you think it's so important for you to tell me about your achievements?"

9. *Therapists label statements that seem to represent the Self-Aggrandizing or Detached Self-Soother modes.* This helps patients learn to recognize their modes when they are in them. When patients are in the Self-Aggrandizing mode or the Detached Self-Soother mode the therapist draws the patient's attention to the mode, and helps the patient to recognize emotionally the experience of being in the mode.

The Therapist Shows Vulnerability

One of the best ways therapists can show patients with narcissistic personality disorder that it is acceptable to be vulnerable is to be vulnerable themselves. Rather than appearing perfect, therapists acknowledge their vulnerability. Therapists *model* vulnerability: They acknowledge when their feelings are hurt and admit mistakes readily to the degree that would be appropriate in a close relationship. They are willing to be imperfect. Even if many of these patients view vulnerability as a sign of weakness, it is still important for the therapist to express appropriate vulnerability. We are not suggesting that therapists discuss intimate details of their personal lives; rather, we are suggesting that therapists share with patients the vulnerable feelings that naturally arise in the course of the therapy session. Generally, it is better for therapists to show more vulnerability as the sessions progress rather than toward the beginning of treatment. If therapists show too much vulnerability early on, the patient may misinterpret it to mean that the therapist is too weak to deal with the patient's difficult behavior. The therapist has to come from a place of strength, having already demonstrated the ability to set limits. Thus what the therapist is trying to convey is really a subtle blend of confidence, strength, and vulnerability.

In the following segment, the therapist expresses vulnerability in order to encourage Carl to do the same. As the segment begins, the therapist is suggesting to Carl that his competitiveness (the "game") is driven by underlying feelings of inadequacy of which he is largely unaware. That is, Carl is compensating for the feelings of the Lonely Child by flipping into the Self-Aggrandizing mode.

DR. YOUNG: Playing this game, what function does it serve for you? What is the underlying function of playing a game like this with someone?

CARL: (*annoyed*) I don't know. It's just a naturally stimulating way to be.

DR. YOUNG: It feels like there's a deeper answer to that question.

CARL: Yes, what would be the purpose of playing that game in general? If I can think about a time when that's the kind of game I would play, that would be the purpose. But if I look at specifically why I would start playing that game with you . . . (*pause*). If, in fact, it does detach me from the content of the interaction, then it is a way of me controlling the conversation, and shifting it away from perhaps the emotional content, which might be a little uncomfortable, to a sphere which is more comfortable.

DR. YOUNG: Yes, that feels right to me. That feels like what was happening. Do you have a sense of what you might be trying to steer away from that's uncomfortable? What would it be like to not play that game at all, and to just be completely emotional with each other? You could share your emotional reactions about me, and I could share my emotional reactions about you. I could ask you questions about what you're feeling at an emotional level, and you would just openly discuss it.

CARL: I think it would be difficult.

At this point, Carl is seeing his motivation accurately—to steer the conversation away from emotional topics that hold the potential to upset him. He chooses detachment and self-aggrandizement to avoid intimacy and the Lonely Child. These avoidant and compensatory modes keep the Lonely Child at bay. Carl has stopped devaluing the therapist. He is shifting into the Lonely Child mode for moments, and then shifting back.

The Therapist Introduces the Concept of the Lonely Child Mode

The therapist then begins to address Carl's Lonely Child mode more directly. The therapist refers to the fact that the interview is being videotaped and asks Carl about his feelings. Carl answers by denying any vulnerable feelings on his part. The therapist responds by expressing his own vulnerability.

DR. YOUNG: How do you feel being here with me, or being here in this situation being taped? Apart from the intellectual analysis of it, what's your gut-level feeling about being in this situation?

CARL: I think that I'm able to ignore it.

DR. YOUNG: There is no emotional reaction or content?

CARL: (*pause*) On my part or on your part?

DR. YOUNG: Both parts. I certainly have an emotional reaction. Here I am, doing a videotape that people will be watching . . .

CARL: (*Interrupts.*) Well, you're a lot more salient than I am, because I'm an anonymous patient more or less, and you are the person who is conducting this (*chuckles*). I won't be judged by what's going on here, *you* will be judged. That's something that's in *your* consciousness. It doesn't have to be in *my* consciousness.

DR. YOUNG: Intellectually that makes sense, but somehow, at a gut level, I don't believe it. I believe that anyone who's in this situation would have an emotional response underneath.

CARL: (*annoyed*) Why don't you talk about how *you* feel!

DR. YOUNG: Well, I think I did. I was saying: to me, I feel somewhat nervous because, here I am in a situation where I have high expectations for myself, the people watching will have high expectations, and there's a real chance that I could make a mistake, it could go badly, and it would be embarrassing.

CARL: (*Interrupts.*) But don't you see, there's no chance I could make a mistake. I'm the patient. I can do and say whatever I want. (*Laughs triumphantly.*)

DR. YOUNG: I'm not saying you're wrong, but are you sure that's what you're feeling underneath, that there's no other level of anxiety or concern about how other people are viewing you?

CARL: Perhaps that's hard for you to understand, because you would expect people to be self-conscious.

DR. YOUNG: Yes. Particularly you: You mentioned you had shyness.

CARL: Yes, but it so happens that I'm really not self-conscious.

Carl is in the Self-Aggrandizing mode, subtly putting the therapist down and simultaneously unaware of his own Vulnerable Child mode. The therapist persists, but it is too early for the patient to recognize what he is feeling underneath.

The therapist begins suggesting to the patient that inside of him there is a Lonely Child—a core part of the patient that feels vulnerable, frightened, inadequate, and lost. The therapist reinforces the patient's vulnerability, while still pointing out the Self-Aggrandizer and Detached Self-Soother modes.

In the following segment, Dr. Young explores Carl's relationship with his therapist, Leah, to see if Carl can acknowledge any feelings of vulnerability or emotional connection with her. Again, Carl shows the same difficulty acknowledging vulnerability.

DR. YOUNG: How do you feel when you're in sessions with Leah, as opposed to this sort of situation? What's your emotional feeling when you're in session with her? Is it different, or is it the same as in here?

CARL: Well, I think that I try to bring whatever capacities that I've learned in my sessions with Leah, to try and be able to apply them here.

DR. YOUNG: No, I meant, when you're in sessions with Leah, what emotions do you have? What emotions are going on in you when you're in a session with Leah?

CARL: Well, I try to keep a detached mien, and be conscious of and mindful of the emotions as they arise.

DR. YOUNG: But there's some sense of not wanting to get lost in emotions, not wanting to get too caught up in them?

CARL: Well, not necessarily. Sometimes I think I like to get caught up in my emotions and discover them and feel them.

DR. YOUNG: But why would you try to maintain a detached mien?

CARL: No, I think that the detached mien is just my natural state. That's the natural state of Carl.

DR. YOUNG: Detached.

CARL: Yes.

DR. YOUNG: Then we're back to that other explanation, that you're detached in order to avoid certain emotional feelings that you don't want to experience.

CARL: You're asking now why I learned to become detached. I didn't start being detached at the age of 37.

DR. YOUNG: When do you think it was that you started developing this separate side of you?

CARL: Perhaps four or earlier, and certainly as a young boy growing up, unquestionably.

Carl acknowledges that he is detached, that detachment is his normal state of being, and that it started very early in his life. Now the therapist has an inroad into his Lonely Child mode. Now the therapist can explore what is underneath his detachment—why at age 4 he started detaching and what he felt prior to detaching that led to the development of this mode.

Dr. Young and Carl call the detached part of Carl, "Detached Carl." In reality, this mode is a blend of the Self-Aggrandizer and Detached Self-Soother modes.

The Therapist Explores the Childhood Origins of the Modes through Imagery

Once the patient is aware of the modes, the therapist moves onto exploring the origins of the modes in childhood, especially the patient's Lonely Child mode. We have found that the best way to accomplish this is through the use of imagery. However, first the therapist must nearly always overcome the patient's opposition to doing imagery.

In the following segment, the therapist explores the origins of Carl's detached mode. The therapist asks Carl to do an imagery exercise, but Carl first expresses a variety of reservations about proceeding and then resists the imagery process.

DR. YOUNG: Would you be willing to do an imagery exercise to get to what you were like before that? Could I ask you to close your eyes and picture yourself as that 3-year-old child, before you detached—so I could get a feeling for what that emotional part of you was like at that point, before you shut off? Would you be willing to try that, and tell me what you see?

CARL: You could try, but I wouldn't be too hopeful, about 3-year-olds (laughs).

DR. YOUNG: Well, try to get the youngest age you can picture.

CARL: You know, I think going back is like, there once was a well that over the years the weather and the dirt has filled it in, and if you want to get down to the bottom, you just can't look down there, you have to dig all this dirt out first, that's what it feels like to me.

DR. YOUNG: Yes, I see what you mean. The image seems hard to get to. But let's try. (*Pause.*) Now close your eyes and get an image of Little Carl, as a child, and tell me what you see. Try to keep your eyes closed until we finish the exercise. Another thing is, try to do it in images. Don't analyze it, or comment on it, try just to tell me what you see, as though it's a movie going through your head.

CARL: Well, generally speaking, I don't see images.

DR. YOUNG: So—keeping your eyes closed—as you try to picture Carl as a child, you don't actually see anything?

CARL: Right. I don't see an image, a cognizable image.

DR. YOUNG: What do you actually see when you look back there?

CARL: Well, I'll try to get some kind of impression.

DR. YOUNG: Yes, that would be good.

CARL: I'll try and just take whatever I get. But it won't be in the form of an image that I can really *see.*

DR. YOUNG: Well, the closest you could get to that would be OK.

Carl is still resisting, but at least he is willing to start. Because he said he was having trouble generating an image of himself as a child, Dr. Young suggests that, instead, he get an image of his mother when he was a child. (Offering the patient increasingly easier tasks is one strategy for countering the patient's resistance to doing imagery.)

DR. YOUNG: How about getting an image of your mother from when you were young, and starting from that. Would that be easier?

CARL: Yes.

DR. YOUNG: What do you feel when you look at the expression on her face in the image? Do you have any reaction to it? What do you feel?

CARL: Well, I feel very sad, because I think I love my mother deeply and dearly, and I just want to be with her and love her.

DR. YOUNG: And does she make that easy?

CARL: (*long pause*) No.

DR. YOUNG: Can you tell me what she's like toward you and how she treats you?

CARL: I can't get an authentic image but, it's as if she's just made of stone. She doesn't move.

DR. YOUNG: Can you tell her right now in the image, as if you were that child, although you couldn't have said it then, what you needed from her? Just say it out loud to her right now so I can hear.

CARL: (*as a child*) "Mommy, I just want you to hug me and love me and pay attention to me and be with me always. And never let me go."

DR. YOUNG: Is it easy for her to touch you, or does she have a hard time showing affection?

CARL: She's stone. She's made of stone in this image.

DR. YOUNG: Yes, and therefore, when you look at her, can you imagine that she's thinking anything? Could you go into her mind?

CARL: (*long pause*) I just think she has a lot of sadness.

DR. YOUNG: And what is she thinking to herself about you, as you're saying to her, "I want to be with you, I want to hold you, I want you to love me."

CARL: I think she can only hear it with just a part of her. I think she's preoccupied with her sadness.

DR. YOUNG: I see. So she's self-absorbed with her own mood.

CARL: Yeah.

DR. YOUNG: Now have her answer you when you say that to her.

CARL: She doesn't really want to talk to me. In fact, I think that she's angry that I'm intruding on her.

DR. YOUNG: How does that make you feel, that she's angry at you?

CARL: It makes me feel terrible.

Here we access the Lonely Child for the first time in the imagery. The patient describes a mother made of stone who cannot give of herself emotionally; and he is a child, wanting her love and having no way to get it.

The therapist has been moving toward this moment all along, trying to get Carl to acknowledge and experience his Lonely Child mode. At last, the therapist has bypassed Carl's detached, self-aggrandizing mode, with whom only a shallow bond is possible. Now the therapist can form a bond with the Lonely Child. The therapist can reparent the Lonely Child and begin the process of schema healing.

The Therapist Does Mode Work with the Patient

The therapist helps patients learn to identify and label their modes and then to create dialogues between them. In the following excerpt, the therapist identifies two modes—"Little Carl" and "Detached Carl." The former is the Lonely Child, and the latter is a combination of the Detached Self-

Soother and the Self-Aggrandizer modes. Beginning with Little Carl, Dr. Young helps Carl connect emotionally to his modes.

DR. YOUNG: I want you to split yourself into two Carls: the Carl that's the little child who wants his mother's love, and then this other Carl, who's got the detached manner.

CARL: OK.

DR. YOUNG: Can you see them both?

CARL: (*Nods.*) Yes.

DR. YOUNG: Describe them both to me, so I can see how they look different, how they feel different.

CARL: Well, the Carl that wants his mother's love is very sad. (*Pause.*) He's so sad he's making the detached part sad. (*Laughs.*)

DR. YOUNG: I see. Is he like, *paralyzed* sad, like he just wants to stay in bed all the time, that kind of sad, like he can barely move?

CARL: (*pause*) No. Almost.

DR. YOUNG: Almost.

CARL: But not quite.

Here the therapist links Carl's depression to the sadness of the Lonely Child.

Once the therapist has helped Carl recognize his Vulnerable Child and Detached–Aggrandizing modes, the therapist moves on to exploring the schemas underlying the modes. The therapist begins asking questions to determine what schemas characterize Carl's Lonely Child mode. Specifically, he investigates whether Carl has an underlying Defectiveness schema, in addition to the Emotional Deprivation schema he has already portrayed in his image of a mother made of stone.

DR. YOUNG: And does he feel insecure, unloved, rejected, or is he just lonely? What's making him sad?

CARL: I think he feels insecure about . . . (*pause*). Well, mostly rejected, I would say.

DR. YOUNG: Does he have any sense of why his mother doesn't want to love him the way he wants?

CARL: No, he's just confused.

DR. YOUNG: Does he think there's something wrong with him?

CARL: No.

DR. YOUNG: What does he think it is?

CARL: He doesn't understand.

DR. YOUNG: He doesn't know.

CARL: No, he just doesn't understand.

DR. YOUNG: He just misses it so much?

CARL: Yeah, and he has *no* understanding why.

DR. YOUNG: Is he lonely? Does he feel isolated or lonely?

CARL: He's lonely for his mother.

Carl indicates that he has an Emotional Deprivation schema, but not a Defectiveness schema. He feels lonely, but not personally deficient.

The therapist educates patients about schema modes. Dr. Young presents the modes to Carl, using Carl's own modes to illustrate.

DR. YOUNG: Looking at your issues, you seem to have two schema modes. One mode is the lonely, vulnerable child, and that's the Carl you connected with at three years old with his mother, who feels sad and lonely, because nobody really gives him the love he needs.

Then there's this second mode, which in your case is an entitled mode combined with a self-soothing mode. And this other mode is designed to hide and compensate for and avoid this more vulnerable little child mode that you don't want to experience.

CARL: (*Speaks in agreement.*) Detached Carl is really not interested in getting close, not at all interested in getting close.

Dr. Young continues exploring Carl's other schemas. Citing Carl's questionnaires, he attempts to determine whether Carl has an underlying Mistrust/Abuse schema. He asks Carl if he views other people as trying to mistreat him.

DR. YOUNG: I feel that, with Detached Carl, from the things you said on the inventories, that there's a more malevolent view of other people, too. It's not just a view that people won't give you love, it sounds like there are views of other people that are even more negative: the idea that they're trying to get you one-down, or expose you, or beat you, meaning "win" over you.

CARL: Well, I think that Detached Carl develops a compensation to have a life and that involves competition.

DR. YOUNG: And that gives him a sense of value and purpose?

CARL: Yes.

DR. YOUNG: The competition is the value.

CARL: Yes. And so this competition, I believe, exists on many planes, not just in the games arena, where it's obvious, but also in just the interaction, as you were able to witness, that Detached Carl is competing there as well. And this could be even with a stranger, potentially.

DR. YOUNG: And is that just because the game's afoot, or is that because he actually views people underneath as trying to get him before he gets them?

CARL: (*Speaks definitively.*) No. He does not view people as trying to get him before he gets them.

DR. YOUNG: It's not a mistrustful view of other people?

CARL: Not at all.

Carl answers that he does not view other people as abusive. Rather, what motivates him to play the game is the satisfaction of winning. Carl's main schema seems to be Emotional Deprivation, not Mistrust/Abuse. He plays the game to fill the emptiness of his emotional deprivation, rather than to protect himself from cruelty or humiliation.

DR. YOUNG: It's just that the game is what gives things a purpose.

CARL: It provides a meaning for life.

DR. YOUNG: Given that there's not adequate connection.

The therapist helps Carl achieve a thorough intellectual understanding of his modes, including the schemas that underlie them.

The Therapist Explores the Adaptive Functions of the Coping Modes

The therapist helps Carl access "Detached Carl" and explore the function the mode serves. Detached Carl exists to distract him from his sadness.

CARL: I think I can get in touch with a nine-year-old Detached Carl.

DR. YOUNG: OK. What's he like?

CARL: Oh, he's kind of impervious. I think he sees this little boy being very sad, and he recognizes that he used to be sad once. If he thinks about it, he could get sad, too, but he doesn't want to.

DR. YOUNG: He doesn't want to think about it?

CARL: Well, he's not in the habit of thinking about it, no. He's in the habit of *not* thinking about it.

DR. YOUNG: What things does he do to distract himself?

CARL: Oh, he likes to read comic books, play chess, and watch TV. (*Pause.*) I don't think he needs to do anything special to be detached.

DR. YOUNG: Is he more with people or more isolated, or can he be in either place?

CARL: He can be in either place.

DR. YOUNG: He doesn't feel any safer, or any less comfortable, one way or the other?

CARL: No, no. He's impervious.

To protect himself from his sadness about his mother, Carl also turned to stone.

The therapist further helps Carl connect emotionally to Detached Carl. Note that Detached Carl initially tries to distance himself by criticizing the therapist's question. He engages in schema avoidance, true to his main function. When Dr. Young asks Detached Carl about his feelings, Detached Carl becomes irritated.

DR. YOUNG: Can I talk to Detached Carl for a second?

CARL: Yeah.

DR. YOUNG: Well, here you are, reading comics, playing chess, watching TV. How does that make you feel?

CARL: (pause)

DR. YOUNG: Do you enjoy doing those things?

CARL: (Speaks in an annoyed tone.) Well, I sort of think your question is silly.

DR. YOUNG: OK. Why don't you come up with a better one? Reword it to make it more reasonable, so it fits the situation better.

CARL: These are just things I like to do. Why wouldn't I like to do them?

DR. YOUNG: So it sounds like Detached Carl, then, has a slightly argumentative flavor to him?

CARL: (Sounds annoyed.) Oh, he just doesn't understand. He doesn't understand what you mean.

DR. YOUNG: But it sounds like there is a little bit of anger in the voice tone—that he's also feeling something . . .

CARL: (Interrupts.) Are you asking Detached Carl to have some feelings?

DR. YOUNG: I'm asking if maybe he has some angry feelings, but not the sad feelings.

CARL: (Interrupts.) I think he's angry if you ask him to focus on himself.

DR. YOUNG: Yeah, that's what I mean. So he is angry.

CARL: Yeah, he's angry if you want him to look at what he's doing or think about what he's doing.

DR. YOUNG: Yes, exactly. And how do you, as angry, detached Carl, how do you feel toward other people in general? What's your connection to them, your beliefs about them?

CARL: Hm. (*Pause.*) Oh, I don't really, I don't like them much.

DR. YOUNG: Why?

CARL: (*long pause*) I don't know why.

DR. YOUNG: Are they stupid, are they selfish?

CARL: Well, some of them are stupid, but some of them aren't stupid. They're not as smart as me, of course.

DR. YOUNG: Do you feel good being smarter than most people?

CARL: (*in an emphatic voice*) Sure.

DR. YOUNG: Why does that feel good to you right now?

CARL: I have to be the best. I have to be the winner.

DR. YOUNG: And why is it important for you to be the best?

CARL: (*in an angry voice*) You're making me angry.

DR. YOUNG: Can you try to explain why you're angry with me?

CARL: Well, you're asking me these questions.

DR. YOUNG: And you don't want to think about these things.

CARL: No.

The therapist helps Carl reach a deeper understanding of Detached Carl. Detached Carl does not like other people very much, does not like to think about his problems, does not like to think about why he does the things he does, and has to be Number One. The therapist helps him understand how Detached Carl feels and operates—an important step toward understanding how Detached Carl negatively affects his life in the long run.

It is noteworthy that Carl describes both the avoidant coping function of Detached Carl and the overcompensating function. As we have said, Detached Carl is both a Detached Self-Soother and a Self-Aggrandizer. One mode serves these two distinct functions: Detached Carl avoids his own negative emotions, and he views himself as superior to other people.

Interestingly, once the therapist identifies Detached Carl and makes him a character in the imagery, Carl's manner toward the therapist changes. He moves out of his Self-Aggrandizing and Self-Soothing modes. He only cursorily engages in a "dance of domination" with the therapist. He only halfheartedly competes and pushes the therapist away. Having been given a voice as a mode, Detached Carl no longer needs to demonstrate his superiority to the therapist, and he no longer needs to distance from the therapist to the same degree.

The Therapist Teaches Modes to Negotiate through Schema Dialogues

Once the patient has identified, labeled, and emotionally connected to the modes, the therapist helps the patient carry on dialogues between them. The therapist teaches the modes to negotiate through schema dialogues. This is a function of the Healthy Adult: to direct negotiations among modes. The aim of the Healthy Adult is to supplant the Self-Aggrandizer and the Detached Self-Soother as protectors of the Lonely Child and to help the Lonely Child get his emotional needs met.

In the following excerpt, the therapist helps Carl conduct a dialogue in imagery between Detached Carl and Little Carl, the Lonely Child. The therapist brings in Danielle, Carl's wife. Danielle's self-absorption echoes Carl's mother, perpetuating the emotional deprivation of his childhood in his adult life. The therapist wants to strengthen the connection between Carl's Lonely Child and Danielle. The ultimate goal is to get Detached Carl to step aside and allow Little Carl to feel and express his emotions with Danielle.

CARL: I think Little Carl wants his mommy. He wants his mommy, and his mommy has a certain quality—maybe a sad quality, maybe a negative quality—but he wants that quality.

DR. YOUNG: So it can either be her or someone a lot like her.

CARL: I think, yes, Little Carl remembers his mother was sad.

DR. YOUNG: So he wants someone sad and vulnerable like his mother.

CARL: Yes.

DR. YOUNG: And how about Danielle? How does Little Carl—

CARL: (Interrupts.) She's sad and vulnerable.

DR. YOUNG: Is that what Little Carl wants?

CARL: (Speaks sadly.) Yes.

The therapist helps Little Carl negotiate with Detached Carl.

DR. YOUNG: Then let Little Carl say, "I'd like to try to get closer to Danielle." What does Detached Carl say back?

CARL: (long pause) I think it's OK with Detached Carl, it really is.

DR. YOUNG: But there are some problems coming up, aren't there? It's not going totally smoothly. So you need to talk about what's interfering with that—how Detached Carl is interfering.

CARL: Yes, you're right. There are problems. Detached Carl's life is being threatened.

DR. YOUNG: Yes, so say that to Little Carl, because you've taken on a separate persona now, and you want to survive, too. You're not just his servant anymore.

CARL: (*as Detached Carl, speaking to Little Carl*) "Yes, Danielle's the one. But, you know, I'm not going to give up *my* life. *I* have a life, too."

DR. YOUNG: Tell him about that life, and the good parts of it.

CARL: "You know, I've got to play chess. I've got to keep the old brain stimulated. You wouldn't want to get bored, would you? Would you want to get bored, Little Carl, would you?"

DR. YOUNG: And what does he say?

CARL: (as Little Carl in a tentative voice) "Uh, no, no."

DR. YOUNG: It sounds like Detached Carl's bullying him a little.

CARL: (*Laughs.*)

DR. YOUNG: Let Little Carl be a bit stronger. Let him grow up a little bit, maybe, so that he's still got those feelings, but he's a bit smarter than that.

CARL: OK. (*as Little Carl, more forcefully*) "OK, you big bully, listen to me. . . . "

Detached Carl is much stronger than Little Carl. The therapist allies with Little Carl in order to even things out. He provides the Vulnerable Child with more ammunition against Detached Carl. It is going to be a fair fight, not a trouncing.

With Little Carl thus strengthened, Little Carl and Detached Carl continue to negotiate. Carl plays both sides, with Dr. Young acting as coach.

CARL: (*as Detached Carl, speaking to Little Carl*) "Yes, yes, OK, you're right, you're right. Family's important, Danielle's important. But does that mean I have to give up everything? Do I have to give up everything? Can't I keep something?"

DR. YOUNG: That's good. Give Little Carl an example, something you would like to keep, without having to keep the whole ball of wax. Negotiate.

CARL: (*as Detached Carl*) "Can I keep my cookies and my chocolate and pizza? Can I keep playing chess on the computer all night?"

DR. YOUNG: How about playing two hours a night?

CARL: That's not enough!

DR. YOUNG: Try and negotiate a little bit here. Don't be quite so hard with him.

CARL: I'm negotiating with Little Carl?

DR. YOUNG: Yes.

CARL: (*as Detached Carl*) "Listen, we'll keep the family, but this is what I need." (*Speaks angrily*) "I need you to leave me alone, and I'll take care of the family."

DR. YOUNG: And what's Little Carl say back?

CARL: (*as Little Carl, speaking mournfully*) "Are you doing it? Are you taking care of the family? I'll leave you alone if you take care of the family, if you take care of yourself. Are you doing it?"

Note that, at this point, Little Carl is actually a combination of the Lonely Child and Healthy Adult modes. Little Carl has taken over the therapist's role of empathic confrontation. He confronts Detached Carl with the current state of affairs: Both Little Carl and Danielle feel lonely and neglected.

The Therapist Links the Lonely Child with Current Intimate Relationships

The therapist helps the Lonely Child connect to significant others in imagery. Dr. Young works to convince Detached Carl to let Little Carl "come out" more with Danielle to give and receive love. This is to Detached Carl's advantage also, because love is something he wants even more than he wants to play games and to win. (In our model, the Maladaptive Coping modes—in this case, the Detached Self-Soother and Self-Aggrandizer— also want love. These maladaptive modes are not there in order to hurt the patient but rather to protect the patient. When these modes are convinced that the Vulnerable Child is safe, they will allow the Vulnerable Child to surface.)

DR. YOUNG: How about having Detached Carl step aside for a while, and let Little Carl and Danielle connect a bit? Close your eyes and let Little Carl and Danielle connect a little bit, just so I can see what happens when the two of them are there without Detached Carl in the picture. What do you see happening now?

CARL: (*pause*) Physically what happens?

DR. YOUNG: Yes. What do you see? How are they relating to each other? Look at Little Carl, but make him a little older, so he's not three.

CARL: Yeah, OK, sure.

DR. YOUNG: What do you see with Little Carl and Danielle? How are they interacting?

CARL: Uh, well, he just crawls into her lap.

DR. YOUNG: And touches her? And holds her?

CARL: Yeah. She holds him.

DR. YOUNG: How does it feel?

CARL: It feels fine, feels good. He looks into her eyes, he looks into her face. . . .

DR. YOUNG: He wants this?

CARL: Yes.

Carl can see that he actually wants to get close to Danielle, something he had not recognized before. It is by getting close to Danielle that the Vulnerable Child can get his core emotional needs met. The therapist brings Detached Carl into the image.

DR. YOUNG: Now, put Detached Carl into the image there, and just have him comment on what he's seeing, from his perspective. What does he feel as he sees that?

CARL: Well, Detached Carl, after all, is pretty enlightened. (*Laughs.*)

DR. YOUNG: (*Laughs.*) So what's he saying as he looks at them?

CARL: (*as Detached Carl*) "Good, good, good. Good work."

DR. YOUNG: (*as Detached Carl*) "Now I'm going to go back and play chess, or I'll sit here and watch television for awhile?"

CARL: No. I wish we could do more of this.

The Therapist Helps the Patient Generalize Changes in Therapy to Life Outside Therapy

The final part of treatment is helping patients generalize from the therapy relationship and imagery exercises in sessions to outside relationships with significant others. The therapist helps the patient select significant others who hold the potential for mutual caring and to emotionally connect to them. The therapist encourages the patient to let the Lonely Child surface in these relationships, to give and receive genuine love.

In the following segment, Dr. Young helps Carl clarify how to generalize from the mode work to life outside therapy.

DR. YOUNG: What do you think is the next step for the "Carls" right now, in terms of making progress in therapy?

CARL: Well, my opinion is that we have to have it so that Little Carl can come out and stay out. I think that we have to focus our attention on and be more mindful of Detached Carl. I think that the dichotomy of

Little Carl and Detached Carl is very powerful with respect to my own self-awareness. And to the extent that we have Little Carl there, Detached Carl doesn't need to be there.

DR. YOUNG: I see, you think Detached Carl actually will recede automatically just by having Little Carl there?

CARL: That's right.

DR. YOUNG: And consistent with that, you seem different right now talking to me than you seemed at the very beginning. Right now you seem more vulnerable, more emotions are coming through than I felt beforehand, and you're not debating the little points of the language anymore.

CARL: That's what Detached Carl has to do.

DR. YOUNG: Yes, exactly, so what you described has already just happened here. You are now less of that Detached Carl than you were earlier. So connecting with Little Carl clearly does change Detached Carl.

CARL: Right. Connecting with Little Carl and connecting to my emotions in general is something I'm not in the *habit* of doing and not used to doing—but it's important for me to have the facility of doing. And, as far as Little Carl is concerned, I think that he really has to just come out and stay out.

Once the patient allows the Lonely Child to emerge and connect to others, then the other modes begin to recede. Their functions as protectors of the Vulnerable Child become increasingly obsolete. Of course, these modes will resurface over time, but the more the Lonely Child emerges and connects to others, the less the other modes will exert the pressure to appear.

To help patients generalize changes in therapy to their outside relationships, we often find couples therapy a useful addition, especially in this stage of treatment. In addition, we use cognitive-behavioral homework assignments to help patients work on their relationships with family members, partners, and friends.

The Therapist Introduces Cognitive and Behavioral Strategies

Although the case example does not illustrate this part of treatment, early on the therapist introduces cognitive and behavioral strategies. These strategies can help patients with narcissistic personality disorder in both the Assessment and Change Phases. Cognitive-behavioral homework assignments are essential to helping patients overcome the avoidant and overcompensatory coping styles that perpetuate their schemas. If patients maintain their self-aggrandizing and entitled behaviors in their current interpersonal relationships, their underlying Emotional Deprivation and Defectiveness schemas will not fully heal.

By writing down their automatic thoughts when they are upset, patients can learn to identify and correct their cognitive distortions. The following are some cognitive distortions common to patients with narcissistic personality disorder.

1. *"Black-or-white" thinking.* Using the tools of cognitive therapy, the therapist helps patients learn to correct the "black or white" thinking of the Self-Aggrandizing mode: "Either I am special and the center of attention, or I am worthless and ignored." The therapist teaches patients to discriminate shades of gray and to respond in more modulated ways to perceived slights. Patients conduct debates between the Self-Aggrandizer and the Healthy Adult or Lonely Child modes.

2. *Distortions about being devalued or deprived by others.* The therapist teaches patients to correct their distortions about how much other people, especially significant others, are devaluing or depriving them. The therapist provides a "reality check" for patients when they feel affronted and asserts the principle of reciprocity: Patients should not expect from others what they themselves are unwilling to give. The therapist guides patients to seek equality in relationships rather than feeling superior or special.

3. *Perfectionism.* The therapist teaches patients to challenge their perfectionism by setting more realistic expectations for performance, both for themselves and for others. With the therapy relationship serving as a model, patients learn to become more forgiving of human flaws. The therapist helps patients identify their inner perfectionistic voice as the voice of the Demanding Parent, who was never satisfied.

4. *Overemphasizing narcissistic gratification over inner fulfillment.* The therapist helps patients examine the advantages and disadvantages of emphasizing success, status, and recognition over genuine love and self-expression. Similarly, the therapist guides patients to examine the advantages and disadvantages of maintaining their entitled thinking and behavior over adopting a stance of empathy and reciprocity. The therapist conducts debates between schemas and the Healthy Adult.

Working with patients, the therapist constructs flash cards that patients use to remain aware of the negative consequences of their narcissism and the positive consequences of practicing "loving kindness" in their lives outside therapy. The therapist helps patients design and conduct behavioral experiments, investigating the consequences of entitled versus loving behavior in their intimate relationships. The therapist acknowledges the patient for behaving in a loving way—for choosing "true love" over temporary narcissistic satisfactions.

The "vertical arrow" technique (Burns, 1980) is useful for helping patients identify the underlying beliefs that drive their endless quest for narcissistic gratification. The therapist helps patients work through "what ifs" such as, "What if you were not perfectly beautiful, brilliant, rich, successful, famous, or high status? What would that mean to you? What would happen? What do you imagine your life would be like?" Working through these "what ifs" with patients is another path to the Lonely Child. When contemplating what life would be like without their narcissistic gifts, patients often get to the loveless place of their Emotional Deprivation and Defectiveness schemas.

Between sessions, patients read flash cards to remind them of what they have learned from doing the cognitive work. The flash cards point them to healthy behaviors that heal, rather than perpetuate, their Emotional Deprivation and Defectiveness schemas.

The therapist combines the cognitive work with behavioral homework assignments. For example, the therapist asks patients to spend time alone for homework, unsoothed and unstimulated, to get to know and understand the Lonely Child. Patients write down or tape-record their thoughts and feelings and then bring them to their next session. The therapist and patient talk about what happened, and the therapist takes the opportunity to reparent the patient.

Patients learn to replace self-destructive impulsive and compulsive behaviors with emotional closeness and authenticity. In social situations, patients carry out experiments in which they resist switching into the Self-Aggrandizing mode. They adopt an observer role for an evening, or focus on listening to others, or refrain from making remarks designed to elicit admiration.

Finally, and perhaps most important, patients with narcissistic personality disorder work on developing their intimate relationships. They carry out homework assignments to nurture others and practice empathy. They reduce the time they devote to impressing others and increase the time they devote to enhancing the emotional quality of their close relationships. They let the Lonely Child come out in suitable intimate encounters to get basic emotional needs met. They observe what happens when they replace addictive, self-soothing behaviors with love and intimacy.

COMMON OBSTACLES TO THE TREATMENT OF NARCISSISM

There are several obstacles to successful treatment of patients with narcissistic personality disorder that we can usually overcome by exercising leverage. Occasionally, the leverage we can bring to bear is not enough.

These patients are more likely than most other patients to drop out of treatment, especially in the early sessions. They might drop out for a number of reasons. The Self-Aggrandizer in the patient might be unable to grasp the goal of therapy—to establish a relationship based on caring rather than specialness—especially if the patient has never experienced real caring. The Self-Aggrandizer may not be willing to tolerate the therapist's frustration of the patient's narcissistic needs for entitlement or specialness, and there is nothing the therapist can do to keep the patient in treatment short of gratifying the patient's narcissistic needs, which would be destructive to both the therapist and the patient.

Patients might drop out of treatment to avoid experiencing the pain of the Lonely Child. They may be unwilling to let themselves become vulnerable enough to trust and become attached to the therapist. If they entered treatment during a crisis, they are at a high risk to leave once the crisis is resolved.

The Self-Aggrandizer might reject the therapist as "not good enough" in some way—not rich enough, smart enough, well educated enough, successful enough, famous enough, and so forth. Alternatively, this might happen later in treatment. Having first idealized the therapist, the patient later devalues him or her.

What leverage does the therapist have to keep the patient in treatment? What does the therapist have that the patient wants? As we have noted, one source of leverage is the negative consequences of the patient's narcissism. The therapist keeps reminding patients that, unless they change, they will continue paying a price for their narcissism in their love and work lives. A second source of leverage is the therapist–patient relationship. If the therapist keeps the patient in the Lonely Child mode and reparents the patient, then the patient's attachment to the therapist can become a reason for staying in treatment.

SUMMARY

We use a mode-based approach with patients with narcissistic personality disorder. We have observed three primary modes that characterize most of these patients (in addition to the Healthy Adult mode): the Lonely Child; the Self-Aggrandizer; and the Detached Self-Soother. The core schemas of narcissism are Emotional Deprivation and Defectiveness, which are part of the Lonely Child mode. The Entitlement schema is an overcompensation for the other two schemas and is part of the Self-Aggrandizer mode.

Patients with narcissistic personality disorder are usually in the Self-Aggrandizer mode while they are with other people; the Detached Self-Soother is the mode they are usually in when they are alone. The Detached Self-Soother can take many forms, all representing mechanisms of schema avoidance. Patients often engage in a variety of activities to self-stimulate. These activities provide drama and excitement. Another group of patients compulsively engages in solitary activities that are more self-soothing than self-stimulating. These compulsive interests focus their attention away from the pain of their Emotional Deprivation and Defectiveness schemas.

We have found four factors that often characterize the childhood environments of patients with narcissistic personality disorder: (1) loneliness and isolation; (2) insufficient limits; (3) history of being used or manipulated; and (4) conditional approval.

In intimate relationships, patients with narcissistic personality disorder typically display characteristic behaviors. They are generally unable to absorb love and view relationships as sources of approval or validation. They are unempathic, especially toward the people who are closest to them. They frequently feel envious of others whom they perceive as one-up in some way. Patients often idealize their love objects in the initial stages of the relationship; and then, as time goes on, they increasingly devalue the partners. Finally, patients display a pattern of entitlement in their intimate relationships.

To assess narcissism, the therapist can observe the following: (1) the patient's behavior in therapy sessions; (2) the nature of the patient's presenting problem and history; (3) the patient's response to imagery exercises and questions about childhood (including the Young Parenting Inventory); and (4) the patient's Young Schema Questionnaire.

Our treatment of patients with narcissistic personality disorder centers on reparenting the Lonely Child and conducting mode work. The therapist helps the patient build up a Healthy Adult mode, modeled on the therapist, that is capable of reparenting the Lonely Child and regulating the Self-Aggrandizer and the Detached Self-Soother modes. The therapist establishes the current complaints as leverage and begins "limited reparenting" of the Lonely Child. When treating patients with narcissistic personality disorder, it is important for therapists to tactfully confront the patient's devaluing or challenging style and assert their rights whenever the patient violates them. Rather than appearing perfect, therapists acknowledge their vulnerability.

The therapist introduces the concept of the Lonely Child mode and helps the patient recognize the Self-Aggrandizer and Detached Self-Soother modes. The therapist explores the childhood origins of the modes through imagery. (Usually, the therapist must first overcome considerable resistance on the part of the patient.) The therapist guides the patient through mode work. The Healthy Adult mode conducts negotiations among the modes, in order to: (1) help the Lonely Child to feel nurtured and understood and to nurture and empathize with others; (2) confront the Self-Aggrandizer so that the patient gives up the excessive need for approval and treats others based on principles of respect and reciprocity, as the Lonely Child takes in more genuine love; and (3) help the Detached Self-Soother give up maladaptive addictive and avoidant behaviors and replace them with genuine love, self-expression, and experiencing of affect.

The final part of treatment is helping patients generalize from the therapy relationship and imagery exercises in sessions to outside relationships with significant others. The therapist helps the patient select significant others who hold the potential for mutual caring and to emotionally connect to them. The therapist encourages the patient to let the Lonely Child surface in these relationships, to give and receive love.

REFERENCES

Ainsworth, M. D. S. (1968). Object relations, dependency, and attachment: A theoretical review of the infant–mother relationship. *Child Development, 40,* 969–1025.

Ainsworth, M. D. S., & Bowlby, J. (1991). An ethological approach to personality development. *American Psychologist, 46,* 331–341.

Alexander, F. (1956). *Psychoanalysis and psychotherapy: Developments in theory, techniques, and training.* New York: Norton.

Alexander, F., & French, T. M. (1946). *Psychoanalytic therapy: Principles and applications.* New York: Ronald Press.

Alford, B. A., & Beck, A. T. (1997). *The integrative power of cognitive therapy.* New York: Guilford Press.

Alloy, L. B., & Abramson, L. Y. (1979). Judgment of contingency in depressed and nondepressed students. Sadder but wiser? *Journal of Experimental Psychology: General, 108,* 449–485.

American Psychiatric Association. (1994). *Diagnostic and statistical manual of mental disorders* (4th ed.). Washington, DC: Author.

Aunola, K., Stattin, H., & Nurmi, J. E. (2000). *Journal of Adolescence, 23*(2), 205–222.

Barlow, D. H. (1993). *Clinical handbook of psychological disorders.* New York: Guilford Press.

Barlow, D. H. (Ed.). (2001). *Clinical handbook of psychological disorders* (3rd ed.). New York: Guilford Press.

Baron, R. (1988). Negative effects of destructive criticism. Impact on conflict, self-efficacy, and task performance. *Journal of Applied Psychology, 73,* 199–207.

Beck, A. T. (1967). *Depression: Causes and treatment.* Philadelphia: University of Pennsylvania Press.

Beck, A. T. (1976). *Cognitive therapy and the emotional disorders.* New York: International Universities Press.

Beck, A. T. (1996). Beyond belief: A theory of modes, personality, and psychopathology. In P. Salkovskis (Ed.), *Frontiers of cognitive therapy* (pp. 1–25). New York: Guilford Press.

Beck, A. T., Freeman, A., & Associates. (1990). *Cognitive therapy of personality disorders.* New York: Guilford Press.

Beck, A. T., Rush, A. J., Shaw, B. F., & Emery, G. (1979). *Cognitive therapy of depression.* New York: Guilford Press.

Beck, A. T., Steer, R. A., & Brown, G. K. (1996). *Beck Depression Inventory-II.* San Antonio, Texas: The Psychological Corporation.

Beck, A. T., Ward, C. H., Mendelson, M., Mock, J., & Erbaugh, J. (1961). An inventory for measuring depression. *Archives of General Psychiatry, 4,* 561–571.

Beyer, J., & Trice, H. (1984). A field study of the use and perceived use of discipline in controlling worker performance. *Academy of Management Journal, 27,* 743–764.

Borkovec, T. D., Robinson, E., Pruzinsky, T., & DePree, J. A. (1983). Preliminary exploration of worry: Some characteristics and processes. *Behaviour Research and Therapy, 21,* 9–16.

Bowlby, J. (1969). *Attachment and loss: Vol. I. Attachment.* New York: Basic Books.

Bowlby, J. (1973). *Attachment and loss: Vol. II. Separation.* New York: Basic Books.

Bowlby, J. (1980). *Attachment and loss: Vol. III. Loss, sadness, and depression.* New York: Basic Books.

Bowlby, J. (1988). *A secure base: Parent–child attachment and healthy human development.* New York: Basic Books.

Burns, D. D. (1980). *Feeling good.* New York: Morrow.

Carine, B. E. (1997). Assessing personal and interpersonal schemata associated with Axis II Cluster B personality disorders: An integrated perspective. *Dissertations Abstracts International, 58,* 1B.

Carroll, L. (1923). *Alice in wonderland.* New York: J. H. Sears.

Coe, C. L., Glass, J. C., Wiener, S. G., & Levine, S. (1983). Behavioral, but not physiological adaptation to repeated separation in mother and infant primates. *Psychoneuroendocrinology, 8,* 401–409.

Coe, C. L., Mendoza, S. P., Smotherman, W. P., & Levine, S. (1978). Mother–infant attachment in the squirrel monkey: Adrenal responses to separation. *Behavioral Biology, 22,* 256–263.

Coe, C. L., Wiener, S. G., Rosenberg, L. T., & Levine, S. (1985). Endocrine and immune responses to separation and maternal loss in nonhuman primates. In M. Reite & T. Field (Eds.), *The psychobiology of attachment* (pp. 163–199). Orlando, FL: Academic Press.

Coleman, L., Abraham, J., & Jussin, L. (1987). Students' reactions to teachers' evaluations. The unique impact of negative feedback. *Journal of Applied Psychology, 64,* 391–400.

Craske, M. G., Barlow, D. H., & Meadows, E. A. (2000). *Mastery of your anxiety and panic: Therapist guide for anxiety, panic, and agoraphobia (MAP-3).* San Antonio, TX: Graywind/Psychological Corp.

Earley, L., & Cushway, D. (2002). The parentified child. *Clinical Child Psychology and Psychiatry, 7(2),* 163–188.

Eliot, T. S. (1971). *The complete poems and plays: 1909–1950.* New York: Harcourt, Brace, & World.

Elliott, C. H., & Lassen, M. K. (1997). A schema polarity model for case conceptualization, intervention, and research. *Clinical Psychology: Science and Practice, 4,* 12–28.

Erikson, E. H. (1950). *Childhood and society.* New York: Norton.

Erikson, E. H. (1963). *Childhood and society* (2nd ed.). New York: Norton.

Fisher, C. (1989). *Postcards from the edge.* New York: Simon & Schuster.

Frank, J. D., Margolin, J., Nash, H. T., Stone, A. R., Varon, E., & Ascher, E. (1952). Two behavior patterns in therapeutic groups and their apparent motivation. *Human Relations, 5,* 289–317.

Freeman, N. (1999). Constructive thinking and early maladaptive schemas as predictors of interpersonal adjustment and marital satisfaction. *Dissertations Abstracts International, 59,* 9B.

Freud, S. (1963). Introductory lectures on psychoanalysis: Part III. General theory of the neuroses. In J. Strachey (Ed. and Trans.), *The standard edition of the complete psychological works of Sigmund Freud* (Vol. 16, pp. 241–263). London: Hogarth Press. (Original work published 1917)

Gabbard, G. O. (1994). *Psychodynamic psychiatry in clinical practice: The DSM-IV edition.* Washington, DC: American Psychiatric Press.

Greenberg, L., & Paivio, S. (1997). *Working with emotions in psychotherapy.* New York, Guilford Press.

Greenberg, L. S., Rice, L. N., & Elliott, R. (1983). *Facilitating emotional change: The moment-by-moment process.* New York: Guilford Press.

Gunderson, J. G., Zanarini, M. C., & Kisiel, C. L. (1991). Borderline personality disorder: A review of data on DSM-III-R descriptions. *Journal of Personality Disorders, 5,* 340–352.

Herman, J. L., Perry, J. C., & van de Kolk, B. A. (1989). Childhood trauma in borderline personality disorder. *American Journal of Psychiatry, 146,* 490–495.

Horowitz, M. J. (Ed.). (1991). *Person schemas and maladaptive interpersonal patterns.* Chicago: University of Chicago Press.

Horowitz, M. J. (1997). *Formulation as a basis for planning psychotherapy treatment.* Washington, DC: American Psychiatric Press.

Horowitz, M. J., Stinson, C. H., & Milbrath, C. (1996). Role relationship models: A person schematic method for inferring beliefs about identity and social action. In A. Colby, R. Jessor, & R. Schweder (Eds.), *Essays on ethnography and human development* (pp. 253–274). Chicago: University of Chicago Press.

Hyler, S., Rieder, R. O., Spitzer, R. L., & Williams, J. (1987). *Personality Diagnostic Questionnaire—Revised.* New York: New York State Psychiatric Institute.

Kagan, J., Reznick, J. S., & Snidman, N. (1988). Biological bases of childhood shyness. *Science, 240,* 167–171.

Kernberg, O. F. (1984). *Severe personality disorders: Psychotherapeutic strategies.* New Haven: Yale University Press.

Kohlberg, I. (1963). Moral development and identification. In H. Stevenson (Ed.), *Child psychology* (62nd yearbook of the National Society for the Study of Education.) Chicago: University of Chicago Press.

Kohut, H. (1984). *How does analysis cure?* Chicago: University of Chicago Press.

LeDoux, J. (1996). *The emotional brain.* New York: Simon & Schuster.

Lee, C. W., Taylor, G., & Dunn, J. (1999). Factor structures of the Schema Questionnaire in a large clinical sample. *Cognitive Therapy and Research, 23*(4), 421–451.

Linehan, M. M. (1993). *Cognitive-behavioral treatment of borderline personality disorder.* New York: Guilford Press.

Maslach, G., & Jackson, S. E. (1986). *Maslach Burnout Inventory manual.* Palo Alto, CA: Consulting Psychologists Press.

McGinn, L. K., Young, J. E., & Sanderson, W. C. (1995). When and how to do longer term therapy without feeling guilty. *Cognitive and Behavioral Practice, 2,* 187–212.

Miller, A. (1975). *Prisoners of childhood: The drama of the gifted child and the search for the true self.* New York: Basic Books.

Miller, A. (1990). *Thou shalt not be aware: Society's betrayal of the child.* New York: Penguin.

Millon, T. (1981). *Disorders of personality.* New York: Wiley.

Noyes, R. J., Reich, J., Christiansen, J., Suelzer, M., Pfohl, B., & Coryell, W. A. (1990). Outcome of panic disorder. *Archives of General Psychiatry, 47,* 809–818.

Nussbaum, M. C. (1994). *The therapy of desire: Theory and practice in hellenistic ethics.* Princeton, NJ: Princeton University Press.

Orwell, G. (1946). *Animal farm.* New York: Harcourt, Brace.

Patock-Peckham, J. A., Cheong, J., Balhorn, M. E., & Nogoshi, C. T. (2001). A social learning perspective: A model of parenting styles, self-regulation, perceived drinking control, and alcohol use and problems. *Alcoholism: Clinical and Experimental Research, 25*(9), 1284–1292.

Pearlman, L. A., & MacIan, P. S. (1995). Vicarious traumatization: An empirical study of the effects of trauma work on trauma therapists. *Professional Psychology: Research and Practice, 26*(6), 558–565.

Persons, J. B. (1989). *Cognitive therapy in practice: A case formulation approach.* New York: Norton.

Piaget, J. (1962). *Play, dreams, and imitation in childhood.* New York: Norton.

Plath, S.(1966). *The bell jar.* London: Faber and Faber.

Rachlin, H. (1976). *Behavior and learning.* San Francisco: Freeman.

Reich, J. H., & Greene, A. L. (1991). Effect of personality disorders on outcome of treatment. *Journal of Nervous and Mental Disease, 179,* 74–83.

Rittenmeyer, G. J. (1997). The relationship between early maladaptive schemas and job burnout among public school teachers. *Dissertations Abstracts International, 58,* 5A.

Rogers, C. R. (1951). *Client-centered therapy.* Boston: Houghton Mifflin.

Rosenberg, M. (1965). *Society and the adolescent self-image.* Princeton, NJ: Princeton University Press.

Ryle, A. (1991). *Cognitive-analytic therapy: Active participation in change.* New York: Wiley.

Sanderson, W. C., Beck, A. T., & McGinn, L. K. (1994). Cognitive therapy for generalized anxiety disorder: Significance of comorbid personality disorders. *Journal of Cognitive Psychotherapy: An International Quarterly, 8*(1), 13–18.

Schmidt, N. B., Joiner, T. E., Young, J. E., & Telch, M. J. (1995). The Schema Questionnaire: Investigation of psychometric properties and the hierarchical structure of a measure of maladaptive schemata. *Cognitive Therapy and Research, 19*(3), 295–321.

Shane, M., Shane, E., & Gales, M. (1997). *Intimate attachments: Toward a new self psychology.* New York: Guilford Press.

Singer, I. B. (1978). *Shosha.* New York: Farrar, Straus, & Giroux.

Smucker, M. R., & Dancu, C. V. (1999). *Cognitive behavioral treatment for adult survivors of childhood trauma: Imagery rescripting and reprocessing.* Northvale, NJ: Aronson.

Suinn, R. M. (1977). Type A behavior pattern. In R. B. Williams & W. D. Gentry (Eds.), *Behavioral approaches to medical treatment*. Cambridge, MA: Ballinger.

Taylor, S. E., & Brown, J. D. (1994). Positive illusions and well-being revisited: Separating fact from fiction. *Psychological Bulletin, 116*, 1–27.

Terence (1965). *Heauton timoroumenos* [The self-tormentor] (Betty Radice, Trans.). New York: Penguin.

Thompson, L. W., Gallagher, D., & Czirr, R. (1988). Personality disorder and outcome in the treatment of later life depression. *Journal of Geriatric Psychiatry and Neurology, 121*, 133–146.

Tolstoy, L. (1986). The death of Ivan Ilyitch. In C. Neider (Ed.), *Tolstoy: Tales of courage and conflict*. New York: Cooper Square Press.

Turner, S. M. (1987). The effects of personality disorders on the outcome of social anxiety symptom reduction. *Journal of Personality Disorders, 1*, 136–143.

van der Kolk, B. A. (1987). *Psychological trauma*. Washington, DC: American Psychiatric Press.

Wills, R., & Sanders, D. (1997). *Cognitive therapy: Transforming the image*. London: Sage.

Winnicott, D. W. (1965). *The maturational processes and the facilitating environment: Studies in the theory of emotional development*. London: Hogarth Press.

Young, J. E. (1990). *Cognitive therapy for personality disorders*. Sarasota, FL: Professional Resources Press.

Young, J. E. (1993). *The schema diary*. New York: Cognitive Therapy Center of New York.

Young, J. E. (1994). *Young Parenting Inventory*. New York: Cognitive Therapy Center of New York.

Young, J. E. (1995). *Young Compensation Inventory*. New York: Cognitive Therapy Center of New York.

Young, J. E. (1999). *Cognitive therapy for personality disorders: A schema-focused approach* (rev. ed.). Sarasota, FL: Professional Resources Press.

Young, J. E., & Brown, G. (1990). *Young Schema Questionnaire*. New York: Cognitive Therapy Center of New York.

Young, J. E., & Brown, G. (2001). *Young Schema Questionnaire: Special Edition*. New York: Schema Therapy Institute.

Young, J. E., & Gluhoski, V. L. (1996). Schema-focused diagnosis for personality disorders. In F. W. Kaslow (Ed.), *Handbook of relational diagnosis and dysfunctional family patterns* (pp. 300–321). New York: Wiley.

Young, J. E., & Klosko, J. S. (1993). *Reinventing your life: How to break free from negative life patterns*. New York: Dutton.

Young, J. E., & Klosko, J. (1994). *Reinventing your life*. New York: Plume.

Young, J. E., & Rygh, J. (1994). *Young–Rygh Avoidance Inventory*. New York: Cognitive Therapy Center of New York.

Young, J. E., Wattenmaker, D., & Wattenmaker, R. (1996). *Schema therapy flashcard*. New York: Cognitive Therapy Center of New York.

Young, J. E., Weinberger, A. D., & Beck, A. T. (2001). Cognitive therapy for depression. In D. Barlow (Ed.), *Clinical handbook of psychological disorders* (3rd ed., pp. 264–308). New York: Guilford Press.

Zajonc, R. B. (1984). On the primacy of affect. *American Psychologist, 39*, 117–123.

INDEX